The Devil's Highway

The Devil's Highway

W.C. Scott

To order additional copies of this book, contact:
Xlibris
1-888-795-4274
www.Xlibris.com
Orders@Xlibris.com
762659

THE WHOLESALER DRESSED in blue jeans, a wrinkled dungaree shirt and an old beat up leather jacket looked just like the ten year old Fleetwood Cadillac he was driving. Tired, dirty, and dented.

It was a long trip up from Boston each week. He had to stop at all the mom and pop dealerships in South Central New Hampshire. And today was no exception, this was the tenth time he had stopped at Johnson's Chevy in Hillbro.

"Here we go again," he muttered to himself. "Friggin Hicksville USA, population two hundred."

Amazed he shook his head eyeing the three hundred new and used cars and trucks. Week after week they just sat there; unsold collecting dust, and they wouldn't even consider unloading one or two to a wholesaler.

Stalling he stayed in his car power smoking a non-filtered Camel, mumbling to himself. "There's got to be something going on here I swear the same damn cars have been here for ten weeks."

"Oh-oh," Dick the wholesaler said louder, "Who's this new asshole coming to run me off?" Quickly he flicked his cigarette butt out the open window and climbed out of the old Cadillac.

Lucky Sullivan the new sales manager had only been at Johnson's Chevy for about ten days, and couldn't get over the laid back approach the two brothers had about running the place.

The brothers kept a huge inventory and paid cash for all their new cars where most dealers couldn't afford that enormous outlay of cash, and opted to pay interest to the manufacture for each day a new car sat on their lot unsold.

Even stranger Johnson's had new cars sitting on the lot that were two and three years old because they wouldn't come down on the price. He couldn't understand it, knowing something wasn't right. He could feel it in his bones.

Carefully Lucky made a list in his small corner office:

Closed Saturday and Sundays.

Paid each salesman a $300 hundred weekly salary + commission.

Free demo for salesman, regardless of number sold.

Extremely high, outdated prices.

Total monthly sales averages: New <u>14</u>, Used <u>17</u>

It was like they had money to burn. He still didn't know what to make of it all, but he did know that if he wanted to make more than his six hundred dollar a week manager's salary he was going to have to change a whole bunch of things to make money out there in the sticks.

Oddly they made it very clear when they hired him ten days earlier that he wasn't to make too many changes right away. No firing of their over the hill sales force, no mandatory weekends, which was unheard of in the car business.

Lucky tried to smile and relax which he found hard to do. Along with being Bipolar his chemical imbalance was triggered by A.D.H.D. which stands for Attention Deficit Hyperactivity Disorder. All this kick back and take it easy approach to car sales was overwhelming.

The greatest perk of Lucky's new job was that he could use any of the hundred of vehicles on the lot, which also included many of the brother's personal vehicles.

All and all it wasn't a bad deal. He just had to sell at least twenty-one new and thirty-three used per month, which was the dealerships best month. This would kick in a bonus of a hundred dollars per vehicle delivered. So if the sales team totaled thirty-four used cars in any one month Lucky would get a bonus check for thirty-four hundred.

But the main problem was that each of the five tired salesmen each averaged only two to four cars a month. Lucky after getting fired from City Corvette in Manchester the biggest city in New Hampshire with a population of only a hundred and five thousand was groomed in high pressure sales where everything you did was based on the number of vehicles you sold per month, and the gross profit per vehicle.

When he got fired Lucky had been salesman of the month for ten months straight selling an average of 19.6 cars per month, which earned him a free demo, sales man of the month bonus of five hundred dollars and a special parking spot next to the front door.

He had been averaging thirty-five thousand a month in gross profit for the dealership which netted him about twenty-five percent, for a total of seven to ten grand monthly. So when he got fired he was devastated, and shocked.

It was over a sexual harassment charge brought on by a jealous husband whose wife had stopped by for a test drive one hot sticky August afternoon. She ended up buying Lucky an expensive room service champagne lunch in a Marriot suite on her husband's Platinum Visa card.

On top of that she traded in her husbands 1968 Fastback Mustang on a triple black forty-thousand dollar used convertible Vette..

Her husband, an attorney having a business luncheon just happened to spot his wife's long blonde hair blowing wildly when Lucky pulled up to the stoplight. Angrily he ran out of Apple-Bees and followed them to the Airport Marriot where Lucky got lucky and proceeded to close the deal.

ONE

Six weeks earlier
Manchester, NH

L UCKY CELEBRATED LATE into the night. The five grand gross profit netted him an easy fifteen hundred on the Vette he sold to the bimbo at the hotel hours earlier.

His first call was to Romeo a Columbian drug dealer who loved Lucky and his fat commission checks. Lucky scored a quarter ounce of powder cocaine for five hundred bucks on credit and would try to make it last a few days, but with his addictive personality he knew it wouldn't.

The sun came up quick.

After only two hours of rest, and feeling like shit, he sipped on a 48 ounce Big Gulp Vanilla flavored Sweet-N-Low coffee as he pulled into his special parking spot at City Corvette.

It wasn't till he got out of his new demo that he noticed the triple black convertible Vette blocking the showroom doors, that he realized something was wrong.

Once inside it only took a few seconds before he heard the loud voices coming from the old mans office down the hall. "Oh shit" he muttered out loud. Lucky knew it was probably the wife's husband in the office causing a scene, which reminded him that he was already on thin ice.

After wrecking two demos and a formal complaint from a father in regards to Lucky's conduct with his daughter when he sold her a car, the timing couldn't have been worse. Especially after a husbands wife used Lucky's charms to get her husband jealous on a test drive and then teased her husband once they got home. That one almost got him fired.

Lucky glanced around the empty managers office nervously and noticed the top pull out draw was unlocked. Impulsively he yanked it open, without thinking he snatched one of the two master lock box keys and shut the door.

Nervous and full of anxiety he hurried to the men's room to do a much needed line of cocaine. The coffee just wasn't getting it done and he needed to be wide awake to face whatever was going to happen in the next few minutes.

For the first time in months Lucky's mood swings were scaring him. He hadn't been down that roller coaster ride since he started working for City Corvette ten months ago.

Sell…Sell…Sell…he told himself working a ton of hours keeping his endorphins racing with a little help from the white lady. "I just need a little bump," he said splashing cold water over his face. After two monster lines and two drops of Visine, Lucky's confidence came screaming back as the endorphins raced in his head starving off the oncoming depression.

Feeling no pain he waltzed back into the quiet showroom like he owned the place because that's just how he felt. "I can sell anyone, anything, anytime," he whispered boldly.

Once outside he anxiously smoked a Marlboro light while he walked the big lot in his Ray Bans. "Hey so what if that prick husband returns the car … I'll just sell another one," he laughed tensely. "No way, the old man wouldn't dare get rid of me; I bring in thirty-five grand a month and sell more than three of these clowns put together."

Nobody can touch me Lucky thought as he grinded his teeth while huffing on another smoke. "I just need to sell another car and quick," he told himself as his dilated pupils scanned the hundred plus Vettes and muscle cars looking for his next victim.

TWO

THE COCAINE HAD him zooming. Things started happening quickly. The lot boy who was actually an old retired cop pulled the classic Ford Mustang up to the front door.

Lucky watched sadly when the old cop pulled the plate off the black Vette and screwed it back on the Mustang. "Oh shit," he could feel the walls closing in. Paranoid, his heart raced while his eyes starting having tunnel vision.

They were all staring at him, laughing and pointing. All the jealous salesmen made him feel like climbing under a rock. He just couldn't believe this was happening. He tried to will it away while he stood there frozen in place. Slowly it penetrated. "Lucky, hey Lucky," someone yelled again louder. He shook his head trying to clear his vision when he saw Tom, the used car manager rapidly waving his arms and calling him. Slowly in a daze he started walking slowly towards Tom.

Impatiently Tom yelled, "Come on Lucky, the old man needs to see you … And I'll tell you bro you really fucked up this time." They both watched as the irate attorney stormed past and jumped into his Mustang slamming the door. Crazily the Mustang engine roared when the angry attorney dropped the clutch and laid rubber all the way to the street.

"Ya well I guess I know what it's about," Lucky responded half under his breath. "You coming with me Tom" he pleaded.

"Of course I'm with you … I just don't think it'll help," he replied shaking his head. *Not this time.*

"That bad huh?"

"Yup … yup … yup … That's one pissed off attorney," Tom said putting an arm on Lucky's shoulder. *Boy I'm gonna miss you.*

"Well you know Tom if I do it … I really do it," he joked jittery. *Boy and his hot wife was so willing.*

"Come on let's go see the old man."

Lucky nodded and followed Tom down the long hallway to the old man's office. He felt the walls closing in, just like walking into the principal's office, but worse.

They were waiting, all of them.

All four managers were seated in a semi-circle around the old mans gigantic oak desk. There were two empty chairs for Tom and Lucky. Lucky ended up in the hot seat the attorney had just vacated.

"Sit down Lucky," the old man ordered. "I'll get right to the point … I gotta let you go"

"Wait a minute," Lucky tried to say before the old man raised his big hand cutting him off.

"Look Lucky this ain't easy son. You're my top gun – my number one ace, shit you almost sold two hundred cars over the past ten months."

He hesitated eyeing his managers, "a fuckin record," he said uncomfortably. "Shit your worth three of those wanna bees sitting out there, "he stated pointing at the showroom. "But I gotta fire you, if I don't that asshole attorney who's wife you fucked the shit out of yesterday is gonna …" he raised his big head. "Shit Lucky he's got the damn motel receipt in his name with two bottles of expensive champagne charged to the room."

The old man rubbed his big paw over his face frustrated. "He's ready to sue my ass if I don't fire you … my hands are tied… I just can't afford another law suit so I gotta turn you loose," he paused. "But if you need a recommendation just let us know," he said looking around the room for confirmation.

"What?" Lucky yelled shocked glaring all around the circle but no one would make eye contact. "I can't believe this shit. I bring you in almost forty grand a month, more than half your sales staff combined … and … and just because some asshole returns a Vette you're gonna shit on me?"

He was getting madder and madder by the second. "I'll … I'll go sell two no three cars today.. is that what you want?" he demanded jerking his head side to side frantically.

He was losing it.

His mind raced faster and faster, as the roller coaster screamed out of control then he realized everyone was staring at him shocked.

"No … no … that's not gonna help. Maybe down the road I can hire you back after all this cools down … say six months or so," the old man said firmly standing up ending the meeting. "But you gotta go today, like now."

Devastated, he tried to stay in control, trying to save face in front of all his ex-bosses that he had worked so hard to impress. Stunned, he stood up and shook the old man's outstretched hand and looked him dead in the eyes and lost it.

"I promise you one thing Sir," he said fuming. "You will regret this – all of you," he scowled wide eyed as the adrenaline surged through his body. Then a mean deep voice came roaring out, "I'm going straight down to Big Mike's Muscle Cars and I will sell every fuckin car he has. And every customer I know from here will know where I've gone and I don't need your damn charity," he screamed as two managers grabbed him.

"Get him out of here now."

Lucky pulled free at the door. "I'll steal every customer I can from you and if you try to stop me I'll tell the union leader the truth about all your shady deals. And make no mistake about it, nobody, I mean nobody fuckin fires, me, Sir," he wailed as he was muscled out the door.

THREE

LUCKY FUMED WHILE he quickly packed up his desk as three bulky mechanics surrounded him. Word spread quickly; Lucky had threatened the old man.

Definitely not a smart move.

It was well known that the old man was very well connected to certain people and that he definitely didn't appreciate being verbally abused in front of his men by some punk salesman with a coke habit.

Swiftly, Lucky stepped outside clutching his cell phone and brief case. Rapidly he dialed Big Mike's Muscle Cars and told him the situation. Eagerly big Mike listened and said he'd be there in fifteen minutes to pick him up because Lucky knew he and the old man were in direct competition and couldn't stand each other.

Angrily he sat down glaring at the three grease monkeys watching him, and lit up a cigarette shaking. Tom squeezed between the mechanics and joined him on the bench.

"Look Lucky, you're the best damn car hawker I've seen in my twenty years in the business, but bro you've got a lot to learn. You can't go around threatening people in this business … especially the old man," he scowled shaking his head smoking a cigarette.

"And one more thing," Tom said dead serious looking all around. "Watch your back bro … I like you … I wish I had half your talent."

"Oh shit, Tom, you know I didn't mean anything. I'm just pissed off and embarrassed. I loved this place," he paused eyeing all the Vettes lined up like soldiers. "It's the best job I ever had and I'm losing it over some horny bitch … that's what gets me the most."

"And, Lucky, another thing watch yourself with Big Mike. Everything over there ain't what it seems, believe me, I know," Tom told him as Big Mike pulled up in a loud classic suped up Burt Reynolds Black Trans AM.

"Later Tom."

"Hey you ever need a recommendation or just someone to talk to give me a ring okay. I'll help you anyway I can, but don't forget your back, you got enemies now."

"Thanks – thanks a lot"

* * *

Over an expensive lunch at the Manchester Country Club Big Mike made it clear he didn't like the way the old man and his cronies thought they ran the town.

He listened to Lucky tell his side of the story while they finished their third Absolute White Russian. Slowly Lucky loosened up his tongue and boasted that he knew plenty of dark secrets on the old man.

Enthusiastically Lucky told him about engine swapping, new cars that had been wrecked, fixed, and sold as new. Then excitedly he bragged about their biggest scam, consignment cars which made up half their inventory.

It was their best moneymaker because they never told the owners how much they sold their cars for so, they always got them to settle for less by flashing a pile of cash, which was always less than the agreed price, pocketing the difference. Or pressure them over the phone to take the lower offer because they might not get a better offer. This intrigued Big Mike and when Lucky pulled out his ten months of sales sheets he was amazed.

"Wow, you sold a hundred and ninety-six cars in ten months … you weren't bullshitting me were you."

"Nope I wasn't."

Big Mike laughed, "Shit, Lucky, I don't know if I got enough inventory to keep you happy. You're a damn gold mine, son … and you say you never sold cars before you worked there?"

"Nope I never have. To be honest I can't tell one motor from the next, and frankly I don't give shit, if the customer likes the car so do I, besides people buy from those they like."

Big Mike drooled over the gross commission payouts and shook his head smiling. "Shit, Lucky, you almost averaged two grand a car in gross profit … that's … uh … almost forty grand a month!" *And you're mine now.*

Lucky nodded. "I made that place a lot of money and what do I get for it? Fired that's what! And it really, really pisses me off – you just don't know how much." *But you'll see.*

"Well listen," Big Mike told him as the fourth round of over sized cocktails arrived. "What's it gonna take for you to come to work for me?" *Blond, brunette, redhead.*

"What took you so long?" Lucky laughed. "First Big Mike I need some wheels, like now, today. And I don't want a shit box. I want a choice demo, one I can be proud of. You know I sold twelve of the demos I was driving. I did crash two of them, but only one accident was my fault."

"Anything else?"

"I'll need a four wheel drive this winter."

Big Mike frowned. "Well that could be a little problem if I let you waltz in and just pick out a car, the other sales guys will be pissed off because they had to earn theirs first."

"What do you want me to do – walk to work?" Lucky barked. "Listen are you sitting here wasting my time? Cause I'll earn that demo in the first week I work for you, but I'm not walking to work or driving some shit box … not with my numbers."

Annoyed, Lucky laid it on the line. "So you decided Big Mike, it's a deal breaker. Otherwise I'll just pick up my phone and call someone else."

"Damn you … what else?" he demanded.

"I want to see your lot, inventory, and your pay scale sheet. No offense, but you hear shit! There's nothing more I want to do right now then put in an eighty hour week and sell every damn car on your lot." *Payback time.*

Lucky continued ranting, "I'm gonna call every City Corvette customer I know and invite them to your place. Believe me, revenge motivates me more than anything. And oh you gotta try to keep your lot full of cars plus keep all your salesman off my back."

Amazed, Big Mike asked "Why?"

"Shit, Mike, it should be obvious. The minute I step on your lot someone will come crying to you about me. They can't handle the competition because I'll be your top gun the first week I'm there and I don't give a shit what any of them say," he said with a devilish grin. "I'm there to make money – not friends."

"Jesus, you're a conceited, confident little shit, aren't you?"

"Yes sir, that's me," he smiled confidently, feeling buzzed. "There can only be one number one." *And I'm it.*

Stunned, Big Mike grinned slowly. "Damn, Son, I like your cocky attitude. Come on, let's get out of here and see what we can do about all your crazy demands."

FOUR

A N HOUR LATER, Lucky left Big Mike's muscle cars driving the black Burt Reynolds T-Top Trans AM with a 454 big block Paxton super charged Corvette motor pushing 600 horse power.

"Bad company, till the day I die" cranked out on the alpine c.d. player as Lucky roared on to interstate 93 and ran it up through the six speed gear box.

Frantically, he snorted a bump of cocaine off the corner of his license as he easily flew past a hundred. Excitedly he watched the speedometer race to one – fifty. With plenty of throttle to go, he backed off grinning ear to ear.

Singing off key to Bad Company, he pulled off the highway into the New Hampshire Liquor Store rest area where he did another bump to keep his endorphins racing in his over tired body and brain.

The state owned all the liquor stores and had smartly located them conveniently on both sides of the highway for the visiting tourists with their own exit and on ramps.

Feeling like a new man after such an emotional day, he jogged into the store and bought a large bottle of Absolute Vodka and a liter of Kahlua.

Back in the car he found Rock 101 on the high-powered stereo and cranked up a classic rock block of Aerosmith.

A few minutes later he pulled into Alexis's apartment. After a quick drink and a few lines they both jumped into the Trans-AM with the T-Tops out. They drove North on I-93 towards Bow Junction, only twenty-five miles away.

Alexis, an adorable five foot four bleached blonde babe worked out constantly. Besides her firm tanned legs and sexy backside, she opted for a superb after market package to the tune of thirty-six double-D's, which gave her a whole new outlook on life.

They had known each other for more than ten years while they were both in their first marriages. Oddly her ex-husband brought Lucky to their place to sell him some cocaine and a month later Lucky received a surprise phone call from Alexis, who had found Lucky's business card he intentionally hid in her couch, during her spring cleaning.

Shortly they became passionate lovers who were both going through messy complicated separations which both ended in divorce. During and after all this, their sex life grew hotter and hotter as they screwed each other's brains out and fell in lust.

Like most backward relationships that started with sex as the only priority, then nothing else matters. This one started with a spark and grew into a burning out of control inferno.

But somehow they had stayed close over the years realizing that what they felt for one another was very special and could be captured by either one in need with just a phone call.

Even though they both had partners in their busy lives they would always make time to sneak away for a naughty luncheon rendezvous.

Horny, manic, and high Lucky had only one thing on his mind as his eyes lusted over Alexis' erotic body. "Let's go celebrate my new job," he cheered as they raced to the car.

On the highway, Lucky called Lung his best friend since sixth grade and invited him to meet Alexis and him at his parents' house for a special get together.

The two of them had shared a few women over the years, including Alexis, and he just happened to be free from his clingy girlfriend. Lucky had given him his nickname years earlier because he was such a powerful guy who played nose tackle on the high school football team and could swim like a fish in the pool.

Unbelievably Lung could swim six lengths underwater at Lucky's parents' private country club and was shockingly fast and fluent in all strokes. They were better than friends, they were like brothers.

Lucky's parents and Lung both lived in the small prosperous town of Bow located just south of Concord, the capital, and twenty-five miles

North of Manchester. Between Bow and Manchester was the town of Hooksett.

His parents were both avid golfers and were gone to Cape Cod Massachusetts for a P.G.A. tournament. They had a stunning three level colonial with four fireplaces. The lower level had a built in Jacuzzi, custom stocked bar, with a big screen TV, and one of the four fireplaces.

It was a lover's paradise. Plants were everywhere.

The house was tastefully decorated with antiques. Even Home and Gardens approached Lucky's Mother about featuring her creative skills as a professional decorator in their house of the month layout.

It was a great place to entertain, which his parents did a lot of, and that's just what Lucky had planned for his two best friends.

FIVE

L UCKY SLYLY GRINNED at Alexis when he hung up his
Nextel phone. "I hope you don't mind a little company do you?"
She smiled embarrassed, "I guess it's too late to say no," Alexis
laughed nervously.

"Yup I guess it is," he yelled over the loud motor and blowing wind.

Once at the house, Lung built a fire while Lucky uncovered the
Jacuzzi and Alexis was busy mixing a pitcher of Absolute White
Russians.

While the Jacuzzi heated up they relaxed on the oversized sectional
sofa watching MTV videos. Slowly they all unwound as Lucky passed
a mirror covered with thick lines of the devils powder and Lung hit up
on a joint of Columbian Gold.

Casually with the lights dimmed, surrounded by tropical plants
they stripped naked except for Alexis who left on her red garter and
matching stockings.

The hot water jets felt wonderful.

And the millions of powerful bubbles set the scene.

"To the three musketeers," Lucky yelled raising his plastic tumbler
high in the air for a toast.

Knowing they all had significant others in their lives made it all the
more special. They had done this before and each time was always better
than the time before. Alexis loved all the extra attention she received,
especially since Lucky and Lung were very comfortable with each other.
They would take turns pleasuring her. Sometimes together, sometimes
alone while the other one watched.

Alexis hopped out of the Jacuzzi to fix another pitcher of White
Russians. She looked hot prancing around in front of the crackling

flames clutching two bottles of Moet Champagne she'd found stashed in the bar fridge. Her wet tanned glistening body made her white firm breasts really stand out keeping them amused.

"I'm ready boys … let's play," she cried out excitedly. "Come on get your cute asses out of that tub and show me lovin' … I'm getting awfully lonely out here by myself."

The guys laughed.

"Go ahead bro – I got the camcorder this time – Ridem cowboy," Lucky kidded.

While Lung was entertaining Alexis, Lucky looked through the camcorder eyepiece set up on the tripod, he was pleased with his novice movie skills.

Then he brought out the mirror and interrupted them as they both indulged in more magic powder. Shortly he joined them on the pull out sofa and kept Alexis' mouth occupied while Lung plunged deeply making her moan with ecstasy.

After swapping back and forth Alexis needed a break. The hot fire had them all soaked in sweet summer sweat and the look on Alexis' face was one of pain and pleasure. "Enough you're gonna kill me. Please Lung tell him to stop," she screamed as she orgasmed again.

He rolled off her totally spent.

Light headed he stumbled towards the shower so he could cool down quickly. With only two hours sleep the night before, Lucky glanced at his Casio "G" Shock when he stepped out of the cool shower and was shocked that it was already three a.m. He came out of the bathroom feeling rejuvenated, and found his friends chilling out in the Jacuzzi.

"Hey guys we might as well finish up that powder on the mirror," Lucky told them with a grin. "Hey what's a matter, you guys all worn out?"

They both leered at him shaking their heads.

"Oh come on … Hey can you guys believe they fuckin' fired my ass … I still can't believe that shit," he said wired grinding his jaw.

"Get over it bro," Lung said ornery. "You gotta start your new job in" – glancing at his watch – "what six hours or so, so chill the hell out okay!"

She nodded, "he's right Lucky, you're wicked high and you can't start your new job looking like that."

He threw his hands up in the air disgusted. "Alright … alright … here you guys split my lines, I've been going strong for two days," he mumbled, plopping down on the couch depressed.

*   *   *

By seven AM the sun started coming up over the mountains and Lucky still hadn't gotten any sleep, and he was really feeling like shit. Alexis was out cold, spread eagle naked on the sofa bed. Lung had left about five AM and Lucky, moody as hell, was still horny.

He eyed her lustfully.

Carefully he slid his manhood inside her hot wet mound trying not to wake her. She stirred slowly the faster he went. And before long her strong firm legs wrapped around him so she could lift up and meet his every thrust. Finally they came together once again, just as the strong morning sun shined through the sliding glass doors.

"Oh Lucky," she moaned. "You fuck me sooo goood. What am I gonna do with you?' she purred. "Please try to get your shit together baby, I'm so worried about you … oh shit … it's almost seven thirty, you gotta get my ass home. It's Friday and I never miss work." *For anybody.*

"Okay," he muttered still inside her.

"Get off me lover boy, I have to take a quick shower." Quickly she tried to get up and realized how sore she was. "Oh God I'm so sore …" She groaned painfully. You guys fucked the shit out of me," she complained.

Lucky laughed at the expression on her face.

"It's not funny."

"Yeah but you loved every minute."

She waved him off and ran for the shower.

*   *   *

After he dropped Alexis off, he stopped for breakfast, which barely made him feel human. Thankfully he only had to spend a few hours at

Big Mike's to learn the inventory and prices before he had to leave to go back and get his last paycheck at City Corvette.

Armed with two large extra sweet Dunkin Donut coffees he figured he could make it through the morning. Big Mike showed him around introducing him to everyone, then gave him a desk and some generic business cards where he could just fill his name in.

He wanted to take the weekend off and catch up on his sleep, but big Mike wanted him to work the weekend, his busiest two days. "You look like you've been partying all night … what gives?" Big Mike demanded. *Another druggy that's all I need.* "Yeah so I did a little celebrating so what?," Lucky responded briskly adjusting his panama Jack shades. "But hey don't worry I'll be roaring to go tomorrow."

"Okay okay, I ain't your damn keeper. Just don't wreck my baby or you're out of here."

"Damn man take it easy, I partied at home all night with a lady friend of mine," he responded defensively lighting up a smoke.

"Well just don't let me down, you don't know how much shit I've listened to giving you my car to use … Just don't make me regret it."

"Just wait and see all the money I make you, then we'll see who regrets what! Just wait and see Boss."

"Good, now go get your last check from those assholes and get yourself some rest. We gotta big day tomorrow." Lucky nodded in agreement.

"Hey how do you like the Trans AM?"

"Man that car has some serious balls under the hood," he joked.

"How much you selling it for?"

"Hey it ain't for sale," Big Mike laughed.

"Everything's for sale Big Mike everything. Watch, I'll sell it right from underneath you."

"Okay, get twenty-five grand for it and I'll kick you three grand cash money."

"Done deal, later." *Boy am I beat.*

SIX

Manchester, NH
City Corvette
Three PM

TWO HOURS LATER Lucky pulled the loud Trans AM into a customers spot near the front door of City Corvette. The clock read 2:59pm. One minute before they started handing out checks at the business office window.

He grabbed his commission payout sheet off the passengers seat and folded it into his sports jacket. Lucky had spent the last hour at AppleBees Bar and Grill having a couple of Captain Morgan and Cokes while he figured out exactly how much they owed him.

Not counting the attorney's wife's Vette, he had delivered four vehicles and his total gross commission equaled $4,168.00 dollars.

He hopped out with a slight buzz and ignored the glaring looks he was getting from the show room glass. Boldly he went inside to get paid. Lucky was very cordial to everyone he saw and was surprised at the few quick smiles he received in return.

Nervous, tired and a little scared, he knew some liquid courage would help him walk in confidently. Once he saw that the old mans Mercedes 500 SL was not in its usual spot, he exhaled in relief. Trembling he stepped up to the window behind a big burly mechanic and waited his turn.

"Hi Joan I came to pick up my last commission check," he said nicely.

"Okay," she mumbled thumbing through the stack of envelopes. "Oh here you are … and … oh … you need to sign this also for me," she said handling him his envelope with a paper attached.

Lucky slid to the side.

He opened the sealed envelope.

The gross was only $1,800.00 hundred dollars. Shocked, he shook his head as he read the attached paper that stated City Corvette owed him no more commissions and that he was paid in full. On the bottom of the page was his name typed under a line for him to sign on.

Angrily he yanked the check stub off and pocketed the check. Impatiently he waited, then he cut the line causing a scene. "Joan look at this," he raged waving his commission sheet in front of her.

Joan eyed the paper tensely. "Wow that's quite a difference," she responded looking at the check stub and Lucky's commission sheet.

"Exactly like twenty-three hundred different," he said hotly blocking the window. "Here, write down these four deals and please check them okay, and tell the old man I'm not signing shit till I get paid in full."

Disturbed Joan shrugged her shoulders. "Well Lucky I can't do anything today because he's not here and I'm not authorized to give you any more money."

"Look Joan, no disrespect, I know you're doing what you're told, but do the old man a favor and give him this message," he stated highly agitated just as a group of employees started to surround him. "Tell him I'll be here Monday at five PM to pick up a gross check for two thousand three hundred and sixty eight dollars and then I'll sign your paper."

He paused for a second. "But Tell him if I don't get my money on Monday in full I'll be calling two customers in particular," he looked all around and nodded. "That's right the Murrays and the Phillips, and they won't be too happy when I tell them a few secrets about their new Subarus."

Shocked she covered her mouth with her hand and nodded.

"Just pass the message and have my check ready and Joan try to have a nice day," he barked sarcastically.

Tom was waiting by the Trans AM.

Lucky came flying out the showroom door agitated and immediately lit a smoke when he spotted Tom.

"Hey Lucky."

"Hey Tom."

"You get all your money?"

"Shit no, they screwed me out of twenty three hundred and sixty-eight bucks ... you believe that shit?," Lucky screeched disgusted.

"Yup I do – but you didn't hear it from me."

"Here look."

Tom studied his check and commission sheet and shook his head. "Looks like you got paid on the first two deals but not the last two. I'll check it out."

"Listen I told Joan to tell the old man to have my check ready by five pm on Monday, otherwise I'm gonna call the Murrays and Phillips, and I will too."

"Definitely not a good idea Lucky, that's a law suit just waiting to happen."

"That's his problem. I want my money."

"I said I'd look into it – now you better get the hell out of here – while you still can."

Lucky looked and spotted the group of mechanics heading his way. "Yup I think I'll take off Tom," he said swiftly climbing into the Trans AM.

"Hey you better watch your ass bro; I've never seen the old man so pissed off after you left yesterday. I'm surprised both your legs aren't broke yet," Tom yelled over the noisy exhausts.

"Later Tom," he said tearing out just as the welcome committee showed up.

His first stop was City Corvette's Bank. This wouldn't be the first time a check had bounced, and Lucky couldn't cash it fast enough.

SEVEN

H E EXITED THE drive thru-window with $1,386.00 dollars. Then he drove back to AppleBees where he ordered the bourbon steak specialty medium rare, steak fries, and washed it down with three more Captain Morgan and cokes.

Wiped out and exhausted, he jumped on I-93 North bound. Cruising at a 100 miles an hour, he called his girlfriend Laura on his Nextel phone to tell her what he was up to.

By seven PM he was sound asleep. He slept like a rock straight through until his high powered alarm clock went off at seven AM blaring Rock 101 and Van Halen's "Jamie's Cryin."

After a huge breakfast at Bow's Famous Rte 3A Truck Stop, Lucky pulled into Big Mike's lot for his first day of work.

Revenge. I need revenge.
I gotta make the old man pay.
Come on think what would really piss him off.
Steal his customers…

City Corvette left a bad taste in his mouth. He was so angry that he worked harder than he ever had. By six pm he had gone on eight test drives and he managed to write up four deals. He was surprised at how busy it was, even though Big Mike's had only half the inventory of City Corvette.

Saturday night he spent with Laura at his parents' house and made love on the same pull out sofa in the lower level that Alexis, Lung, Lucky had indulged on only two nights earlier.

Very rarely did Lucky ever do any drugs around Laura. She wasn't into drugs and always tried to be a good influence. Occasionally she would drink alcohol. She was his good girl, his angel.

They met at an over thirty dance club in Concord called the 'Take Five Music Hall' and both fell madly in love. She was a gorgeous Greek goddess, with dark flowing hair, and olive toned skin which was always deeply tanned. She was everything Lucky wasn't, faithful, committed and serious.

When they were voted the best dancers their first night together they both knew they were for each other.

It took two months till their first fight.

He never asked directly and she never gave her age. Months later when Lucky found out she was twenty years older than him, he went ballistic and moved back to his parents.

Two weeks later they were back together dominating the Music Hall's dance floor. He was a very experienced lover, where she'd been married for over twenty years before getting a divorce. The problem was, her sex life was non-existent until Lucky convinced her to let him teach her.

Before long the teacher taught his willing student how to achieve an orgasm. After that their love life thrived as they held regular classes often.

Things were going well as they shared a bottle of California Chardonnay, while they ate delicious jumbo fried prawns from the popular Back Room Restaurant in Hooksett.

"So how did your first day go honey?," Laura asked sexily lying in front of the fireplace.

"Pretty good Angel. I wrote up four deals … but I don't know how many will get bought … but I guess I can't worry about that since I have no control over what the bank says."

"Hey that's super honey."

"Mmm-mmm … Big Mike was pretty pleased because no one wrote over two deals and on my first day I dominated," he laughed slyly.

"I knew you'd do well," she paused. "So honey tell me what happened Thursday night, I was all packed and ready to come here and spend the night?"

"Oh, shit Thursday night, ya I was wicked upset … you know after all that shit went down at work, I needed to unwind … and you don't wanna be around me when I'm like that." *Getting high and fucking Alexis.*

"Okay, but you've got a lot to make up for so get over here," she ordered patting the silk coverlet. "And show me teacher how much you missed your student," she purred sexily.

They cuddled and made mad passionate love through out the night, enjoying each other's company. It wasn't till the next morning, Sunday while he was in the shower, that Laura folded the sofa bed away and found Alexis' red garter stuffed under one of the cushions.

She started looking around.

Then she noticed the antique mirror was put back crooked. She eyed the dried finger smudges and cocaine residue and immediately she felt lied to. When she found the three dirty champagne flutes, and two empty bottles of champagne she was furious.

Enraged she started throwing her clothes into her carry-all as Lucky came out of the bathroom smiling.

"So what the hell's this?" she hollered holding up Alexis' semen stained red garter belt angrily. "Your mothers … huh … And don't even try to lie to me … I know this wasn't here last weekend … so who's is it, and I want the truth now?" she raged hitting Lucky in the face with the airborne dirty garter.

"Oh shit," Lucky mumbled. "Honey it's not like you think – listen I'll tell you alright?" he said raising his voice while he watched her throw her stuff recklessly into her bag.

Shit. "Alexis and Lung came over Thursday night after they found out how upset I was … and … well … uh … we ended up in the Jacuzzi drinking Mom's champagne … and –"

"And?" she screamed. "I'm not stupid Lucky."

"I know – I know … okay … Yes we had sex with her, but she's just a good friend … It didn't mean anything. Listen, she's got a boyfriend. It just happened," he said dejected as he followed her up the stairs to the main floor.

Impatiently, he yelled at her. "She doesn't mean anything."

Laura spun around and jabbed him in the chest.

"You lied to me … right to my face … then you chose to be with your so called sex friends over me, how do you think I feel," she cried, angrily racing to her convertible Camaro he had given her to use. "I just don't know anymore," she sobbed tearing out of the driveway.

*　　*　　*

Rejected, he ran upstairs to his bedroom.

In a whirlwind he started tearing books out of his bookcase looking for his last stash. "Fuck it, fuck it, fuck it," he screamed just as he found the gram of cocaine hidden inside an old algebra test book that he had cut the center out of.

Manically he dumped the gram onto the book cover and snorted half of it in one blast. "Aah," he shrieked into his bedroom mirror out of control. "Who does she think she is … stupid bitch … walking out on me … nobody walks out on me … nobody," he growled snorting up the other half gram.

Zooming, he drove to work at noon after scoring more cocaine off Romeo. He managed to write up three more deals on Sunday afternoon while he kept sneaking into the men's room to do small bumps of cocaine.

Feeling rejected and depressed, he knew better than to call or stop by Laura's because she was still probably too angry to deal with. Without a second thought he called Alexis and told her to get rid of her muscle head boyfriend because he was on his way over.

They spent the next few hours doing lines and drinking screwdrivers, and then he took out all his sexual frustrations in her bedroom and finally he started to relax.

"Ooops," she laughed naughtily when Lucky told her about Laura finding her garter belt under the cushion. "Oh shit, I'm sorry … I was wondering where it went to … Oh dear she must have been really mad. Shit I had to tell my boyfriend I spent the night at my sisters and I was so damn sore I couldn't let him touch me Friday night," she giggled. "Boy was he mad."

EIGHT

I T WAS MONDAY, about two pm.
He was walking the lot at Big Mike's when Tom pulled up beside him in a new Jag Convertible. "Hey got anything decent for sale, all I see is a bunch of dogs," Tom joked grinning. "Hop in," he ordered pushing the passenger's door open.

Lucky glanced around, then hopped in the expensive car.

"Here take a look."

Lucky eyed the sealed envelope… watching Tom, he ripped it open and saw the check. Smiling he eyeballed the gross $2,368.00 dollars. Enthusiastically he kissed the check. "Hey alright," he yelled.

"Read this and sign it then I'll endorse your check," Tom said handing him a different piece of paper than Joan had tried to get him to sign.

Carefully he read it out loud.

"I Lucky Sullivan of Bow, New Hampshire in accepting this commission check for two thousand, three-hundred and sixty-eight dollars in gross commissions, agree that City Corvette has paid me in full and no longer owes me any money.

Also I agree to have no further contact with any customers and or employees of City Corvette. Nor will I make any derogatory statements or comments to any former or future customers of City Corvette. Failure to comply with any or all of the above terms stated, I realize that a possible defamatory liable suit may be pursued against me. By accepting this check and signing below I Lucky Sullivan agree to abide by all the above terms."

"Holy shit … Wow …," Lucky said shaking his head. "I guess I really did piss the old man off huh Tom?"

Tom nodded. "You sure did. I came over here myself after I finally talked the old man into paying you off, plus deliver you a message. Stay the hell away," he ordered.

He dropped the fancy glove box and signed his named and pulled off the second carbon copy for himself handing the top copy to Tom.

"Listen, Mr. Lucky, I like you … but you stirred up a hornets nest. They want to teach you a lesson for all your disrespect … Especially now since you're finally over here selling cars for this asshole … but –" Hey I warned them, I told those assholes they'd regret it and I meant it," he grinned pocketing his commission check.

"Yup you did! I was there remember? Anyway I don't blame you, but take some advice and let it go unless you want to get seriously hurt over this," he said earnestly. "Hey you hear what I'm saying?"

Lucky nodded, "I'll let it go, Tom. I actually kind of like it over here, and I'm not doing too bad."

"How bad?"

"Lets see four Saturday, three Sunday, then I wrote two today … so what's that make … only nine in three days," he laughed sarcastically.

Tom, amazed, shook his head lighting a smoke. "Figures … I knew you were really pissed off, and I told them you'd come over here and take revenge by kicking ass."

Lucky agreed smiling. *Exactly.*

"Hey you remember that one crazy Saturday when you sold six Vettes in six hours and we just kept turning you lose on more customers. Man what a day that was," Tom burst out laughing remembering all of Lucky's customers lined up outside the Finance office.

"Ya … ya … that was pretty funny wasn't it."

"Damn, Big Mike must be shitting all over himself, he's so damn happy stealing you away."

"Hey so far he's pretty amazed, but I'm just getting warmed up. Can you say thirty maybe forty cars in a month," he said confidently. "Yup I'll make him double his inventory."

"Lucky, isn't that Big Mike staring at us from the showroom … probably thinks I came over to steal you back," Tom laughed.

"Fat chance ... fuck him ... hey you brought me my check which I've been stressed out about all weekend. Plus you saved me a big hassle of going back over there tonight."

"True, true ... well I better get out of here before he throws me out. Hey you take care, buddy, and do me a favor stay away for a while will you!"

"Don't worry Tom I'm too damn busy making money", he said hopping out of the Jag. "Hey thanks Tom."

Tom pulled off and waved getting a nasty look from Big Mike while Lucky slowly walked towards the showroom gloating over his fat check. As he got closer Big Mike yelled out impatiently, "hey what the hell did he want?"

"Take it easy Big Mike – can't my old boss come by to say hi?"

"Yeah right ... let me guess ... he was just driving by."

Lucky had a shit-eating grin as he pulled out his commission check and showed Big Mike.

"Ah now I get it ... your check ... don't want you bothering them no more, huh," he laughed heavily. Relieved.

"Nope they sure don't. Here read this while I run to the bank and cash this check before they change their mind," Lucky said eagerly running for the Trans AM.

"Hey I don't blame you, but don't get lost on me," Big Mike pleaded.

"I'll be right back."

"Hey did he ask you how many cars you've sold?" he asked with a big smirk.

"Of course he did ... I told him it was kinda slow ... that I only sold nine since Saturday," Lucky yelled out the window as he roared off the lot.

NINE

O N WEDNESDAY LUCKY sent a dozen long stem pink roses to Laura's office with a note begging her to meet him for dinner at her favorite restaurant, The China Dragon.

By eleven pm they were back at her condo making love. She was everything he wanted and needed... Beautiful, sexy, reliable, and devoted. But somehow he felt unworthy even though he knew his angel would make a wonderful wife. The problem was every time they got serious Lucky would do something stupid to screw it up.

Between his manic work pace, chasing skirts, and doing drugs he had little time for anything else. Besides visiting his V.A. hospital psychiatrist once a month to renew his psychotropic medications for his chemical imbalances, which made him extremely compulsive, his quick decisions based on spur of the moment impulses from addictive irrational thought patterns, usually resulted in poor decisions, getting him in trouble.

The first week at Big Mike's he worked manically at a very fast pace obsessed with selling twelve cars in six days. Because a car wasn't considered sold until it was actually delivered. Lucky learned quickly that Big Mike's finance department wasn't nearly as good as City Corvettes finance guru at getting questionable credit bought by the banks.

This meant less loans approved and less commissions for Lucky. By Friday, payday, he had delivered his eighth car. The other four were turned downs, but it still gave him a sixty-seven percent delivery ratio. Aggravated he couldn't match his eighty percent ratio from City Corvette, he realized he would have to work harder and sell more cars to hit the magic thirty delivered in thirty day goal that he set for himself.

It was five pm, check time.

Excitedly, he picked up his first commission check, then sat down at his tiny desk to go over his sales sheet to check the figures. His total gross exceeded twenty grand for the eight cars he delivered for an average of $2,600 hundred per vehicle, which put him in the thirty percent range of the total gross commission for an average of $770.00 dollars per car net.

Immediately he noticed something was wrong when he saw his total gross of $20,800.00 dollars reduced by six grand to $14,800.00. Alarmed Lucky glanced over the pay stub looking for an explanation.

Then he found it in fine print on the bottom of the check stub. "For every vehicle sold a lot fee of $750.00 dollars will be subtracted from the vehicles total gross before your commission is calculated."

"Holy shit," Lucky said out loud. "A six grand lot fee you gotta be kidding me," he yelled angrily, as one of the other veteran salesman walked over.

"What's the matter?" *Hot shot.*

"What's this shit … you telling me this is for real … a seven hundred and fifty dollar rip off fee for every vehicle you sell, no matter how many you sell?," he demanded an answer raising his voice pointing at the six grand figure deducted from his total gross.

The salesman, not a fan of Lucky's answered with a shit eating grin. "Yup sure is, Big Mike gets his right off the top," obviously pleased that the new star was pissed off.

"Unbelievable … I … I used to pay two-fifty per car for the first ten cars a month, then the rest were no charge … but seven-fifty is absurd," Lucky roared.

"True … true," the salesman laughed backing up a step. "But just ask him to explain it, and he'll tell you, two-fifty for prep, two-fifty for advertising, and two-fifty for the house."

"That's fucking bullshit," he screeched, slamming his fist onto the cheap desk causing a scene. "I ain't payin that shit … that … that comes out of his profit not mine," he wailed jumping to his feet angrily.

"Hey – hey take it easy," the snotty salesman told him, alarmed at Lucky's sudden hostility.

Lucky stepped quickly towards him seeing nothing but red, the old mans face, and Big Mike laughing. "Fuck you punk ... you take it easy ... I sell eight fuckin cars in six days and I get taxed six grand ... no way ... no fuckin way," he hollered as he pushed off and punched the arrogant salesman in the nose sending him sprawling to the carpet.

Out of control, Lucky, spun around and noticed everyone was frozen in place staring at him in shock.

"Where is he?" Lucky demanded angrily.

Luckily, Big Mike was at the gym or he would have seen a side of Lucky he didn't like. And even though Big Mike was six foot five and two hundred and sixty pounds who spent his off time at Gold's Gym five days a week, Lucky wasn't anything nice when he lost total control.

At five foot eleven and a hundred and eighty-five pounds, Lucky was skilled in martial arts. He was equipped with a fast pair of feet and hands, which gave him the option of kicking or running depending on the situation. He probably wouldn't have stood a chance against Big Mike, but it wouldn't matter because Lucky had to make a stand. Because this was the second time in two weeks he'd been screwed over by a greedy owner.

"What's wrong?", the sales manager demanded eyeing the bloody salesman still on the floor. "What the hells going on in here?"

He was in a zone.

The only thing running through Lucky's mind was that they were all laughing at him, and he could see Tom telling him I told you so. "Damn right there's a big problem," Lucky stormed heading outside he slammed the showroom glass door into the wall cracking it.

Rapidly he moved towards the Trans-Am blinded by rage. He tore out of the parking lot laying a nice patch of rubber for Big Mike to see. He was supposed to stay till eight p.m. and it was only five, but he was done for the day.

"Fuckin' asshole," he cussed as he raced to Big Mike's bank before it closed. "Nobody fucks me out of my hard earned money, nobody," he swore as the teller sent him his cash. Rapidly he counted out thirty-four hundred dollars.

With AC/DC cranked full throttle he raced through Friday's rush hour traffic recklessly thinking of only one thing. Getting high and escaping from all the disappointment.

Thankfully, Laura always went out with her girlfriends on Friday nights because there was no stopping him now, as he continued to break every rule of the road. It was calling him, come get me I'll take you away.

Once on the seedy side of Manchester he decided wisely to slow down seeing more and more cop cars cruising the streets. The way he was feeling he knew there was only one substance strong enough to escape the pain.

Oddly he had met the Colombian through another car salesman who had sold the drug dealer a used caddy for nine grand cash, all in small bills, keeping it under the notorious ten grand I.R.S. reporting figurer that car dealers had to file paperwork when any customer purchased a vehicle in excess of ten grand with cash. Lucky had eyeballed the Columbian piling fives, tens, and twenties on the salesman's desk.

Eagerly he paid a hundred bucks for the Columbian's pager number for future use.

The bad thing about New Hampshire was that unless you knew exactly where the drug dealers lived, you'd have a tough time trying to get high.

Because unlike Florida, where crack and other designer drugs were sold out in the open on many street corners, New Hampshire was exactly the opposite where most transactions took place behind closed doors.

Eagerly he dialed his Nextel phone.

From memory he entered the Columbians pager number, remembering to enter his own code on the end, 007.

The closer he got, the worst it became.

Anxiety.

He could feel the rush from that first hit of crack. His mouth salivated, his pulse raced as his mind remembered the devils evil smoke. His phone rang. Anxiously he grabbed it on the first ring, "Hello?"

"Hey Gringo whas up wit you?"

"Hey Romeo, I need to see you … like now!"

"Man what you be lookin for Gringo?"

"Heavy pizza bro, say five large pies to start with."

"Mmm … okay no problemo amigo how soon?"

"Well I'm only five away … you want me to pick up pizzas or you delivering curbside?"

"I'll come out … but you better make it ten, I gotta finish baking the pies first … what you got for wheels?"

"Black loud Trans-Am."

"Okay Gringo you know the drill, cruise by slow one time so I scope you, then on the second pass pull in next door."

"Got it – later."

His next stop was the corner grocery store that sold little tiny roses inside glass stems for $3.99 a piece. He bought four of them. A box of Choir Boy brillo and a six pack of Bic lighters. Impulsively he grabbed the latest Hustler, Penthouse and High Society off the rack to go along with a carton of Marlboro Lights.

He knew he'd be very horny later, but too wired to be with anyone so he'd keep himself amused with the girly magazines.

Back in the Trans-Am he pushed the rose out of the glass stem, then he pulled off a piece of brillo. Recklessly holding the ripped piece of brillo with his expensive gold tie clasp, he burned the brillo with three Bic lighters held together with a rubber band. The coating gave off an awful smell. Satisfied he balled up the chunk of brillo and pushed it into one end of the stem. Presto, instant crack pipe sold right at most corner stores.

Romeo was waiting on the porch.

He cruised by slowly making the mandatory pass.

They made eye contact.

Casually, Romeo watched him cruise by looking for a tail or anyone around who shouldn't be.

After Lucky made the second pass he saw the signal to pull in next door. He knew because Romeo had removed his Tommy Hilfiger hat on the second pass by.

He waited shutting the noisy car off. His pulse was racing. He was in the zone. The drug zone, and if anything bad was going to happen, it would happen soon. He waited anxiously for Romeo who would casually make his way over to the car and get in. But if on his way over Romeo eyed something suspicious he'd put his hat back on and walk by. Lucky would wait five minutes, pull back out the drive way and wait for his Nextel phone to ring.

"Hey Gringo … nice wheels bro …" Romeo grinned flashing his two gold capped teeth as he climbed into the Recaro racing bucket seats. "Man you must be up to no good again; you look like you're ready to get busy."

Lucky nodded nervously expecting the cops to come flying out any second. "Hey let's do this. You got my package?"

"Yup … as they say show me da money."

Lucky whipped out five new Ben Franklins.

"Okay, okay don't I always take care of my suit and tie customers?" Romeo laughed pulling out a bag full of twenty dollar rocks. "Here take a look. Thirty fat twentys. Six per hundred, so you got five free."

Lucky stuffed the baggy in his suit jacket pocket. "Okay, okay listen Romeo, you know once I start smoking this shit, I'll probably need more later so don't run out on me. My money's long and I know its Friday night," Lucky paused thinking. "Let's say midnight or so, all right?"

"No problem Gringo you're first rate with me, I'll be ready, just call me first. You know them pigs be cruisin heavy on Friday night, so be careful."

"Okay, Adios Romeo."

"Later Gringo."

TEN

HE COULDN'T WAIT.
 Lucky pulled into the first safe place he saw. The Donavan's Country Club parking lot. Quickly, he opened his back pack and pulled out his 9mm Baretta and stuck it in between the center console and the passenger's seat. Then he pulled out his weekly pill holder which held his seventeen pills per day. Between the Prozac, Wellbutrin, Lithium, Trazadone and Bendedryl, the new pipe was neatly hidden amongst the colorful pills. Shaking he pulled the stem out and tossed the pill case back in the pack. He glanced around while he took a twenty dollar piece of crack and snapped it in two. Impatiently he crammed the crack into the end of the four inch glass stem on top of the burnt brillo. Expertly, he melted the devils drug on to the brillo.

Satisfied it wouldn't fall out, he exhaled deeply. Then he raised the other end to his trembling lips. Lightly he hit the flame over the melted crack while he inhaled slowly. The devils smoke filled his lungs as he continued to inhale deeply filling his lungs with the delicious poison.

Instantly the drug raced into his blood stream straight to his brain. Everything stopped. Bells, trains, alarms were all screaming inside his head as he held the smoke in till the last second.

Nothing else mattered.

Then he exhaled slowly letting out the devils smoke. "Holy shit … oh my god," he mumbled wide-eyed as the train screamed into his head, faster and faster.

Immediately, he became another person.

Paranoid.

Schizoid.

Afraid.

They were closing in on the car. Nervously he fired up the motor and pulled off.

That one delicious hit turned him into a hallucinating, over suspicious, uncaring crack addict. He put his Ray bans back on when he pulled out in traffic.

Immediately aware of his surroundings he glanced down at the gauges and saw the thirsty motor had drained the gas tank.

His mind raced trying to think of a full service station where he didn't need to get out of the car to pump gas.

Minutes passed.

Frustrated he pulled off the main road into a nice residential neighborhood.

Another quick blast, he told himself.

He left the Trans-Am idling as he jammed another chunk of crack into the stem. Shaking, he hurriedly lit the other end and greedily inhaled the evil smoke.

While he held his hit in all his senses were on full alert.

A door slammed loudly. *Oh no.*

An outside light came on at the nearest house. *Go, go there coming.*

Bug eyed, he exhaled the scented smoke as the demons rushed in and tried to trap him. Panicking he let the clutch out and hit the gas.

Lucky still had twenty-nine more rocks to smoke and it was only seven pm.

Finally, he found a full service Sunoco station. He had the gas attendant fill it up with 105 Octane Racing fuel. Eighty bucks later he was back cruising the country roads outside Manchester and Keene smoking crack trying to outrun the imaginary demons.

Sometimes he could get three maybe four hits from a twenty. But never would he pull over for long and just park. No way. Only long enough to take a hit. His biggest fear was getting caught. Every time he stopped he could feel them getting closer and closer the longer he sat still. Every car behind him was following him, chasing him, after him.

Swiftly he continued to smoke, his mind hallucinated telling him they were out there. Regular cars all looked like cop cars. Then he imagined that every car tailing him had to be an unmarked cruiser. He kept telling himself that if he didn't speed or stop too long then they'd never catch him.

Two hours later, by nine pm, he had smoked fourteen rocks. Hit after hit he grew more unstable, wishing he wasn't driving such a loud noticeable car. "Fucking assholes" he muttered thinking about how they were all out to rip him off. "Steal my money … fire me … will ya, no fuckin way," he screamed over Bachman Turner Overdrive.

By ten thirty he ended up over by City Corvette on Elm Street, pulling into a small abandon lot across the street. The dealership was closed, and there was no one around. Just sitting there he got madder and madder by the second. Intoxicated on the crack, weird evil visions and thoughts flashed through his mind until he couldn't stand it.

Disgusted, he hit the stem again.

Lucky started the car and crossed the street.

Slowly he cruised through the neat rows of Vettes and muscle cars grinding his teeth violently. On his way out fuming he spotted the 1970 Chevelle SS 454 up on the display rack by the road. It was the car of the week and the spotlights gleamed off its polished chrome. A bright reflection caught Lucky's dilated eyes for a split second, blinding him. Then he saw what it was, the lock box key box attached to the drivers window.

"Oh shit … oh shit, that's it … that's it," he yelled with excitement slapping the brushed chrome dash board with his hand. Faster and faster his mind thought of a plan as he recalled the master key still stashed in his work boot at home.

Hysterically he started laughing.

Sweat poured out of his pores from all the drugs.

"I got a key to all these beautiful fuckin' cars and the old man doesn't know it." Uncontrollably he growled at the top of his lungs, "I'll get you mother fucker, I'll get you … it's pay back time."

Even with the A/C on high he was still sweating like a pig. By eleven pm he couldn't wait any longer. He called Romeo. Ten minutes later his Nextel phone rang.

"Hey Gringo, you're early."

"Well you know me, I'm ahead of schedule," he whispered softly into the phone trying to drive. "And I don't like running out … so you got me or what?"

"What ah we talking, Gringo?"

"Same order, just add two large soft drinks with that order."

"Man you sure that's enough, Hombre?" Romeo laughed sarcastically.

"Who knows," *how much I'll need.* "But let's do this now so I can get the hell out of this city. If I call you later, than I do … If I don't, I don't."

"Jesus, bro why you whisperin'. You alright?"

"Huh … uh … I will be … same spot or what?"

"Yup that'll work, just watch out for five-o. They're cruisin' hard, see you in ten."

"Okay."

*   *   *

Lucky hung up the phone just as he came up to a major intersection and was first in line in the right lane waiting for the red light to change. A Manchester cruiser pulled up beside him in the left lane and both cops eyeballed the loud rumbling muscle car.

Nervously, he tried to keep his eyes straight ahead.

Oh shit, oh shit he thought as he pushed the butt of his gun sticking out between the seats lower. "Come on, come on turn green," he pleaded. They know, they know his mind kept telling him. *No they don't, no they don't, stop it.*

Green light.

He wanted to tromp the accelerator and race away, but timidly he pulled off slowly and let the cruiser blow by in the other lane. "Whew that was close," he told himself, making the turn towards Romeo's busy neighborhood.

Just as he turned into Romeo's neighborhood, a cruiser turned on his lights, right behind Lucky. "Oh my God, fuck what am I gonna do," he mumbled pulling to the side. The cruiser raced past almost giving him a heart attack. He made the next turn and he saw two cruisers pulled over. Slowly he drove past, and spotted four drug addicts spread eagle against the car. "Holy shit." *Man oh man.*

He coasted by, eyeing the cops and the bright lights. *Man that was too close* he exhaled looking back in the rearview mirror while he continued towards Romeos mumbling "Man I'm glad that wasn't me."

Now he was in the seedy neighborhood, right near Romeos. Slowly he cruised by his front porch making the mandatory first pass. On the second pass he pulled in next-door and waited clutching his gun.-

He was so tense and jittery that when Romeo rapped on his driver's side window he jumped smacking his head on the roof of the car.

Slowly, he lowered the window.

"Jesus Gringo, man you be flyin high man," Romeo said shaking his head.

"You know it," he whispered looking all around. "So what's up you got my shit?"

"Gringo put your piece away man you don't need that shit with me around, my boys are all over this area. Nobody would be stupid enough to fuck with you in our territory.

"Now come up to the crib, five-o's cruising heavy and it's been hot as hell … Come on, come chill out for a while."

"Okay … okay," he replied reluctantly throwing his gun and phone into his pack.

Romeo lived on the top floor. They trucked up the four sets of steep stairs while Lucky clutched his backpack in one hand and a warm twelve pack of Budweiser in the other, he'd bought hours earlier at the corner store.

At the top of the stairs Romeo quickly gave a coded knock on the heavily reinforced door. Rapidly the door bolts slid open.

"Hey Lucky."

"Hey Sasha," Lucky responded to Romeo's gorgeous girlfriend.

"Come on in and relax … you look like you could use it," she laughed, raking her sexy long blonde hair with her hand." Lots of cops out tonight huh."

"I'll say. I'm glad to be out of that damn race car I'm driving." *And looking at you.*

"Man, Gringo I can't believe you been driving around all this time smoking that shit ... Come on in here and I'll hook you up."

The three of them walked into the old fashioned kitchen and sat down. "Why don't you take off your jacket and tie and relax," she purred taking the warm beer from Lucky and started filling the freezer.

There was a large dinner plate on the table with a monster size cookie of crack sitting on it.

"Now that's a serious cookie," Lucky said enthusiastically.

"No shit, amigo, that's five grand sitting there in just my cost. If you was anybody else I wouldn't have let you in here with no gun," he said pointing at Luckys pack.

Lucky eyed the ten millimeter glock sitting on the table, then his buldging eyes went back to the cookie.

"So what you want, Gringo?"

"Give me a good deal on an eight ball of powder and twenty rocks and if it's all right I'll hang out in the back bedroom till the cops cool down, I'm sick of driving around."

"We can do that," he said, as Sasha walked back into the kitchen wearing a thin silk robe with nothing underneath. Only twenty-one, she had a hard body and her long blonde hair hung all the way down past her ass, and when she looked at you, her deep blue eyes sparkled.

"So you've been up to no good, I see."

Lucky snickered trying not to stare at her perky breasts. "You got that right." *God this shit gets me so damn horny.*

He couldn't believe that Romeo was living with a Supreme Court judge's daughter. He watched her strut around the kitchen gracefully teasing them. "So did you bring me a treat Lucky," she asked smiling.

"Jeez, I don't know ...," he replied digging into his back pack knowing Romeo and Sasha were both pot heads and never touched crack, only once in a while would they snort a few lines.

"Ah look what I just happened to find stashed away in my side pouch," Lucky teased pulling out a fat ounce of green skunk bud, that Lung had bought for him two weeks earlier. The weed was very expensive costing $350 an ounce, and it was very powerful. The buds were sticky and loaded with red and gold hairs full of THC.

He pulled out a nice bud and handed it to Sasha. "Try that out," he said grinning, noticing her nipples poking through her robe.

"You got any smokes, Lucky," she asked eyeing his Marlboro Lights.

"Would I forget you beautiful?"

"Not yet you haven't," she giggled.

He pulled out a new pack of Marlboro Lights and handed them to her, "All yours."

"Oh isn't he sweet, Romeo, he always brings me gifts … make sure you take extra good care of him."

"Of course I will baby," he told her cutting off a chunk from the thick cookie. "You want me to break it up for you or you like it like this?"

"Just like that."

"Oh here's your eight ball, three and a half grams of decent powder. Let's see that's five bills on the crack and two fifty on the powder, that's seven-fifty," Romeo paused waiting while Lucky pulled out his fat wallet and counted out seven hundred and fifty dollars.

Romeo grabbed the money off the table and counted out seven Franklins and left fifty on the table. "That's Sasha's discount," he grinned.

Surprised Lucky scooped up the fifty, "thanks guys."

"Hey you're a good tie customer and Sasha don't like many dudes so you're cool … Hey baby Lucky's gonna chill out in the back bedroom for a few hours till five-o chills out … okay wit you?"

"Yes baby, you know how I feel about Lucky, he's always welcome here."

"Go ahead, Gringo, make yourself at home."

"Okay thanks," he said putting his new purchases into his back pack.

ELEVEN

THE BACK BEDROOM was sparsely furnished. A queen size mattress sat on the floor with dirty sheets and nasty blankets. In one corner was a stack of grubby adult magazines. Beside the bed was a rickety table and lamp with no shade. In the center of the room sat an old wooden rocking chair that looked like it was ready for kindling.

After his first hit he realized that anyone outside could look through the thin soiled curtains and see him getting high. No matter where he sat they could still see him, and he just knew someone was out there.

Watching.

Nervously he loaded up the four stems with crack while he set his gun on the bed beside him. He really did trust Romeo and Sasha, but he had no idea who else might stop by.

It was a crack house, after all!

He finished the last four rocks from the thirty he'd bought earlier, the paranoia came screaming back and toyed with his over stimulated mind. The faster he smoked the quicker his brain hallucinated. Fearfully, he listened to every little noise.

Getting up and down, up and down.

Continually clutching his gun he went to the windows, sweating heavily he peeked out the ratty curtains. He could feel it. All the buildings close by were the same height, and he just knew they were out there watching him from across the street in the next building over.

Finally he sat down and hit another blast. The devils smoke played with him filling his mind with fear. Wired he stripped naked and grabbed a handful of girly magazines. Page after page he tried to get a hard on but nothing worked, his mind was racing a hundred miles an hour.

Frustrated he knew he was too wired. The next thing he knew he was back at the window, trying to hyper focus he stared down into the parking lot four stories below and swore he could see movement around the Trans-Am. "Oh shit they're down there," he said scared. "What am I gonna do?"

Trembling he clutched the Baretta in his right hand. "Fuck it," he muttered. There was no way he was going out there to confront who ever it was. Everything important to him was right there with him. His pack, cash, drugs and gun. He still had over two grand in cash in his wallet, but he'd already spent twelve hundred tonight on getting high and the night wasn't over.

After two more hours he had to pee really bad and the only bathroom was located off the kitchen. He slid his underwear and pants on, then glanced at his Casio "G" shock. Just after two am. Shit its getting late he thought as he tip toed to the kitchen clutching his back pack with his gun tucked into his waistband behind his back.

Romeo and Sasha were busy at the kitchen table breaking up the large cookie. Sasha was actively filling up little tiny blue baggies with twenty dollar pieces of crack as Romeo continued to cut chunks off the cookie with a surgical blade.

Lucky glanced into the bathroom mirror after he flushed the toilet. "Holy shit … who the hell is that?" he mumbled. You got a serious buzz going he told himself as he continued to splash cold water onto his sweaty face. His pupils were fully dilated and his teeth and jaw were going a mile a minute. "Slow down," he ordered himself breathing deeply, he wiped his face, then walked back into the kitchen to grab a cold beer from the ancient icebox.

"Wow," Lucky said noticing the hundreds of blue baggies lined up like soldiers in formation on the kitchen table.

"Man, bro, you lookin very high … here pull up a chair and chill out."

He sat down and sipped the frosty Budweiser while he watched them in action. His heart was beating out of control as he tried to sit still. Impulsively he reached over and snagged the fat roach from the ashtray and lit it, inhaling the strong weed hoping it would help calm him down. He noticed how bloodshot their eyes were, "Hey this is good shit huh."

"I'll say Lucky," Sasha grinned beautifully.

"Man Gringo, you didn't smoke up all that shit I gave you already did you?"

"No … no … shit I only made a little dent in it … but I don't think I can get much higher so I'll just chill out before I try to drive."

"Good. That weed will take the edge off, it's grade A shit," he laughed trying to count the rows of twenty five rocks. "That makes five hundred baby … ten gees worth and we still got all that to go," Romeo said eyeing the chunk on the plate.

"Hey I see you got your nine on you, why you carryin in my crib?" Romeo demanded sharply.

"Shit, man, relax. Here," Lucky replied defensively setting his Baretta on the table.

"Easy Romeo," she warned him.

"Ya well I don't like no other guns in here other than mine, so when you packin heat, you tell me."

"No problem, I won't forget next time."

"You know Gringo, all this shit will be gone in thirty-six hours … twenty grand in rocks … unbelievable huh," he laughed evilly.

"Jesus, that's a lot of shit to sell."

"Well me and the boys each got a territory to cover and the city's pretty dry right now, so it might be gone in twenty-four."

"Wow." *So I'm not the only one addicted huh.*

"So Gringo, you wanna trade some of that grade a weed for some more hard?"

He hesitated, enjoying the reefer buzz.

"Oh come on, Lucky I only took three hits off that joint and I'm baked," she giggled. "Please Lucky we don't have any, and we'll give you a super deal won't we Romeo."

"Gringo, what you want … hard … soft? Come on Gringo make my lady happy."

I'd love to. "Shit, alright … alright," Lucky said pulling out the fat ounce from his pack. "Give me some of both, but I'm keeping a bud for later to come down with. You know what this shit cost me?"

"No but I know it sells for a hundred a quarter bag," Romeo said confidently.

"Good guess … so show me this super deal since I already spent twelve Franklins with you."

"Damn, no wonder you sell so many damn cars."

"Somebody's gotta do it."

"True that."

"I'll do the deal," Sasha stated standing up giving Lucky an eyeful. A minute later she returned. "Here Lucky here's an eight ball," she said setting the three and half gram ball of quality powder cocaine on the table. Then she reached over to the dinner plate and cut a fifteen-rock boulder. "And this goes with it, satisfied!"

He nodded, knowing she was giving him almost six-hundred dollars worth of stuff. "Yup, that will work."

Quickly she wrapped up the cocaine and crack into a sandwich baggie and then put it inside a brown lunch bag. "Deal?" she asked handing it to Lucky.

"Deal, deal," he responded shaking his head. "Well, I think I'm out a here, I'm feelin much better now."

"You sure? Well be safe and don't shoot nobody," Romeo joked.–

TWELVE

OUTSIDE IT WAS pitch black. The sliver of moon was hidden by a blanket of clouds. Lucky nervously struggled to unlock the dark Trans-Am. Once unlocked he eagerly climbed into the car and locked the door.

The clock on the dash board said two forty-five am.

His first thought besides getting out of there was of Alexis and he wondered if just maybe she was at home, and alone. *Fat chance.*

He fired up the noisy car and winced at all the noise. Jesus, this fuckin' car's loud, he told himself. Without revving the motor, he pulled out as quiet as possible trying not to draw the police's attention.

Rapidly he vacated the seedy section.

Before he got on the highway home he took a chance and called her hoping her muscle head boyfriend didn't answer the phone. On the sixth ring she picked up. "Hello?," she whispered.

"Hey Alexis it's me, you alone?"

"You know what time it is Lucky? What the hell you doing calling me so fuckin' late?"

"I'm sorry, I'm sorry, I'm just a lonely, lonely man and I got all these party goods and no one to share them with."

"You really are crazy … oh God what am I gonna do with you?"

"Invite me over," he pleaded. *I'm so horny.*

"God, my boyfriend just left here like ten minutes ago pissed off, he could come back over any time, though I doubt it, but … we can't party here and I'm not going all the way to Bow. So what else can we do?"

"Hotel close by … I'll be there in five minutes or so."

"Listen if you get me up for nothin I'll kill you … I'm half drunk and half asleep so you better have something for me to wake up with."

"Don't worry I got you ... be ready, I got a black Trans-Am, you'll hear me."

*   *   *

Five minutes later he pulled up to the large apartment building that Alexis's parents' owned. She was already on her way out looking sexy as hell even at three am in the morning.

He shut the loud car off.

She climbed in grinning. Alexis laughed. "It looks just like Burt Reynolds car in 'Smokey and the Bandit.'"

"You always loved Burt".

"I guess I do ... hey what's that?"

"Your wake up present," he told her pulling a mirror out of his pack. Then he dumped a fat pile on the mirror from one of the eight balls. Expertly he crushed the small chunks of cocaine with his Bic lighter and using a razor blade he made three big lines.

"Here twist this up," he said handing her a new hundred dollar bill.

While she was busy snorting up her two lines he pulled out two stems and packed each one with a big crack rock.

"Shit Lucky, you trying to fuck me up or what?"

He laughed. "You could say that, no I just don't want you falling asleep on me."

After they finished the lines he handed her a lighter and a stem. "Are you sure? You know I don't like this shit."

"Go ahead, I won't tell anybody."

"Okay here goes," she whined lighting the stem and inhaling.

He was busy with his own blast. Now they were both zooming, he couldn't sit still, so they pulled out of the parking lot.

"God Lucky, that's some powerful stuff," she whispered sexily, looking hot as hell in her short mini skirt.

All he could think of is how horny he was thinking about how Sasha kept flashing and teasing him in her flimsy see through silk robe.

"Lucky, this shit is wicked strong," she moaned in ecstasy licking her red lips. "God, you're so bad." *Lover boy.*

They pulled into 7-11 to buy some O.J. for the bottle of absolute she brought along in her overnight bag. They went into the store together, holding hands.

While they were inside waiting in the check out line, a group of punks pulled up in a dark mustang GT with out of state plates and parked next to the Trans Am.

Alexis and Lucky started coming out the door with a bag of groceries when they watched in horror as the Mustang backed out rapidly at an angle scraping the passengers side of the Trans Am with its front bumper. The punks yelled and laughed pointing their fingers at Lucky, then they took off, squealing the powerful Mustangs tires.

"Shit," Lucky screamed angrily eyeing the green crease of paint down the side of the car. "Get in, get in," he yelled at Alexis while he quickly ran around the car and climbed in.

Rushing, he started the big motor.

"Put your belt on," he ordered backing out rapidly in hot pursuit. The Mustang already had a good lead, and he burned the tires tearing out of 7-11 parking lot in a cloud of smoke.

The big suped up engine roared to life. He mashed the accelerator in first gear red lining the RPM gauge, speed shifting into second, the high octane Sunoco racing fuel poured into the fuel injectors kicking in the paxton supercharger.

At seventy-five he hit third gear. They raced on catching glimpses of the Mustangs taillights ahead. Lucky blew by the 30 mph speed limit sign doing eighty-five.

He was a completely changed man.

All the suppressed anger came screaming back into his head. Between the cocaine, crack and adrenaline, his endorphins in his brain were maxed out. The Mustang slowed for a busy four way stop sign, and hesitated almost hitting one car, it took off to a flurry of blaring horns.

He came screaming up to the four way down shifting, hard on the brakes, scanning both ways wildly he ran it with the Mustang only 400 yards ahead, and heading for the highway.

Lucky was so caught up in catching the Mustang he forgot all about the illegal drugs he had on him.

But nothing else mattered.

The Trans Am responded like an eager thoroughbred closing in for a win, "Yes, yes," he screamed elated. "They just made their first mistake," he yelled manically. "There's no way they can out run us on the highway."

Loudly he heard Alexis respond for the first time over the deafening motor. "Just don't kill us," she pleaded scared out of her buzz she was clutching the dashboard with both hands.

He pushed the big car through the long sharp looping on ramp trying to keep pace with the better cornering Mustang that was now pulling away.

"Oh shit ... oh shit," she cried. "I shoulda stayed home."

The Good Year Eagles squealed violently in protest as the heavy car tried to brake free. Barely, just barely the Trans Am clutched the pavement. Every time the heavy rear end started to break free, he'd feather the throttle while the Mustangs lead grew.

Once on the highway the Mustang had at least a half-mile lead. He grinned crazily, *Go get em girl* flooring the big 454 supercharged engine in 2nd gear, sixty ... seventy ... eighty ... red line. Third gear, ninety ... hundred ... 110 ... red line fourth gear.

"We're gaining," he yelled excitedly. 120 ... 130 ... 140 ... red line fifth gear.

"Oh my God ... oh my God we're gonna die," she hollered, crying as she glanced at the speedometer.

In a trance he reached over and pushed in the AC/DC Back in Black cd and cranked it all the way up. Quickly they were gaining. His mind was overloaded with stimulus pushing his brain faster and faster. 150 ... 155 ... 160 ... 162 ... 165 ... sixth gear.

They came over the rise surprised to see two state trooper cars pulling out after the Mustang with their laser lights blaring.

"Fuck ... fuck," he yelled angrily swerving to the right around the two slower accelerating police cars.

He didn't even hesitate. 166 ... 168 ... 170 ... 172 ... one hundred yards and closing. 173 ... 174 ... 175 ... eighty yards ... 176 ... 177 ... fifty yards.

Thirty yards.

Twenty yards.

Ten yards.

One foot off the Mustangs bumper he eased off giving them a tap letting them know he was there. The Mustang swerved to the left, Lucky accelerated out to the right while Alexis was screaming at him to pull over and let her out.

"Shut up ... shut the hell up," he screamed at her wildly. "Let me concentrate," he glared at her, possessed.

He pulled up beside the Mustang and put down his window shaking his fist out the window, enraged, Lucky screamed at the punks, "pull over motherfucker, pull over."

The Mustang window went down quickly on the passenger's side, and before Lucky could react, a gun came out of the back seat and fired off a shot at his front tire. Then another shot rang out rapidly.

"Holy shit," Lucky screamed, swerving away down shifting into fifth gear then back into sixth gear to pull ahead of the Mustang.

Another shot rang out.

"Fuck this," he wailed, swerving to the left cutting off the Mustang. Things were happening fast. When he tapped the brake peddle on the Trans Am it sent the Mustang driver into a panic.

The driver over reacted by cutting the wheel hard to the right trying to avoid running into the back end of the Trans Am. Lucky glanced back in the rearview mirror and freaked when the Mustangs rear-end slid around losing control. Wildly the car started to flip and roll and flip some more. *Holy shit.*

Quickly Lucky swerved to the left and hit the brakes as both he and Alexis watched in horror out the passenger's window as the Mustang flew past them on the highway upside down, then right side up shredding parts everywhere.

"Oh my God ... oh my God," Alexis pierced the air screaming over AC/DC's 'Hells Bells.'

They were only a mile from the Hooksett tollbooth. Suddenly he realized that they'd have some kind of roadblock up ahead at the tollbooth. He snapped out of his shocked state when he spotted the blue lights coming fast off in the distance in the opposite lane, right at them.

Realizing he had only seconds to move before they were boxed in, the fear came rushing back.

"What are you gonna do, what the hell are you gonna do?" Alexis demanded hysterically.

Rapidly he downshifted slowing to seventy. "There it is," he hollered out, seeing the next U turn sign for police cars and snow plows.

The two cruisers behind him came flying over the knoll. The net was closing quickly. He down shifted into second gear and shot through the U turn road as fast as humanly possible, turning back south away from the toll plaza and the two approaching high speed cruisers.

He didn't waver. Every second counted. Heavily, he accelerated, while the cops closed swiftly. Alexis was screaming again, beating on his shoulder for him to pull over.

"Shut up ... shut the hell up ... let me drive," he roared. "Shit ... oh shit," he said watching in the rearview mirror as they closed in rapidly. 60 ... 70 ... 80 ... 90, the two cruisers were less than four hundred yards back and coming on fast.

The first two cruisers chasing him in the other lane were pulled over next to the totaled upside down Mustang. 100 ... 110 ... 120 ... "Shit, come on, come on baby," he pleaded. Two hundred yards ... Now less than one hundred yards. 130 ... 135 ... 140. Fifty yards, forty yards. 145 ... 150 ... 155 ... Slowly the distance held at thirty yards. Fifth gear ... 160 ... 162 ... 165. Slowly the Trans Am pulled away. That's it baby, "come on, come on," he whispered feeling the big motor respond.

167 ... 169 ... 171 ... 6th gear. 173 ... 175. They were flying down the deserted highway pulling away. 176 ... 177 ... 179 ... 180 ... 181 ... 182.

It didn't matter anymore. He'd never driven this fast ever, and the adrenaline surge pumped through his veins. One tiny mistake and he knew they were dead.

White knuckled, Alexis clung to the dashboard whimpering for dear life. The roadside whipped by so fast it was blurry. He glanced down at the speedometer 185 and holding. "Shit we gotta get off the highway before they set up a roadblock ahead," he said desperately shutting off the radio.

"You're fuckin crazy," she yelled starting to ball again, afraid to let go of the dashboard and wipe her mascara running eyes.

Lucky glanced back one more time relieved he couldn't see any blue lights or headlights anymore. "Here we go," he said swerving over to the right lane and downshifting to make the next off ramp. At the bottom he ran the red light thankful there was no one around he accelerated again.

They took a bunch of side streets over the next two miles before he finally slowed down to the posted speed limit. Every turn he glanced back, expecting trouble. His heart pounded in his chest, but there was no one back there.

They came out to a major intersection on the west side of Manchester. Nervously they waited, for the red light to change. He looked all around and spotted the Howard Johnson's Motor Lodge sign and didn't hesitate.

The light changed and he pulled into Hojo's driving all the way around back before he parked. "Whew," he said exhaling shutting down the noisy hot motor. Relieved he glanced over at Alexis, "I think we're okay."

"Ya ... well you're fuckin crazy," she mumbled wiping her eyes. "They're probably all dead back there you know ... I swear I saw a guy come flying out the window ... oh my God Lucky what are we gonna do?"

"Come on," he responded firmly grabbing her arm. "Let's get out of this car now."

THIRTEEN

THEY RENTED A suite out back and also rented a few in house adult movies. Alexis was badly shaken up, so Lucky went back to the car and carried in their gear and groceries. Then he moved the Trans AM down twenty spots so if the cops showed up they wouldn't be near it.

Swiftly he filled the ice bucket and mixed two strong absolute screwdrivers. He handed one to Alexis who was still shaking. She chugged it down. "I can't believe it," she sighed. "I just can't believe all that just happened. Can you?"

Lucky plopped down heavily on one of the queen beds shaking his head in disbelief. "Yeah unreal huh?" Stunned he grabbed his back pack and broke out the mirror. "Let's do a line."

She nodded, yes, and he dumped about a gram on the mirror. Silently he chopped up two fat lines and pushed the rest into a pile. "Here baby do one of these," he said handing her a rolled up Franklin.

Daintily she sniffed while Lucky held the mirror. Then she switched nostrils and finished the other half. "God, this shits pretty good," she said with a little smile.

He sat the mirror on the table and in one quick blast he snorted up his whole line, "Whew, man, I needed that."

While Alexis went into the bathroom Lucky set the four stems up with hits and laid 'em on the table. She came out looking delicious, wearing black thigh high stockings and matching crotchless panties. On her feet were six inch black stiletto fuck me pumps.

Her enlarged chest was nicely displayed in a matching Victoria's Secret half-cup laced bra and her nipples hard as buds were boldly exposed.

Lucky eyed them lustfully through the black sheer silk robe she wore over her outfit.

"Boy you look good," he commented sweetly.

"Thank you. I'm still shaking from all that shit."

"It's okay baby," he mumbled staring at her tanned hard body.

"Wow, where, the hell did you get a rock like that?," she asked amazed at it's size. "Okay never mind ... I don't wanna know ... just don't go getting all geeked out on me and barricade yourself in the bathroom or I'm out of here."

"Now why would I do that?"

"Oh don't even go there ... how many times ... huh? ... oh just forget it."

"I know, I know but let's party okay ... shit, its already four am."

Over the next hour they partied hard drinking multiple screwdrivers, snorting lines and watching the pay per view adult x-rated channel.

"Oh Lucky can you believe all that stuff just happened?," she asked sipping her fifth screwdriver.

"Screw it baby," he responded holding up his sixth drink in a toast. "We got away, either they're dead or they wish they were. Christ we were doin a buck fifty or better when they lost control. Stupid fuck should have never swerved and hit the brakes at that speed," he said shaking his head. "Yup, that was the wrong move for sure ... oh well, we'll see if there's anything on the six am news."

They both took a hit of crack and moved onto the bed He had her lie on her stomach with two pillows under her waist, facing the movie. Slowly he started massaging her toned hard legs. They had a light coat of Hawaiian Tropic Coconut smelling oil on them and he inhaled the sweet odor while he caressed her calf muscles.

He was obviously excited as he worked his hands up the back of her now stocking-less legs watching the seduction scene on TV.

She moaned passionately. Slowly he spread her legs exposing her inner thighs to his hungry hands. Then he squeezed her firm buttocks working his fingers lower into her crack, feeling the heat of her womanhood. Lightly he rubbed back and forth till his fingers were slick with her juices.

Tenderly he teased her love button before entering her with his fingers. She responded with a low moan. Expertly he worked her into a frenzy. His love muscle ached in his boxers so he freed himself. Alexis reached back and squeezed him with her tiny petite hands slowly stroking him.

Eagerly, he increased the speed of his fingers, feeling her respond willingly clutching his fingers with her muscles. She was close and he knew it.

He couldn't wait any longer so he climbed up on the bed and entered her quickly from behind. Slowly he thrust deep inside her clutching her tiny waist. She arched back to meet his thrusts. Hungrily he reached around with both hands. One hand went to her button so he could help stimulate her, while the other one squeezed and milked her large firm breasts.

They both moaned in ecstasy. In a frenzy they climaxed together grunting and groaning till they collapsed onto the bed in weakened pleasure.

"God Lucky," she whispered tenderly. "You're gonna give me a heart-attack ... mmm baby that felt sooo-good."

"Mmm yes it sure did," he answered back kissing her neck lightly. Then they cleaned up the mess they made and tried to catch their breath.

"You are crazy. First of all you wake me up at two thirty in the morning, twenty minutes after my friggin boyfriend leaves. Then ... you get me high and take me for a ride from hell in that thing you call a car, and of course you gotta outrun four police cars like you're Dale Earnhardt, bringing me here to watch dirty movies, do illegal drugs and have earth shattering orgasms,!" she said with a grin. "Unbelievable, lover boy."

He shut her up with another line of coke and hit of crack. It was already five AM.

By five-thirty they were finally trying to relax sipping another strong cocktail. Lucky restless wandered outside to take another look at the scratch.

"Man that scratch is wicked bad," he told her, shaking his head disgusted.

Alexis was tuning the TV to channel nine to try to catch the local six am news updated. She turned it up just as the top story flashed across the screen in big letters. 'LATE NIGHT CAR RACE ENDS IN DEATH.'

"Good morning New Hampshire, I'm Lynda Paris, a high speed car race late last night on interstate 93 left one dead and three critically injured. The state police are still looking for a second vehicle that fled the scene with state police in high pursuit. We go to Steve Johnson for a live update, Steve." "Lynda this is what's left of the stolen late model souped up Mustang that Lt. Frank Brooks, from the state police, says rolled numerous times. According to Lt. Brooks late last night around three am two vehicles were racing northbound just south of Hooksett toll plaza on I-93 in excess of one hundred and fifty miles an hour, when the Mustang you see behind me lost control and flipped over multiple times.

The occupants in the stolen Mustang apparently were all gang members called Northern Kings, who fired gunshots at the second vehicle before the Mustang lost control and crashed.

The driver died at the scene, while the other three passengers are at Manchester General Hospital in critical condition. The second vehicle was described by police as a dark colored two-door coupe. Possibly an older muscle car. It fled the scene, out running the police at extremely high speeds.

Police say there's a reward for any information on the second vehicle that, according to police, must be souped up or modified because they clocked it in excess of a hundred and seventy-five miles an hour. Back to you, Lynda."

"Holy shit, Alexis, unbelievable ... three of those punks are still alive ... and the police don't have a clue who we are," he laughed excitedly feeling like a celebrity. "Yes sir."

While she went into the bathroom, he cut off a chunk and set it on the TV. Quickly he hid the rest.

"Hey honey look what I found," he said pointing at the TV.

"I knew it, I just knew you were holding out on me like you always do," she laughed ruffled, but relieved, she could pick her head back up.

They continued to get high. And lucky told her about the plan he had come up with about missing work and getting the car fixed before Big Mike found out.

By six thirty am he had pieced a plan together. They would drop the Trans Am off at Buddy's Automotive. It was the same body shop that he had used while he worked at City Corvette, and had referred a lot of extra business his way.

Then he'd call in sick to work and make Big Mike sweat because he robbed his check for six grand. He knew he was going to quit anyway on Sunday, when he returned the car all repaired.

Lucky reminded himself how pissed off he was about letting another crooked dealer rip him off, some way some how he was determined to get his revenge.

After talking it over they decided to both go over to Buddy's to drop off the car, and then they would come back to the hotel to party some more and crash.

He also asked her to remind him to call his girlfriend, later on, to cancel their Saturday night dancing date at The Music Hall in Concord . Lucky had already decided that he wasn't going anywhere with a large boulder, an eight-ball of powder hidden in his pack and a hard body blonde to party with.

FOURTEEN

AT EIGHT AM both armed with sunglasses and Dunkin Donuts coffee, they pulled up into the alleyway next to Buddy's Automotive. She waited in the car while Lucky went inside to see Buddy alone.

After a brief discussion he came back outside followed by a short fat balding middle-aged man with long bushy side burns and oversized ears. His tiny John Lennon glasses were hanging from his thick neck on a shoestring.

He watched as Buddy put on his tiny spectacles and carefully ran his fat pudgy finger down the length of the scratch. Buddy was totally absorbed with the scratch rubbing his chin he gave it one more look. Surprised he finally noticed Alexis sitting in the Trans Am in her scantly petite bathing suite top sipping her hot coffee.

"Oh my," Buddy replied.

"Buddy that's Alexis ... Alexis, my main man, Buddy."

She smiled blowing out a cloud of cigarette smoke. "Hi Buddy," she responded friendly. "Can you fix it for us ... please?" she pouted. "Oh these are for you, I thought you might want something sweet to eat," she teased using her fingers to get him to come over to the car. "Here buddy."

"You got me donuts," he said excited.

"Of course we did ... will you fix it?"

Buddy stared at her thirty-six double D's barely covered in her small top and drooled licking his lips.

"For you little lady I can fix anything."

Lucky explained he needed it the next day, how it was his bosses demo, and that some punks had scratched it last night.

This wasn't the first time Buddy had done a quick repair job on one of Lucky's demos.

"I know who's car it is … I'm the one who painted it the first time … it's Big Mike's … He's such an asshole," Buddy told them while they all laughed nervously.

"I need it tomorrow, Buddy, how much you gonna charge me?"

"Well how bout three fifty and a nice look at those tits of hers?," he laughed heartly.

"Shit, Buddy … I think I can arrange that, can't we Alexis?," he asked her pleading.

"Well only if it's a real good job Buddy," she grinned.

"Oh it'll be first rate … you'll see."

"I bet it will, I bet it will," Lucky mumbled smiling. "Hey Buddy I need to borrow some wheels til tomorrow, whatcha got for us?"

"Shit Lucky, this ain't no damn car lot ya know. Man I got eight military Hummas I'm paintin for the National Guard," he paused. "Shit I guess you guys can take my car and I'll use a Humma to get home. It's over there," he pointed at a mint Buick Grand National.

"I don't want no lady like Alexis to be driven around in no stripped out Humma," he replied helping Alexis out of the Trans Am he held her hand while he walked her over to his Cherry clean Buick. "There you go little lady," he said grinning holding the door open for her.

"Oh thanks, Buddy," Alexis answered sexily letting him get an extra long look at her scantly clad breasts.

They said good-bye and told him they'd be back around nine am Sunday morning.

"Well shit, honey, that was easy. We got wheels and the car's getting fixed. Now I just need to call work and tell em I'm not coming in, then we'll be straight."

It was already past eight-thirty am in the morning, so he quickly dialed the number for Big Mike's. The dealership didn't open till nine, but it was Saturday, the busiest day of the week, and people usually came in early.

He was hoping to catch a secretary or a salesperson, anyone but Big Mike. "Hello Big Mike's Muscle Cars this is Jennifer how may I help you?"

"Hey, Jennifer, this is Lucky, let Big Mike know I won't be in today 'cause I'm sick ... but I'll be in tomorrow at noon, okay?"

"Hold on Lucky," she said putting him on hold. A few seconds later she came back on the line. "Hey Lucky, Big Mike just pulled up you wanna tell him yourself?" *Hell no.*

That's the last thing he wanted. "No ... no ... Jennifer just pass the message along ... and hey, thanks," he said rapidly hanging up his Nextel phone. "Shit, that was close." Quickly he shut his phone off in case Big Mike tried to call him back.

"Wanna eat before we party ... I haven't eaten since lunch yesterday?"

"Sure. What a we gonna eat?"

"How bout steak and eggs at Stephanie's? That sounds pretty good to me," he told her.

"Mmm ... that does sound good, doesn't it!"

"He lit up a joint to help their appetite along. After a couple of hits they were both stoned so they put it out and saved it for later.

Stephanie's Restaurant was packed as usual on a Saturday morning, but they managed to grab a booth in the smoking section. He ordered them both filet mignons medium rare, with onion and cheese omelets. And grilled English muffins with two sides of smoked bacon. Of course all breakfast plates came with Stephanie's famous home fries.

"Oh can we also have two large premium O Jays and two vanilla bean coffees, please."

He loved the place because they carried everything top shelf, and you could customize your order. Finally their food came and they were much hungrier than they thought. All the delicious food helped energize their tired bodies.

"God Lucky, let's go ... I'm so full!"

"Me too ... let's get out of here."

They swung by the New Hampshire Liquor Store to stock up. He handed her a Ben Franklin. "Get us some Absolute and Kaluha," he told her while he waited in the Grand National. "God, she's got such a nice ass," he whispered to himself, watching her strut inside.

While she was in the store he called Romeo and waited for a call back.

"Hey Gringo you still up?"

"Shit, you know me bro ... I'm still up ... I got some company can you help me out?"

"For you no problemo. What you talkin about now?"

"Say two large pizzas and two large sodas?"

"Okay Amigo. Sashas still asleep so you come on up and pick up your pizzas real quiet like and I'll have em ready. Better make it ten minutes ... in and out real easy."

"See you soon."

They left the liquor store and on the way to Romeo's he told her how she was gonna drop him off and go around the block and then pick him back up as he walked down the street.

"You sure this is okay, Lucky, I don't need to get in any trouble."

"Yes it's early ... there's no one around ... just do it and we'll get out of here okay. I'll be right back ... if I'm not just go around the block again okay?"

"Okay, okay I'll do it," she said as they switched places. She dropped Lucky near Romeos dilapidated apartment building and then drove off.

Lucky bolted up the stairs, winded he handed Romeo four crisp Ben Franklins "Later Romeo," Lucky whispered, pocketing the package Romeo handed him.

"Sssh be cool, now get outta here before you wake up my princess."

Lucky saluted then tore down the steep stairs. He came outside and started walking up the street just as Alexis was making her first pass by. He hopped in the passenger's side smoothly. "Let's go baby – let's go."

On the way back to the motel they stopped at Ashley's Grocery Store and bought some half and half for the White Russians, a half-gallon of Tropicana premium with chunks and smokes. He also grabbed a box of Tijuana small cherry cigars and six more lighters.

By ten-thirty they were back at Hojo's where they stopped off at the front desk and paid for another night.

*　*　*

Big Mike had heard all about the car race on the highway. In fact it was big news all around the city of Manchester at all the various performance shops. Everyone was trying to guess what kind of car the high-speed mystery car was. After all it had to run at least a hundred and seventy-five miles an hour.

He was more than just a little suspicious.

Lucky had called in sick and wasn't answering his Nextel phone. It was when the state police stopped by Saturday afternoon and started asking all sorts of questions about his muscle cars, especially regarding a Black Trans AM they heard he owned, that was capable of very high speeds.

Big Mike's anger grew until he wanted to snap Lucky's neck.

The State Police learned about Big Mike's badass Trans Am from talking to City Corvette where they had just come from. Now they wanted to know where the car was.

Big Mike tried to explain that his top salesman, Lucky Sullivan had the car, and was out sick. But that the car would be back on the lot by noon. Tomorrow.

Trooper Brooks wasn't pleased. "Big Mike you make sure the car and the driver are both here by noon tomorrow, is that clear?"

"Yes sir." If that little shit put one scratch on my baby or had anything to do with this shit I'll break his skinny neck, he thought slamming his huge fist onto his desk.

"Jennifer," he barked. "Get that asshole on the phone I need to talk to him now."

"Big Mike, he must have his phone off cause it just keeps ringing," she responded sweetly.

"Damn it. Keep trying."

*   *   *

Buddy also caught the news updates and it didn't take him long to realize he was looking at the mystery car. The more he thought about it the more it made sense. "Yup, knowin Lucky this just might be the beast they're lookin for," he laughed thinking about Alexis and Lucky out running the cops.

W.C. SCOTT

Then he thought about Big Mike and what a real pain in the ass he'd been over the years and how Lucky had done nothing but send him car after car.

*   *   *

Back in the motel they continued to party looking for news updates. Alexis mixed two Absolute Kaluha half and half White Russians with lots of ice. While Lucky cut up a bunch of lines on a glass-framed picture he took off the wall with his leather man tool. After that he cut off ten hits of crack off the large boulder and set them on the mirror.

He pushed all the stems with a coat hanger. Back and forth he pushed scraping the sides with the caked brillo. After such heavy smoking there was a lot of powerful resin built up on the sides.

This was always the most powerful crack, and usually he didn't push the brillo till very last when he was completely out. Coming down from the crack buzz was known as jonesing. And that's when most addicts started pushing their stems when they were out of money and rocks. But the stems needed new brillo so after Lucky made them ready they both enjoyed smoking the potent brown caked brillos.

After they both snorted two lines they were buzzing along again. "Honey, this is so much fun hiding out like this, I feel like Bonnie and Clyde," she giggled.

"Hey Bonnie, make sure you put out the do not disturb sign will ya."

"Okay Clyde, but don't you think we need some clean towels?"

"You're right Bonnie, okay when she knocks give her a few bucks for towels just don't let her in okay. Go out in the hallway and get em," he told her throwing a five spot on the table.

"We don't need a noisy maid in here with this shit all over the place," he explained, seriously, turning back towards the TV to catch the eleven AM news update. A minute later a sexy brunette named Carol chimed in:

"Latest reports on the deadly car chase last night on I-93 are that two stolen handguns were found at the scene of the totaled stolen Mustang. One of the two handguns whose serial number had been filed off was recently fired and three bullets were missing from the clip. The three shells found at the scene matched the other bullets found in the gun. The four occupants in the stolen Mustang, including the deceased driver, are all members of the Northern Kings. The police have traced the car and the gang members to the high crime area of Roxbury Massachusetts.

"The state police are still trying to piece together what happened last night. The latest has the stolen Mustang fleeing a downtown 7-11 off Bridge Street around three am late last night with a dark colored muscle car in high pursuit. With the latest on the injuries of the other three gang members we go live to Danny."

"Carol, the latest update is that there were four occupants in the stolen Mustang, the driver, a Oscar Rodriguez died, at the scene when he was thrown from the high speed flipping Mustang.

"The passenger in the front seat is in critical care and is not expected to make it through the day. While the two passengers in the back seat suffered multiple injuries including internal bleeding, compound fractures and broken bones. Both are expected to survive according to the emergency room doctors.

As you can see from this picture of what's left of this expensive stolen Mustang G.T. they are indeed Lucky to be alive. I'm Danny Henry, live at Manchester General, back to you Carol."

FIFTEEN

"HOLY SHIT, THIS is turning into a real nightmare," Lucky mumbled pacing back and forth nervously in front of the TV.

"It doesn't make sense Alexis ... Northern Kings Way up here in a Stolen Mustang deliberately scratching my car ... to get us to chase them. Then ... they fire three shots at us," he told her concerned rubbing his stubble. "There's something more going on here, I can feel it in my bones."

"Listen Lucky, just calm down. Everything will be all right, once you return the car tomorrow. They don't have any idea it was us, so stop worrying so much you're making me scared."

But Lucky wasn't listening. His mind was racing a hundred miles an hour, and all types of warnings came flooding back. "Watch your back, you're lucky your legs aren't broken," Tom had warned him more than once but he had shrugged it off.

"Shit, shit ... shit," he yelled angrily when it dawned on him. "It's gotta be the old man ... It's gotta be."

"What the hell are you yelling about? Look at yourself. You're ... you're worrying so much you're ruining my buzz. Now get your cute ass over here and party," she demanded, patting the bed beside her.

He nodded and moved to the bed. "Okay, okay but please just listen to this," he asked softly. "I think those punks intentionally scratched my car on purpose so we would get mad and chase them. Then they deliberately got us out on that highway and tried to shoot out my tires so we'd crash."

Shocked, she responded, "What ... what are you saying that ... that was all planned out? Come on Lucky this isn't some TV show. You actually believe that shit?", Alexis asked doubtfully shaking her head. "Here, drink your drink and lets do another line. I'm starting to come down and it really sucks, so wake me up before I decide to go home."

*   *   *

Buddy continued to work his magic on the scratch. It was already filled, sanded and coated with primer.

His TV, a customer gave him towards partial payment, sat up high on a huge red Craftsman Professional toolbox. Buddy watched the latest news update at the same time as Alexis and Lucky, and he couldn't help smiling eyeing the Trans AM. That's when he decided to check out the motor.

Carefully he opened the hood. "Holy Moly a big block 454 Vette engine," he whistled enthusiastically. His helper was deaf so buddy was always talking to himself. "Ah a Paxton supercharger, modified headers, Holy four barrel, man, this things pushing six hundred horsepower, easy," he mumbled admiring the chrome valve covers and chrome alternator.

Scott-85

His paint stained hands ran over the shiny clean motor giving him a thrill. Then he saw it. "And what's this big asshole,?" he muttered following the thick cable from the battery post to the back of the speedometer to a tee joint. From there the cable continued underneath the motor.

"Now I'm curious," he said grabbing his droplight and floor crawler he slid underneath the jacked up car. Easily he found the cable again and followed it to the passenger's side. It led right to a small black box hidden neatly between the four large exhaust pipes.

He shined his shop light and read the cover, "speedometer recorder ... oh shit Lucky if that was you last night I gotta feelin this little baby will tell all ... mmm let's just see what it says you've been up to shall we."

One of Buddy's hobbies was electronic gadgets and gizmos, so it only took him a second to recognize the evil black box from one of his high tech popular mechanics magazines, where they called the device the 'teen-manager' because a parent could monitor their teenagers' speeds, abuses and habits.

Within a few minutes he found where the computer hook up was located conveniently right at the tee. Buddy went into his office and brought out his high-powered IBM Laptop ThinkPad. He set it on top of his workbench and ran a secondary adapter cable from the laptop to the tee.

He turned it on and booted it up. The program from the black box showed up on the color screen, and he clicked on download. Excitedly, he waited while the information was downloaded from the recorder inside the box to the think pads powerful memory. "Holy shit Lucky," he screeched eyeballing the screen. The date, the time and the speed were clearly displayed.

Scott – 86

"Wow, you've been hauling ass ... let's see he's got this set to record at any speed over a hundred and according to this Lucky you were doin one-eighty-five last night at three-twelve am."

He whistled wondering what he should do. "Jesus Christ, Lucky, you're gonna owe me big-time." Within minutes he erased the last five days information. He smiled as it disappeared off the screen. "There, that should at least get you out of this scrape," Buddy laughed, quickly re-connecting the cable and shutting the hood.

*　　*　　*

They continued to party, having wild sex in the shower drinking white Russians. But the higher Lucky got the more paranoid he became. He just couldn't relax. Back and forth he went, from the curtains where he peeked out, to the TV so he could turn it down and listen for any noises.

Impulsively, at six pm, he called Buddy's shop. "Hey Buddy it's Lucky, how's the car coming?"

"Well my good friend it looks good as new. It just needs to sit overnight so the clear coat can cure. You okay you, sound funny?"

No shit I'm high as a kite. "Ya, I'm feelin better now."

"Good so I'll see you tomorrow morning and Lucky I saw the news, you're damn lucky to be alive!"

"Jesus Buddy, you don't miss a thing do you?," he responded hesitantly.

"Nope, I don't, but I do know how to keep my mouth shut, and make sure when you come tomorrow you bring that sweet rack with you so I get to see'm all natural okay."

"I'll be there and Alexis will gladly show you her beautiful rack," he laughed. "Oh and by the way you're car is nice and safe cause we're laying low."

"Well that's good to hear, you've had enough excitement for one night ... listen I'll see you tomorrow."

"Thanks Buddy."

He pumped his fist excited. "Good news baby, the car is lookin like new."

"See, I told you everything would be alright."

"I know ... I know ... he said he can't wait to see your rack. I told him you'd give him an eyeful tomorrow, so you gotta do that for me okay?"

"Alright, I said I would. If it gives little Buddy a hard on, but he ain't touchin any part of me, and I mean it."

Lucky smiled watching her facial expressions. "Okay, don't worry ... just let him see how gorgeous that boob job of yours is, and give him a quick thrill, then we're outta there."

She smiled motioning him to the bed with her index finger. He knew exactly what that meant and quickly he responded standing in front of her.

Alexis eyed his bulge. Teasingly she tugged down the front of his silk black boxers and eagerly took him inside her mouth while he milked her firm breasts. Lustfully, he caressed and pinched her hard erect nipples. Promptly he responded to the pleasure of her mouth and they wasted no more time on foreplay.

Scott – 88

Again, he entered her doggy style reaching around to feel her swollen breasts while his other hand clutched her tiny waist. He moved inside her slowly at first. Then he increased his speed as she egged him on with moans of ecstasy. Spryly he reached around with his long arm and stroked Alexis's love button while he continued to increase his speed. They climaxed simultaneously. Afterwards they collapsed onto the bed, exhausted, covered in sweat.

"Whoa baby, you're gonna kill me," he exhaled climbing off her and collapsing on the other bed. "I need to rest, I'm so light headed."

"Boy, and I was just getting warmed up," she purred. "What's wrong with you ... gettin' old? ... Too many drugs huh ... or you just can't handle me anymore," she teased, raking her long red nails down his back, she slapped his cute ass.

He had hit the wall and was feeling really sick. The lack of sleep over the past two nights was catching up to him.

Thankfully, he had called Laura's answering service earlier, letting her know he couldn't make their dancing date because he was tied up trying to get Big Mike's car fixed. He also remembered telling her he was gonna quit on Sunday and they'd drive up to the White Mountains in the convertible.

The moans he heard coming from the TV caught his attention and he rolled over to watch. Alexis's eyes were glued to the screen as two hunky construction workers worked over a naughty secretary. Immediately, Lucky's first wife came to mind as he watched Alexis masturbate with her vibrator. Slowly he crawled closer to get a bird's eye view. Stopping off to do another bump off the mirror.

She started groaning, "oh ... oh yes ... I'm gonna ... oh I'm gonna come," she mumbled huskily. Her eyes closed as she bucked the vibrator, "oh yes ... oh ... oh yes ... aah yes," she screamed while she climaxed.

That did it. He was hard again. Immediately he climbed on top of her and made her hold the vibrating toy on her sensitive love button while he pumped her wildly. She was so hot and wet that he just couldn't resist any longer. His orgasm came ripping out of him quickly.

After a short rest they ordered pizza and shared a joint while they waited for the Pizza Hut delivery truck. They munched on the meat lovers pizza and watched the latest Stephen Segal movie on the pay per view channel.

The last time he glanced at his watch it was ten pm. The next thing he knew he was being shook awake. Groggily he glanced at his "G" shock, eight am.

"Let's go, sleepy head. You gotta shower and shave and get ready lover boy. You gotta big morning ahead of you. Come on get up so we can go eat some breakfast before we pick up the car."

He mumbled and stumbled into the bathroom and found a fresh cup of coffee and all his clothes laid out neatly.

After a quick shower and shave he came out of the bathroom decked out in his Calvin Klein suit. "You're too much M&M," he said smiling.

"Boy, you haven't called me that nickname in years; you must be feeling pretty good."

"Yes … yes I am feeling much better thanks to you."

After they stopped at Denny's for two grand slam breakfasts they headed for Buddy's to pick up the Trans Am.

The car was perfect. Lucky paid him the three-fifty and Alexis kept her promise and gave Buddy a long hardy look at her knockers. After they left an excited Buddy Lucky dropped Alexis off at her apartment giving her the rest of the drugs to hold till they could get together again.

"Thanks M&M for everything," he grinned.

"You're welcome, be careful and please call me," she told him watching him pull off in the Trans Am. *I hope he's okay.*

Fifteen minutes later he pulled up to Laura's condo and fixed his hair with styling gel and splashed on some Dakar glancing in the rearview mirror.

Anxious, he knocked on her door.

"Hi there stranger," Laura said with a sneer. "You finally fixed the car?"

"Yes, it's all fixed. I'm going to return it when they open at noon, and then quit."

Laura shook her head. "I don't know, it sounds like trouble to me."

"Not really he shorted my check six grand, so he can stick his job," he mouthed angrily.

"Okay, well I guess you already made up your mind. So where do I come in?"

"I'd like you to pick me up in the convertible as soon as I call you on my Nextel. Please try to be ready so I can get out there and then we can take a nice ride up to North Conway through the Kangamangus Highway. How's that sound?"

"It is a beautiful sunny August day for the top down ... how soon is this all going to happen?"

"I'll leave here in a few minutes, it's eleven ten now so by the time I get there Big Mike will be in, and it doesn't take long to quit so," he said giving her a hug and a kiss.

He could tell she was still angry over last night, but right now he had a lot more on his mind to worry about. "Oh would you please bring me something to wear ... I still have some clothes here don't I?"

She nodded. "Okay, we'll go, we need to talk anyway."

"You know where it is right," he asked nervously.

"Don't you remember you took me there before?"

"Oh yeah that's right ... okay then I'll call you soon honey ... bye."

"I'll be waiting. Good luck."

SIXTEEN

H E GLANCED AT the gas gauge. Barely above empty. Lucky chuckled, "Fuck em he can fill it up himself." The closer he got to Big Mike's the more his anger started to flow. "Nobody rips me off like that and gets away with it," he told himself in the rear view mirror.

He pulled into Big Mike's lot and parked next to Big Mike's corvette. He looked over and noticed the dark green and silver New Hampshire State Police cruiser with Area Supervisor lettered on the side.

"Oh shit, stay cool," he mumbled taking a deep breath and exhaling before he climbed out of the car.

"Here he is now," Big Mike yelled loudly to the state trooper who was following him out of the showroom. Pointing Big Mike added, "and that's my car."

"Lt. Brooks introduced himself to Lucky and asked him to remain while he inspected the Trans Am. Slowly he and big Mike walked around the car.

Nothing.

Then he started asking Lucky questions opening a small green notebook and pulling a gold cross pen from his uniform chest pocket. "So you're name is Lucky Sullivan and you live in Bow and according to Big Mike you've been the only one using the vehicle since a week ago Friday, is that correct?"

"Yes, sir Lt., that's correct," he responded respectfully remembering his Coast Guard breeding. Then casually he fired up a Marlboro Light and waited for more questions.

"So Mr. Sullivan do you know anything about the high speed race out on I-93 early Saturday morning around three-am just south of the Hooksett Toll plaza?", Trooper Brooks demanded staring hard at Lucky.

"Yes sir, I saw it on the news yesterday, something about a stolen Mustang full of gang members," he said nonchalantly adjusting his Ray Bans. "But why are you asking me about this," he shot back at the Trooper confidently.

"I'm glad you asked Mr. Sullivan, a car just like this one was seen racing after the Mustang at speeds of a hundred and eighty miles an hour ... and there aren't too many cars in the area capable of those kinds of speeds. So do you see my point now," he asked raising his voice.

"Sure Lt., I get your point loud and clear. But it certainly wasn't me," he paused. "Shit I wouldn't dare push his pride and joy that hard," pointing at Big Mike. "Why he'd break my neck."

"Okay hot shot," Big Mike barked. "But since it's my car and you've been implicated and there's at least one death involved I say we find out if you're telling the truth or not."

Lt. Brooks smiled, "I think that's a good idea. Now that we've got the car maybe your mechanic can get us some straight answers."

Lucky wondered what the hell they were talking about.

"Hey Tony," Big Mike bellowed to his head mechanic. "Pull the Trans Am out back and hook her up to your computer."

"No problem, Big Mike," Tony said hopping into the Trans Am.

They all watched the car drive off. Big Mike just grinned viciously at Lucky. "You got no idea what I got hooked up to this baby, do you?"

Lucky just shrugged wondering where he could hide.

"Come on," Big Mike roared, "I wouldn't want you to miss out on all this excitement," he told him putting one of his large paws on Lucky's expensive Calvin Klein suit jacket.

Unwillingly, Lucky followed Big Mike and Lt. Brooks back into the garage. He got very nervous watching Tony undo a cable and hitch it up to the back of his computer.

He tried to maintain his composure. Unbelievable, he thought. He just couldn't believe his eyes. What the hell was going on he told himself lighting another smoke skittishly.

It took Tony about five minutes to hitch everything up, and it was the longest five minutes of Lucky's life. After a few more minutes Tony downloaded what was on the black box and sent it to the printer located on the work bench.

"You know what this is, Lucky? ... No ... Well this little contraption will show me if you've been abusin' my baby ... plus it'll tell me how fast you been driven on what day and what time. Pretty neat stuff huh," Big Mike smirked looking over at Lt. Brooks who stood between Lucky and the exit.

Oh shit, what the hell am I gonna do he thought, feeling the walls closing in. Instantly he recalled the article he read in Motor Trend magazine about a gadget parents could hook up to the family car to see if their teenagers were driving responsibly or not. His pulse quickened, his heart raced. He tried to control his breathing but he knew he was scared. The sweat started slowly dripping down his back. *And I almost pulled it off.*

"All set, Boss," Tony said.

Big Mike nodded. "Well let's go see what we got here, he said as everyone in the garage, except Lucky and Lt. Brooks, moved closer to the print out.

He just stood there waiting for the bad news.

"Interestin' Lt., Lucky here drove one fifty one for one minute last Friday, the first night he had my car. Then on Saturday he drove one eleven for three minutes ... hmm but I'll be damned since last Saturday he ain't broke a hundred," he stated, looking up, amazed, he shook his head.

"Here look for yourself Lt."

Trooper Brooks walked over and took a hard look at the print out. "Let's see. According to this ... your boys clean ... he couldn't have been driving over a hundred miles an hour this past Friday," he paused studying the printout. "How accurate is this contraption you've got here, Big Mike?"

"It says it's ninety-eight percent accurate and I've tested it out a few times before I let no show for work use my car," Big Mike said sarcastically. "But it's workin fine or it wouldn't have recorded these fast speeds over a hundred last weekend."

Lucky kept stone faced still not believing what he was hearing. He just couldn't believe that he might actually get away with it after all.

A sense of relief overwhelmed him. Pumped he whipped out his Nextel and called Laura. "Hey baby, come get me ... yup, now would be great."

"And where the hell do you think you're goin?" Big Mike demanded raising his deep voice.

Lucky started to walk out of the garage until he heard Big Mike's loud voice. He stopped and spun around angrily.

"I don't work for crooks," he screamed. "Yup, that's right you robbed my paycheck, six grand. Don't you remember what I told you. Nobody fires me ... I quit." He spun around with a smirk on his face and walked outside while Lt. Brooks just stood there in the garage with his mouth open.

Immediately Lucky was glad that Trooper Brooks was present because he could tell Big Mike was ready to blow a gasket, but couldn't.

Lt. Brooks and Big Mike followed him outside. Big Mike pleaded, "come on Lucky I just saved your ass with this here speed reader ain't that so Lt.?"

"That's true, Lucky, he did clear the car of any involvement."

He tried to ignore Big Mike, then his Irish temper got the best of him. "Just remember, Big Mike, you stole from me and you tried to fry my ass on some shit I had nothing to do with. Fuck that, adios ... I'm outta here," Lucky shouted striding away rapidly towards the troopers car.

"Hold up Mr. Sullivan. I got a few more questions," the Lt. said quickly catching up to Lucky while they continued walking towards his cruiser.

"Let me get this straight, you say you weren't involved in all this and Big Mike's contraption shows you weren't," he paused. "But I want you to know how serious this is, we've got two dead men ... the second one died this morning."

Lucky puffed his cigarette impatiently listening and looking for Laura.

The Lt. continued, "so I would greatly appreciate if you hear anything ... and I do mean anything you give me a call," he told him handing him his card. "And I suggest you get out of here as soon as possible if you know what I mean."

"You can count on it."

"I'll stick around till your ride shows up, but how can I get a hold of you? ... Through your parents in Bow?"

Shit No ... Don't bother them. "Here, call my cell phone I always have it with me and if I don't answer just leave a voice message and it will signal my phone," he said, handing him an old City Corvette business card with his cell number and he also wrote Laura's home number on the back.

They turned to see Laura pulling up in the Camaro convertible with the top down and the Doobie Brothers cranking on the local rock and roll station, Rock 101.

He smiled, remembering buying the car off an old couple whose son died over in Desert Storm fighting Iraqi soldiers for Uncle Sam. Laura looked hot dressed in a skimpy white summer dress with lots of her dark tanned body parts exposed.

She grinned behind her sexy sunglasses showing a full set of white straight teeth. "Hi," she said, turning down the radio slightly.

He felt better already and shook the Lt.'s hand. Quickly he jumped into the passenger's seat and leaned over to give Laura a kiss.

"Thanks Lt., have a nice day."

"You too Lucky, and do me a favor stay away from here."

"You can count on it."

SEVENTEEN

H E UNDID HIS tie and slid off his suit jacket and shirt. Then he eagerly slid off his dress pants and put on the shorts she brought him.

Laura pulled over so they could switch places. "So what was that all about," she asked holding his hand.

He exhaled cigarette smoke. "I'll tell you all about it later … let's just cruise okay."

"Okay."

"Oh and by the way you look absolutely gorgeous today," he said with a devilish grin.

"Why thank you kind sir," she replied pushing the Tracy Chapman CD into the stereo player. They cruised up I-93 North past Concord with the smooth voice of Tracy Chapman playing loudly over the Alpine speakers.

Ninety minutes later they got off the highway at Loon Mountain Ski Resort. After they passed through the small town they continued further into the White Mountains until they entered the world famous Majestic Kangamangus Highway.

The elevation rose quickly, and the temperature dropped. The scenic winding curvy two lane highway, famous for it's mountain vistas and cold water mountain streams, was the perfect setting for any romantic interlude.

They pulled over on one of the many rustic sightseeing lookouts. Holding hands they breathed in the fresh mountain New Hampshire air. They walked into the woods till they found a small deer trail to follow. He carried the picnic basket that Laura made while she toted a blanket.

A short way down the tiny trail they heard the pleasant sound of a babbling brook. Shortly, they came into a wild meadow with waist high tall straw grass, blowing in the breeze.

Excitedly, they followed the deer path down through the meadow to the stream where the hearty deer came to quench their thirst. They looked all around and the view was breathtaking. Eagerly, they found a perfect spot to lay out their blanket.

Laura set out chunks of Vermont Cheddar and wheat thin crackers while Lucky poured cool white Zinfandel into Dixie cups. Even though it was close to ninety degrees out, there was just enough of a mountain breeze to make it comfortable.

No words were spoken.

The soothing sound of the stream and the clean mountain breeze put them in great moods. It was a natural state of serenity.

Slowly he started to massage her shoulders and neck. Lovingly he worked his way down her long lean back. She was lying on her stomach and he could smell her clean womanly scent while he worked his skilled hands lower and lower.

Her sexy light summer dress had ridden up high on her tanned thighs and he couldn't resist touching them. Lower and lower he went down to her firm calves.

She moaned slightly trying to sip her wine. Gently he lifted her sundress and exposed her cute white cotton panties. Smoothly he slid both index fingers into her waistband. Then he slid both fingers out to her hips, and tenderly lifted. In one slick motion she was panty less.

Hungrily, he kissed her legs teasing her womanhood with his tongue. He felt her arch her back to meet his kisses.

They made love passionately while the hot summer sun beat down fiercely making them sweat. The mountain wind stirred the tall straw grass as their hearts melted together. Anxiously they clung to one another feeling the intensity build and build until they both felt a thunderous explosion completing their lovemaking.

"Oh Lucky if I could only straighten you out," she whispered, wiping the sweat off Lucky's brow. "You know I love you Baby and I'm always here for you," she sighed into his ear when he collapsed beside her.

Her hands felt wonderful on his back. "I love you Laura. You know I do … I guess I Just get scared cause I love you so much," he whispered from his heart.

They washed up in the cool stream enjoying each other's nakedness. Within minutes a swarm of hungry mosquito's attracted to the sweet sweaty human smell and the carbon dioxide they breathed out, attacked in force. They had all they could do to make it back to the Camaro without getting eaten alive.

Over a late lunch on the rustic porch of the old Conway Country Inn they ogled the beautiful panoramic mountain views while he told her all about the car chase, the shooting, and Big Mike stealing from his check. Lucky also told her about Buddy. The only thing he failed to mention was Alexis.

"Wow, you're damn lucky to be alive … how the hell did you manage to get away from the police? … Okay, never mind," she paused taking it all in. "I just don't understand how that computer gadget didn't show you speeding the night of the chase when it showed you speeding at other times?"

"I know, I know, it's very strange isn't it. I can't figure it out. I guess someone was looking out for me or the damn thing malfunctioned cause I was going so fast," he laughed. "Because it sure saved my ass."

"Yes and such a cute ass," she joked.

"You should have seen the look on Big Mike's face after he tried to nail me to the wall in front of the state trooper. Boy, was he livid."

As they finished their gourmet lunch and sipped the delightful California White Zinfindel he decided to open up to her further about his theories. He told her how he felt it wasn't a random act. That it was done on purpose and he asked her if she would talk to her father about the old man.

Her Dad had been in the wholesale car business for over twenty years, and he knew everything about everyone.

"So what do you think really happened?"

"Well I think I was set up by the old man. That either he or someone he knows, hired that gang, to purposely hit my demo and get me mad enough to chase after them out on the highway, so they could shoot out my tires at a high-speed so I'd crash. That's what my gut tells me and that's what all the evidence points to."

"Okay, I'll talk to him."

Laura told him she'd check with her father and see if he had any dirt on the old man. She knew her Dad didn't particularly care for City Corvette or the way they did business in the city.

EIGHTEEN

O N MONDAY WHILE Laura went to work, Lucky played golf with his father at Concord Country Club.

Lucky had played golf and swam on the country club swim team since he was ten years old.

The club was private and too expensive for Lucky to join now that he was out of college. And of course his father had plenty of good advice about employment opportunities. But Lucky was stubborn and always wanted to prove he could make it on his own.

Monday night he attended a Narcotics Anonymous meeting and took all his prescribed psychotropic medications for the second day in a row. He came back to Laura's, where he was officially spending the week feeling very good.

The wonderful smell of Baklava wafted through the condo. Laura was making her specialty. And the Greek pastry melted in your mouth and also your waist.

She had conveniently laid out the New Hampshire Sunday News classifieds for him to look through. He smiled enjoying a hot piece of Baklava scanning the sales ads she had so expediently circled.

Tuesday morning he interviewed at a Toyota Super store and also at a brand new BMW dealership. They both offered him a sales position but he decided he liked the high end BMW's. The sales training class was set for two weeks and was mandatory. It paid a flat hundred bucks a day. During break, on the very first day of sales training, Lucky went outside for a much-needed cigarette.

He had answered almost every question the sales trainer had thrown at the class of green horns and because of his advanced Joe Verdi sales training seminars that City Corvette had so freely paid for, gave him a serious advantage.

While he ate a chili dog from the Roach Coach he watched a car carrier unload seven brand new Z-3 convertibles. The sales trainer, a sharp dressed car pro stepped over with Lucky to have a smoke. "You seem to know a little bit about the car business Lucky."

"Yes sir, I guess so."

"Oh come on, you knew the answer to every single question I asked ... so what gives ... why's a car pro like you wasting time in my sales class?"

"Hey I'm ready to sell today, but that's what BMW requires so-"

"No, why are you available at all?"

"Shit, honestly I'm still asking myself the same question. I guess I'm just sick of all the bullshit. You know ... robbing my commission check ... not backing me up," he shook his head in renewed anger thinking about Big Mike and City Corvette. "Sir, I sold twenty cars a month for ten straight months, you'd think I could get a little management support."

"I know what you mean. Hey listen even though I'm here training, I'm still an independent contractor, and I was just thinking you just might be perfect for another position somewhere else," he said as they locked eyes.

"Really ... what are you talking about?" *Not again.*

The trainer smoked his Camel and sipped his coffee. Casually he glanced around. "Listen, say we meet after class today at three-thirty. You know where the Eighty-Eight Lounge is?"

"Sure do."

"Okay then we'll meet there and I'll buy you a drink and we'll talk. I kind of feel a little guilty talking about it on their dime, if you know what I mean."

"I'll be there."

NINETEEN

Hooksett, NH
3:30 PM
88 Restaurant

Purposely, he took the long way to the restaurant. Not wanting to arrive too early and seem over eager about what the car pro had to say.

But in reality he had been extremely excited all afternoon trying to figure out what he was going to talk about. When he finally strolled in to the lounge he saw the trainer sitting comfortably in a booth relaxing. Smiling, Lucky slid into the other side.

"Ah glad you could make it, Lucky," he said eagerly shaking Lucky's hand. So what can I get for you?"

Lucky eyed the empty Martini glass. "A Molson Golden would be great."

The trainer snapped his fingers and the cute bar maid came to the booth. Within minutes she brought a cold Molson Golden and another Vodka Martini shaken, not stirred with olives.

"So tell me a little more about yourself Lucky, consider this an informal interview because I've already reviewed your BMW application, and according to your sales sheets you attached, you've been a super star your first year in the business."

Lucky nodded, sipping his Molson from the bottle, skipping the glass.

"But you haven't been very stable, bouncing around. So what's the story with that?"

"There's not much to tell. I can sell cars anywhere. Anytime a new guy comes on boards and kicks ass it causes problems amongst the sales team. You know that."

"True I do. I did take the liberty and called Tom at City Corvette because you put him down as a reference, and he had a lot of positive things to say about you, as well as a few things he said you needed to work on," he paused, sipping his Martini.

"But overall he did say he would love to have ten of you, and that statement alone, coming from Tom, is a very strong recommendation."

He went on to explain about the job opportunity he had in mind. It was a sales manager's position at a large country dealership. Which included a decent base salary with incentives and bonuses. And then he went on to ask Lucky if he'd ever been a sales manager before?

"Sure, sure, I have, insurance, real estate, restaurants. And I am flattered you're considering me for this opportunity ... but to be honest I'm not sure it's really what I'm looking for at this point in my life, because I really do enjoy selling cars. And I'm not much of a paper pusher."

"Okay, but let me tell you about the dealership. It's in Hillbro and it's called Johnson's Chevy. It's right on the main drag and it's pretty big ... they've got about three hundred new and used in inventory and a huge service department."

The sales pro stopped and ordered another round of drinks.

"I think I can get you a thirty-grand base salary with incentives, of course. Listen, why don't you take tomorrow off from class and take a ride by the place before you decide," the trainer hesitated, watching Lucky.

"Don't worry, I'll excuse you from class. Just call me on my cell phone when you get back. So if you decide you don't want to consider it, you can just rejoin the class, and of course you'll get paid ... but it never hurts to look at other opportunities. Isn't that true?"

He sat there sipping his beer listening impatiently before he responded boldly. "Okay, let me be frank with you, why me, and what's in it for you?"

"Wow, you get right to the point don't you. I'll tell you why. First of all I get a great feeling about your abilities and I think you'd be a good fit over there," he paused again munching an olive.

"And secondly, what's in it for me is a commission when I fill the position with a decent manager ... but hey, I'm not looking to just stick anyone out there as I've handled their account for years ... so I need to find someone exceptional."

Lucky nodded. "Alright sir, I'll go by in the morning and check it out, and then I'll give you a call tomorrow afternoon on your cell phone ... and hey, thank you Mr. Pelton for all your confidence in me, and the cold beverages," he told him, standing up offering his hand.

"Listen Lucky, you can call me Rick," he said shaking his hand vigorously. "Oh, and do me a favor, keep this between us. I don't think the BMW owners would be too pleased with me stealing a potential star."

"No problem Rick, it's our secret."

TWENTY

H E WAS EXCITED, but confused on the ride back to Laura's condo. She wasn't home yet so he went inside to relax.

"Hey Taffster, what's up boy," he stated to Laura's cute dog giving him a milk bone.

"Wanna go out, boy?"

Taffy came running back with his leash in his mouth and dropped it on Lucky's two hundred dollar leather oxford shoes. "Good Boy, Taffster, Good boy!"

Off they went with Taffy leading the way. Bush to bush, tree-to-tree Lucky was jerked along Taffy's usual routine. Eagerly he sniffed out his old territory, lifting his little leg, and re-marking his spots.

Slowly, they passed by the condos pool house, and Mark the assistant manager, from City Corvette pulled up, beside Lucky and Taffy, in a late Model Vette. Mark also lived in the complex and he and Lucky were so-called friends, but due to their direct competition for salesman of the month at City Corvette they tried to tolerate one another.

And now that he got fired, their rivalry should have ended because he knew Mark was very glad he was out of the picture. Now Mark could be the top dog once again. Lucky had beaten him ten months straight causing some serious jealously and embarrassment.

"Hey Lucky, what's goin on bro ... a little dog sittin," Mark asked, with a big grin.

"Yeah, Mark just out for a little stroll with Laura's beast," he joked watching Taffy stop to sniff some fresh dog shit left by one of his competitors.

"Hey, I hear you're over at Big Mike's and sold eight in seven days ... not bad ... not bad at all bro ... you're still kickin ass I see," he said slyly letting him know he knew exactly what time it was.

"Ya well, it was actually twelve in eight days, but I could only deliver eight of them," he bragged rubbing it in.

"Really, wow. For what it's worth bro I was sorry to see you go even if you did cut into my sales, the competition was good ... but shit, now I'm so damn busy cause I inherited all your customers too ... it's plain crazy things are lookin wicked good," he bragged with sarcasm. "But hey, I am glad you're doin well over there."

Lucky nodded, grinning. "Me too, bro, me too. Hey it ought to feel good for you to finally be salesman of the month again huh! Shit what I beat you ten straight months in a row," Lucky responded laughing. "Hey, catch you later Mark."

"Sure Lucky, no hard feelings," Mark yelled pulling away quickly.

"And fuck you too," Lucky mumbled, getting pulled along by Taffy. He had to finally yank on the leash because the dog had stopped to admire a huge turd that the resident Great Dane, who lived somewhere in the complex, must have unloaded.

"Make your own pile, stud," he laughed watching Taffy reposition himself and back up near the Great Danes pile and raise his tail, squeezing out a tiny turd.

"Good boy, Taffster."

By the time they finished Taffys tour of the complex, Laura's Lincoln Town Car was in its spot.

TWENTY ONE

"HI BABY."

"Hi honey," she replied giving him a quick hug and kiss glancing at Taffy who wasn't going to let her forget about him.

"How's my baby boy ... ya oh ya," she cooed rubbing Taffy, who was jumping up to greet his master while she hugged him affectionately.

"And where have my two boys been off too huh, a little walk, yeah ... and mommy's got some news for daddy."

After stopping by her fathers shop on the way home from work and telling him almost everything that Lucky had told her, she had learned a few tidbits from dear old pops. The first thing she told him was that her father agreed with him about the old man being the one responsible for the gang and car chase. Also he advised Laura that Lucky should lay low, and maybe find a job out of town till he could find out what was really going on.

Then he told Laura that Lucky should take any threat seriously and they also discussed if he would be endangering Laura by staying with her, but he agreed with Laura that everyone in the car business knew Laura's father and knew she was off limits.

He listened carefully to everything she told him while pacing back and forth in her living room.

"Yup, your dad's probably right ... no one will dare come here ... uh, uh ... everyone knows not to mess with your dad, I heard that before I even met you."

They sat down on the leather sofa together. She kicked off her high heels and Lucky loosened his new Jordan Marsh silk tie.

They cuddled together while Taffy attacked his Lucky Dog brand dog food that Laura set out for him.

"You'd think he never ate before," she laughed, watching him inhale his favorite wet food slowly pushing his dog bowl across the kitchen tile.

Finally the air conditioning started to cool the condo. He exhaled and told her about his first day of training at the sleek new state of the art fancy BMW dealership. He went on about how he excelled in class answering all the questions and then he explained how the class trainer asked him to meet him after class at the 88 Restaurant for a drink.

Laura was listening, resting her pretty head on his chest, while he held her and stroked her with his long arms.

"So what did he say?"

"Talk about strange. This guy, Mr. Pelton, he's like this highly polished car pro who's a private contractor. And I guess he goes around doing training seminars for various dealers. Anyway, when I get to the 88 he's drinking Vodka Martinis James Bond style, right? Then he buys me a Molson and after he sweet talks me he offers me a sales manager's job at some way out in the woods Hicksville Chevy dealership. I think he said it was out in Hillbro. You ever heard of it? I think the name of it is Johnson's."

"Oh yeah, my dad took me there when I was little. If I remember the place is pretty big. And it's been there forever, so what did you say?"

Well, at first I said I wasn't interested. He offered me a thirty grand base salary plus bonuses... but shit, I was making seven to ten grand a month, that's like ninety grand a year. Anyway, he wants me to take tomorrow off and take a ride by the place to check it out." *Big Deal*.

"So – are you gonna?"

"Yes, I'm going to. Afterwards I'll give him a call with a yes or no", Lucky responded flatly thinking about all the money he'd be losing every month.

"You know honey, this might be really good for you working out of town and all, with everything that's going on."

"I know honey, but I really do love selling cars. No sitting in some stuffy office pushing paperwork."

"I'll tell you what. Why don't I take tomorrow morning off and we can ride up together. It's only like a two hour round trip right, then I'll go to work in the afternoon, how's that sound?" she asked thinking

Go with him.
Get him out of town.
Talk him into the job.
Keep him safe.

"Okay, that sounds fun. Yes I'd love to have you come along, besides I value your expert opinion," he laughed much happier, "I really do love being with you."

"You do huh? Well let's just see how much you love being here .. come on," she said pulling his arm. "Come with me young man. I need some help getting undressed."

"I thought you'd never ask." *Is she really taking the lead or am I dreaming?*

TWENTY TWO

THE FOLLOWING MORNING they were on the road early. After driving by Johnson's they stopped off for a nice country breakfast at one of the oldest inns in all of New England, the Maplehurst Inn in Antrim.

"Well, what do you think – it's big isn't it?"

"Sure is … strange all those cars and trucks way out here in the sticks," he mumbled sipping the delicious tasting coffee.

They had driven into the dealership on the way to breakfast and made one complete circle around the large complex. They were both amazed by the rows and rows of vehicles lined up for sale.

"Jeez, I guess route 4 and 202 running over to Keene is a lot busier than I thought."

And a long way from her condo.

Almost an hour commute each way.

But it's a long way from the old man.

What are you, afraid?

You know you are.

"This could be a whole new start for you way out here, away from all those slimeball city dealers trying to get back at you."

Oh, oh. Here it comes.

You knew she came for a reason.

Now you know why.

I love it when I'm right.

He sat there quietly, not saying anything, sipping his coffee, enjoying his western omelet with home fries. The homemade toast and blueberry muffins served with fresh homemade jelly and preserves made the meal all that more special.

Laura looked radiant, so full of life. Her brown bedroom eyes sparkled every time she smiled between bites of food. "Even though I agree with my dad, you probably don't have anything to worry about now, especially since you stopped working for Big Mike," She paused thinking. "Now the old man has no reason to be mad at you because you're no longer selling for his main competitor, right?"

"Yeah, that's true. So let's take another look on our way back, but I don't even have the job yet ya know … I still have to go for an interview," he grinned.

She just smiled back warmly and put her warm hand over his and said, "Lucky, they'd be fools not to hire you, and you know it."

"I guess, but let's just wait and see, okay?"

She stopped him out on the Maplehurst's porch and asked, "Do you want me to talk to my dad?" You know how well connected he is, I'm sure he knows them too…"

"No – no, I need to get this on my own – If I decide to take it", he responded, shaking his head, wondering what he'd do once he had to actually make a decision.

"Oh, I understand. I just want to help out if I can."

Maybe they won't hire me and this will all blow over. "Thanks babe, but they're either gonna hire me or they're not. That's the way it's got to be. Hell, I'm qualified anyway. We'll just have to wait and see," he boasted opening the passenger's door for Laura.

On the way back, they pulled into Johnson's Chevy and immediately noticed how busy the service department was. And even seeing the vast inventory of vehicles for a second time he was astonished at the quantity. "Unbelievable," he muttered driving around the enormous complex.

On the long ride back to Hooksett, he couldn't help but notice how upbeat Laura was. She was so excited and pumped up that he seriously started considering trying to get that manager's job. He made the call to Mr. Pelton and told him he was interested at thirty grand plus incentives.

Rick responded by saying he would make a few calls and try and set up an interview for sometime this week. He also added that Lucky would still be able to collect his weekly training pay either way.

Laura was in his arms, so pleased that he really didn't care where the job was. If it made her this happy, he'd do it. The more he thought about it, the more he really loved staying at her place, playing house and pretending they were married. She was his angel. It was very strange, she always seemed to know what he was thinking. It was like she could read his mind and know exactly what he was feeling.

Lucky couldn't help but laugh thinking how she'd been married for twenty years and had never experienced an orgasm till recently. And now that he had her in training, her skills in the bedroom and self-confidence were through the roof.

But her inexperience made her all that much more attractive. They made a game of it. She would say "Teacher, is it time for school?", with a naughty grin and he would respond that once the student was properly dressed in her school clothes that were laid out in the spare bedroom, the student's next lesson would begin.

She left for work at noon excited, giving him a hot kiss and a hug, with a look that said you better watch out later on.

So after she left, he and Taffy went into the bedroom and started carefully going through her extensive wardrobe for classroom tutoring later on that night.

He carefully laid out a white sexy garter belt with matching thigh high white stockings. Then he found an expensive Victoria Secret white push up bra that was cut low enough to leave her nipples exposed. In the bottom of her closet, he found a pair of red six-inch stiletto fuck-me heels he had bought her, and set them on the bed.

Into her skirts he ventured until he found a very short cute plaid skirt and a white silk see-through blouse that buttoned daintily up the front. Carefully, he laid out everything in the spare bedroom adding a pair of horned rim secretarial glasses with clear lenses. Already he was starting to get excited thinking about how sexy his angel would look in her school clothes and he was having a hard time waiting for later.

He fantasized about what he was going to teach her and how he was going to seduce her. He couldn't wait to see her all dolled up after a hot bath so he could tenderly kiss her long sexy neck, teasing her stiff nipples with his finger nails while he blew lightly in her ear, rimming it with his wet tongue.

He could picture it, he could see it, and he couldn't wait to hike up her little plaid skirt and kiss his way up her long tanned legs to her well-trimmed mound and taste her sweetness.

Then he shook his head to break the fantasy. Glancing at his watch, he realized he had four more hours till she'd be home.

TWENTY THREE

IN A MUSCLE shirt and cutoff jeans, he jumped into the convertible Camaro with Taffy along for the ride. It was another fine hot sunny August New Hampshire summer day and his first stop was at Danny's Beer Depot.

He picked up a cold case of Miller High Life bottles, a small box of Milk Bones for Taffy, and a pack of Cherry Tijuana small cigars.

Taffy absolutely loved the top being down. He would run between the two front bucket seats into the back seat. They stopped at Buddy's Automotive where he and Taffy went inside armed with beer, cigars, and dog bones.

Buddy had just finished spraying one of the National Guard Humvees and he was covered with Desert Storm camouflage paint and when he took his goggles off he looked like an owl smiling.

"Hey Lucky, that for me? Hey, who's your little friend?" he asked, reaching out for the cold beer Lucky held out to him.

He patted Taffy and Lucky slipped him a couple of milk bones so they could make friends. "Hey, put the rest in the old fridge will ya.., and oh, did I say thank you? It's even my brand," Buddy roared while Lucky went off to fill the old Kenmore Ice box with Miller High Life bottles. Then Lucky walked over to Buddy's mute helper and handed him a beer.

The mute just grinned and nodded thank-you.

"So tell me, how'd it go with Big Mike…any problems?" Buddy asked with a wolfish grin after downing half his beer.

"Well, the good news is the car passed with flying colors, but somehow I think you already knew that," Lucky grinned slapping Buddy's shoulder. "But hey, listen to this…the strangest thing happened

Sunday when I returned the car, there was a state trooper waiting for me with Big Mike," he said, stopping and staring at Buddy.

"No shit, I was like oh oh, here we go when they both started looking over the car and questioning me. After that, Big Mike took the Trans Am back into the garage and when his mechanic hitched it up to a computer, I started shittin' bricks," he laughed, remembering the sneer on Big Mike's mug.

"Anyway, Big Mike's fucking with me, staring at me like my machine's got you cold. It was awful Buddy, standing there with that big state trooper blocking me," he told him, tossing the empty Miller bottle into the trash can. When Lucky returned with three cold ones, Buddy was laughing so hard he had tears in his eyes.

"Hey, it's not that funny! But listen to this, that speed contraption device of Big Mike's ended up saving my ass. There I was standing there waitin' to go to jail when the trooper looks at me and says I'm free to go, huh! How about that shit?"

Buddy grinned, guilty.

"Whew," Lucky sighed. "Scared the living shit right out of me, Buddy," he stated, looking up from Taffy.

"So how'd you do it?"

"What ... do what Lucky?" Buddy answered, confused. "I ain't got no ideas what you be talkin' about...not me...uh-uh, I ain't seen no cawr ... and man, it's been awhile since I seen you...shit, only thing I remember dreamin' about is some bodacious titties on a little blonde filly that looked good enough to eat," he roared with laughter, doing sign language to his deaf helper.

"Come on," Buddy ordered, walking towards his tiny office where he opened up his expensive laptop. "Here, take a look." Lucky sat on the corner of Buddy's desk and watched his pudgy nimble fingered friend fly over the keys, then halt. With a grin, he spun the laptop screen so Lucky could see it.

"Holy shit," Lucky mumbled, eyeing the screen vividly seeing his top speed displayed. "One eighty-five, oh my god." *What the hell happened?*

Buddy came back swiftly armed with two more cold Millers and handed one to Lucky. "Seen enough, Dale Earnhart?"

"Oh yeah." *More than enough.*

"Good," he mumbled, saluting the screen. Just as he hit the delete key, the computer screen went blank. "Adios."

"Man oh man do I ever owe you…I mean anything you ever need, just let me know okay…you saved my ass big time!" *Boy did you ever.*

"Yup, that's true, but hey, I couldn't let that big prick fry your ass. Shit, you've sent me a lot of fuckin' business, and besides, you're good people," Buddy grinned, messing up Lucky's curly hair.

"I won't forget this Buddy." No *way, not anytime soon anyway.*

"You better, cause it never happened! Now get outta here before I get too drunk. I gotta wicked lot of work to get done yet."

*   *   *

Now it all made sense. He just couldn't believe it. Eagerly, he pulled back into Danny's Beer Depot, where both he and Taffy went inside.

Lucky made a deal with Danny, the owner, a former car customer, giving him a Ben Franklin for ten cases of Miller Highlife and a carton of non-filtered camels which both Buddy and his helper smoked.

The beer filled up the trunk and backseat. Their next stop was at the best pizza in all of Manchester, Vinnies Pizzeria, where he ordered three large pies.

The manager of Vinnies, a foxy brunette also knew Lucky from City Corvette because of all the pizzas the sales staff had ordered. Lucky told Nicki he needed two pies delivered to Buddy's Automotive, along with the beer.

"How many cases of beer do you have Lucky?"

"Only ten, Nicki, but I'm a good tipper," he smiled.

"Yes-so I've heard," she replied, pointing at her delivery driver and telling him to load the beer into the delivery truck.

Lucky followed him outside so Taffy wouldn't freak out. After the muscular kid unloaded the beer, Lucky handed him Buddy's card, the carton of Camels, and a twenty spot. "Make sure he gets it okay."

The kid's attitude changed immediately when he pocketed the cash. "I deliver, no problem," he smiled, eagerly going back inside.

Lucky followed him in and paid for the three pies. One thing about Vinnies Pizzeria is that it was the most expensive anywhere, but absolutely delicious.

He put the extra cheese, Canadian bacon, and onion in the trunk. There was no way Taffy was getting the opportunity. It smelled too good.

Back at the condo, they had a little while to kill before Laura would arrive so he put the wonderful smelling pizza in the oven on warm.

The smell was driving them both crazy so he took Taffy for another neighborhood stroll. While out on the walk, his Nextel phone rang. Mr. Pelton enthusiastically told him he had an interview set for Friday morning.

Impulsively, Lucky called Alexis, but she was still at work, so he left a message on her machine. "Alexis, this is Mr. Sullivan, your mechanic. Just wanted you to know I looked over your engine and after a few minor adjustments it's purring better than ever. I hope you agree Alexis, adios."

Damn, he was feeling so good for a change. His psychotropic medications were really keeping his mood swings in check, and playing house with Laura was wonderful for his ego.

"Screw them," he mumbled. Thinking about how some of them were giving him evil looks and whispering sly remarks about him not being clean because he was taking all those prescription pills, which really irked him. Half of them think a fuckin' aspirin will make you relapse he thought, shaking his head.

It didn't take long before he stopped going to Narcotics Anonymous (N.A.) meetings altogether, telling himself that he'd be okay as long as he took his seventeen pills everyday and stayed with Laura, he could stay in control.

Laura strolled into her condo with a smile, and said, "That's right, Honey, you keep taking your pills and stay off that other shit." She paused, kissing him affectionately. "Otherwise, your cute ass is out that door and I mean it." *Mmm, what's that delicious smell?*

She peeked into the oven, watching him put a Caesar salad together. "God that pizza smells good." She pulled out two long red candles out of the closet and a cold bottle of California White Zinfandel from the fridge. "You mind?"

"No…no pour it baby."

She filled each crystal-stemmed glass a quarter full and handed him a glass. "To you Sweety, for a wonderful week together and to your job interview." she smiled, jokingly. "May it last longer than the last one."

Very funny. "Ha ha," he laughed. "And to you my beautiful, sexy student who has class tonight…may you learn your lessons well," he grinned devilishly, lightly toasting her glass.

Immediately she knew he must have laid out an outfit for school or he wouldn't have brought it up. She loved it when he took control and made her feel like such a woman in the bedroom.

She talked to him while he expertly mixed the salad together. "So, Friday's the day … what do you think … are you excited?"

He was in such a good mood and he just smiled when he said, "Yes Baby, I guess I am. I think getting out of this crazy town for a while would be nice, just like you suggested."

She came back over and put a splash more wine into his depleted glass. Recklessly, he leaned over smelling her thick hair while he whispered naughty secrets into her ear. "I guess I can drive an hour away to spend a glorious night with you," he said, tenderly licking her ear lobe.

She shuddered and pulled away, wiping her ear off with a paper towel. *Oops, a little too wet.* "But I don't want to get too excited about it, because if I can't get a decent incentive package, then I'm gonna go try out BMW, agreed?"

"Whatever you want. As long as you're happy and behave yourself. I know exactly how you are, you can make money anywhere. I just want you to try something different for a change, and of course you have to keep teaching me," she added, poking him in the ribs with a laugh. *I love my lessons.*

She looked him in the eyes with her long Greek goddess eyelashes batting away. She told him without blushing, "The student needs another lesson tonight. Does the teacher have anything new to show the student or should we get a substitute teacher?" She giggled, wrapping her arms around his waist from his backside.

"Oh, I'll think of something special...I wonder if I could find a qualified female instructor...what?" *Boy, wouldn't I love that.*

"Stop."

"Okay." *Just thought I'd mention it, you never know.*

"It sounds interesting professor. But let's eat our delicious meal before class starts because this student plans on taking a nice bath before her new lesson begins."

She lit the candles while he served the Caesar salads and pizza. In no time, the delicious pizza was gone because they were both very hungry.

After dinner, she bathed in exotic oils while Lucky cleaned up the kitchen. Then when she emerged wrapped in towels, she headed straight for the spare bedroom to see what crazy outfit her professor had picked out.

While Lucky was in the shower, she dressed smiling, making sure to put her long black hair up into a secretarial bun to go along with the horned rim glasses. He changed in the master bedroom into black leather biker chaps with nothing underneath. Then he put on a black leather snap vest over his bare chest. Carefully, he slid on a black thong over the chaps and a pair of black leather weightlifting gloves for his hands. Watching in the mirror, he tied his Harley Davidson bandana on his head grinning. His spit shined Coast Guard boots and mirrored ray bans finished his outfit.

The lesson that night was how long you could go without touching the other person masturbating. Of course he provided the proper adult movie to set the mood and casually he selected his shy Greek goddess a vibrating friend to help her achieve success.

The key was getting her to use it while he watched instead of participating. After a lot of encouragement and teasing on his part, she finally relented. Watching the movie, she relaxed and gave him the show he wanted.

It sure didn't take too long before they both achieved orgasms separately. Shortly after he attacked his sexy pupil in his leather garb, teasing her into another frenzy before they made love in their crazy outfits.

TWENTY FOUR

FRIDAY MORNING, LUCKY met Rick the trainer and they rode up to Johnson's Chevy in Rick's new Lincoln Town Car. "It's not mine Lucky. Just another dealer perk," he said with a grin. "I enjoy big cars and this model happens to be one of my favorites. Plenty of power, floats down the highway, and room to move around."

He paused driving with his knee to light an expensive humidor cigar. "Yup, I'll take a big car any day over all that foreign crap they're pushing now."

Lucky quietly just listened and lit up his own cigar, a twenty-five cent plastic tipped cherry Tijuana small.

"Listen, these brothers are a little strange, okay? Nothing probably like you're used to in the city. These guys wear jeans to work and drive old, worn out cars, but don't let the country poor look fool you," he glanced over between puffs.

"Yup, they're loaded with dough. Their great uncle built the place like eighty-years ago and it's been in the family ever since," he paused daydreaming. "Shit, I knew their old man for years, but he's dead now, and the sons are pretty laid back. They're just different, not all gung-ho like you're used to. So what I'm saying is, just take it slow. You don't need to oversell yourself. I did all that trust me. Just the fact you're meeting them means they're very interested, okay?"

"I hear you. I guess I just feel a little strange about working way out here in the sticks, but hey, a change of pace might be just what I need." *At least my angel thinks so.*

The big interview didn't last too long. Lucky felt like it was over before it really got started. They told him if he wanted to give it a go, he had the job. After they agreed on an incentive plan, they told him to go out and pick out a demo.

"Sheeeit," the older brother said with a grin, glancing at his younger brother. "Sonny there's like three hundred of 'em out there… you oughta be able to find somethin' you like"

"Just don't touch my truck. That be the old Chevy parked on the side," the younger brother yelled as Lucky walked out of their plush offices excited, but very confused.

He came out in the bright sunshine to pick out a decent demo when he spotted Rick the trainer leaning up against his Lincoln smoking another stogy bullshitting with one of the sales staff.

When Rick spotted Lucky looking at the cars, he knew what time it was, and shook hands harder with the salesman then started walking towards him with a smile.

They walked the big lot together looking for something he liked while they discussed the brief interview. Lucky picked out a late model Pontiac Bonneville SSEi. Satisfied, they walked back towards Rick's town car. Slyly, Rick pulled out a sealed envelope out of his suit jacket and handed it to Lucky. "Congratulations."

Stunned, Lucky asked, "What's this?"

"Oh, that? That's your week's training pay I promised you," he stated climbing into his car. "Oh, and by the way, if you need anything. Just let me know, you've got my number."

Johnson's Chevy
Two weeks later

It was the end of his second week at Johnson's Chevy when he finally met the Notorious Dirty Shirt Dick, the Boston Wholesaler.

He spotted him from the showroom glass just sitting there in an old caddy chain smoking a cigarette with his car door wide open.

"How are you doing today sir? Anything I can help you with?" Lucky asked walking right up to him.

Dirty shirt Dick stepped out of the old caddy, crushing his cigarette butt with his cowboy boot. "I doubt it," he responded, loaded with sarcasm. "See, I stop by every week, sometimes every other week to buy cars, but those two in there," pointing at the showroom, "don't sell to no city wholesaler."

Dirty shirt paused looking all around the big complex full of vehicles, and then he continued talking," And it looks to me like they don't sell to no one," he exclaimed with a hacking smoker's cough.

"Yes, you have a valid point there, but hopefully that will all change. At least that's what I think they hired me for," he shot back, sticking out his right hand. "I'm Lucky Sullivan, the new sales manager, and you're?"

"Dick, but my friends call me Dirty Shirt. Get it? Dirty Shirt Dick," he guffawed shaking Lucky's hand firmly.

They walked the lot while they talked and smoked because Lucky could feel all the reckless eyeballs from the showroom burning his back.

"So you buy cars do you?"

"You bet! I buy em all over New Hampshire for a guy out of Boston who puts em on different lots all around Boston. Shit, last week I bought twelve cars on my trip through the good ole Granite State. But I never could get one outta here"

"Well Dirty Shirt,that might just change. I got most of the say so and as you can see, I sure got a shitload of cars to sell," Lucky laughed heartily. They stopped behind a big Chevy Dually.

Dirty Shirt Dick told him how he just couldn't understand how the owners could sit on all this inventory, because it really looked like to him, that over the past twelve weeks not much had changed in the huge inventory. It was like they didn't give a shit or something.

"So you buy late models…cash I presume and then resell them in the big city right?"

"Yup. Something like that, it's by cashier's check, but basically that's it."

"Listen Dick, let's be up front here," he said glancing all around. "I'd just as soon sell you a bunch of cars so I can turn over my inventory… but if the owners haven't dealt with you yet…that kind of ties my hands…you get my drift?"

"Yeah, yeah Lucky, we all need a little incentive in life."

Lucky glanced into the big truck and on the drivers seat there was a crisp hundred dollar bill. He didn't hesitate getting into the truck and climbing behind the wheel. Smoothly, he pocketed the yard.

"You know Dirty Shirt, I think we can work something out," he smiled. "And I've got an idea how you can get in better with the staff here since I already heard all about you long before I met you, so-," "Lucky grinned."

"How's that?"

Obviously this dude's not too bright, Lucky thought.

He told him he should come by and take him and his five salesmen out to lunch on him of course, and Lucky would say that it was Dirty Shirt's idea. Also, in the mean time, he would go through the inventory to see if he could come up with a few vehicles they owned right that they could possibly sell to him.

"So what days good for you?"

"How bout this Friday? I gotta pick up a car down at the Ford garage?" he said, thumbing his hand towards Lucky's competitor.

"Great, I'll set it up. We can go to the Maplehurst Inn, they have great food. You know where that is over in Antrim?" Lucky asked him.

"Yeah, ain't that the old joint right on Main Street?"

"Yup, that's the place," he smiled wondering if Dirty Shirt Dick would actually show up. "So come by here around noon time Friday and we can all ride over at the same time. The guys will love it," Lucky laughed excitedly.

"Shit, I'm sure they will Lucky," he responded sarcastically. "I hope all this shit is worth it!"

"Dirty Shirt, where's your faith brother?" Lucky roared. "No seriously, you'll get your share, just keep these coming," he commented, tapping his coat pocket. Then he got back out of the truck and they both lit another cigarette while they walked to his old caddy.

"No problem with your pocket, just as long as you look out. You know I gotta buy em right or I can't deal, but I guess you know that already, huh?"

"See you Friday, Dick," Lucky said, pocketing the wholesaler's business card.

TWENTY FIVE

H E WALKED BACK into the showroom and one of the good ole boys that had become part of the furniture caught Lucky's attention, waving him over. "So I see you finally met old Dirty Shirt, the wholesaler. What a guy," Billy laughed.

Lucky waited patiently till Billy stopped chuckling. Then he surprised him. "Yup, and good ole Dirty Shirt's taking us all out to lunch Friday at noon, so be hungry," he said, walking away quickly, leaving Billy stunned.

Before Lucky got far, Billy recovered. "Jesus Lucky, well that's awfully nice of him. Okay, never mind, I won't even ask how you got him to do it."

Over the next few hours he went over the vast inventory trying to pick out a couple potential wholesale pieces that he might be able to sell to Dick and still make a profit. He focused on a few of the cars Dick had pointed out. The main problem was most of the vehicles on the lot they owned for so long that the value had depreciated back down to what they owned it for.

Not a good situation to be in. But after getting depressed, he finally found a gem they owned right and was well below wholesale.

*　　*　　*

Friday's lunch was a huge hit with the guys. They all had expensive cocktails in the old fashioned lounge before they moved into the formal dining room where they all had shrimp cocktail and prime rib, the house specialty.

Dirty Shirt actually looked presentable in a new shirt with an old stained tie and a new pair of Levis that he must have just bought recently because a piece of the Levis tag was still attached to the back pocket.

After a few potent cocktails, the guys started to warm up to Dick's corny used car jokes and after a terrific lunch they all thanked him before leaving Lucky and Dick at the table.

They both moved back into the cozy lounge and ordered another drink. An adorable waitress left a visa book on the table containing the big check.

Dirty Shirt sipped his Bacardi and Coke while Lucky stirred his Absolute and O.J. Lucky was very aware that if he drank anything other than Vodka, his breath would stink like booze and that wouldn't go over too well with the customers back at the dealership.

He watched Dick frown when he glanced at the bill. "What's the damage?"

"Too damn much, but hey, look at all the new friends I got," he chuckled, almost hacking up a lung. "And of course you got good news for me, right?"

"Well, yes and no. Yes, I found a car we own right, but no I haven't cleared it with the owners yet, and I won't till you and I get a firm price down," he said seriously.

"Hey, don't give me that look…You're buying a car…it's just which one and how much," he went on pulling out a handful of psychotropic medication and swallowing them down with his screwdriver.

"Jesus, you're a walkin' pharmacy."

"I guess so," but if I don't take'm I get crazy, at least that's what my girlfriend says, so hey, fuck it, I take em most of the time." *When I'm not getting high.*

Then he sat back down and got down to business. Carefully, he pulled out a neatly folded sheet of paper and laid it on the small bar table, lighting up a Marlboro Light, while Dick fired up enthusiastically eyeing the paper on the table. Slowly, Lucky unfolded the paper and folded it flat with his hand.

"So, you like that Ninety-five Buick Grandmaster, one owner, older couple, low miles, real clean, right?"

Dick nodded, waiting to hear the numbers while he pulled out his black wholesale N.A.D.A. book and started thumbing to Buicks.

"Okay, now we own it for six grand and I gotta put a profit on it to make the deal go down, plus something for me, so I'll sell it to you for sixty-five hundred," Lucky said, looking over at Dick to see his reaction.

"I know, I know the numbers; sixty-eight wholesale, seventy-six trade-in and eighty-five retail," Dick paused thinking. "How many miles?"

"Only forty-five k. Christ, I saw you drooling over it. It's fuckin' clean and I'm selling it to you at three-hundred below wholesale for Christ's sake."

"Alright, alright, you think they'll go for it?"

"Hey, that's my problem, right? I gotta good buzz going now, so I'll try to get it done today because I could use two yards from you when you take delivery," he grinned as they got up to leave.

"No problem on my end. Sixty-three hundred to them and two bills to you," Dick laughed. "Hey, you're the one who's gotta convince those two assholes to sell one of their precious cars," he stopped, holding the door open for two of New England's classy, elderly ladies out for lunch at the Inn.

"God, I wish I could see their faces when you tell 'em," Dick grinned, lighting another cigarette.

"Shit, thanks a lot. I guess that's my problem," Lucky mumbled climbing into Dick's old caddy.

TWENTY SIX

LUCKY TRACKED DOWN the older brother figuring he would be easier to approach, boldly he knocked on his office door, getting right to the point, he told him he was going to sell the Ninety-Five Buick Grandmaster to the wholesaler.

"And why would you want to do that? We don't give cars away here Lucky. I thought we were very clear on that!" he said, firmly taking his feet down off the desk.

"Well, we make three-hundred on the deal. No commissions paid and you've owned the car for ten months without even a test drive or an offer," he paused for effect, still standing erect, slightly buzzed, he went on. "And we really do need to turn over some of this inventory. It's old and stagnant. Customers continue to see the same vehicles every time they drive by and that's the problem," he stated, catching his breath, figuring he better say what he had to say while he still had his attention.

"Also sir, we need to take a good look at most of our prices, because sure they might have been competitive when you originally set them a year or two ago, but as you probably know, these vehicles are depreciating every day they sit out there. For example, that Ninety-Five Silverado four-by-four plow truck," he hesitated, opening his small black book. "You own it for twelve-seven. You had it priced at seventeen-five twenty-seven months ago, well today retail is only fourteen-seven…but it's still priced at seventeen-five, so no one in their right mind would even consider buying it at almost three grand over market value. And that's just one example, sir," he said compassionately waiting for a response.

The older brother just sat there impatiently eyeing Lucky, while he slowly paced back and forth telling him the real deal about his inventory.

Then he looked up. "Well Lucky, you have a good point. I guess I never really thought about it in those terms, but I do know my kid brother does get attached to the inventory and is stubborn about selling them," he exclaimed, rubbing his hand through his well-styled beard. "Listen Lucky, your points are all valid. It's just that you really have to move a little slower here, he hates sudden changes."

Shocked and amazed at what he was hearing, he wanted to scream. *Don't you want to make any damn money, if I move any slower I'll be crawling!*

"I personally would like to see some cars gone and some new inventory, but it's him you gotta walk softly with."

"Why the hell did you hire me," he almost said, pissed off. "Okay sir, this is what I'm gonna do," he told him starting to pace again. "I'm gonna have a car and truck special each week until it sells. I'll put 'em out by the road with the sale price clearly marked with some type of roof sales marker."

"Also, I will have a picture each week in all our ads of the car and truck of the week, plus we are gonna move the vehicles around every two weeks, and I want to hang up some string banners over the sales lot."

"Okay…Okay…that sounds terrific! So tell me, how is everything else going?" *Is this guy listening to anything I'm saying?*

"Well, I'm glad you asked. What I really want to do is hire another sales person, as I'm not allowed to dismiss anyone you have already, so let me bring in one of my own." *So I can make some damn money!* "All your guys average two to four cars a month and it's just not getting done. I really feel some new blood other than me who will produce, will help lift the sales numbers of the other guys."

He was all fired up with a few cocktails in his bloodstream, and he knew he only had his attention for a few seconds longer, so he stopped to let the owner absorb all he had told him when the crafty owner took advantage of the silence.

"You got someone in mind?"

"Yes sir, I sure do. He's a solid ten to twelve car guy month after month."

"Where's he from?"

"He works at City Corvette."

"Why don't you have him stop by sometime okay? And listen, I'll talk to my brother and see if I can get him to loosen up, alright? Oh, and go ahead and sell your Buick."

Lucky just stood there frozen, amazed at the change.

"Is there anything else?" the owner demanded, slightly annoyed.

"One last thing sir. David, your salesman needs to go, he's terrible. He won't listen or follow my very simple requests and I'm fed up," he told him, raising his arms to show him how disgusted he really was. "Sir, his attitude really sucks…sir."

"Whoa..Whoa…," the owner roared standing up. "Shit, I'll talk to him okay." *Sure you will.*

"Okay sir, one final thought."

"Hurry up, I'm leaving. I suddenly got a headache."

"Alright, I think we need to be open at least noon to six on Saturday and Sundays. We are completely missing out on prime selling time."

Jesus, this guy never quits. "We told you we don't want to over work our sales staff…but maybe you can work it out so it's voluntary or optional or something," he said, leaving his office hurriedly.

"Okay sir, I will work it out." *And thanks…thanks for nothing'.*

TWENTY SEVEN

H E PHONED DIRTY Shirt Dick. "Hey, when ya coming to get your Buick? Huh, it's taking up valuable space on my busy lot," Lucky snickered.

"Shit, you really did it! I had my doubts."

"Me too-but the sooner the better. I caught the right one alone and I'd like you to take delivery before the other one finds out so-"

"Hey, I'll swing by the bank and pick up a cashier's check for $6,300 right?"

"Right."

"And then I'll be right over."

Good, hurry up...and remember those two yards."

"I gotcha Lucky, see you in a few."

Sitting at his desk, he called City Corvette. He asked for Ryan and waited for him to be paged. He already knew he wanted to steal him away and that Ryan admired him, so the first thing he told him about was the three-hundred a week salary and weekends free.

It was in Lucky's nature, when he really wanted something, he found a way to get it. "Ryan, I'll give you a sweet demo on day one, and of course I'll throw you all my own sales since I can't make any commissions."

"Jesus Lucky, where the hell is this place at?" Ryan asked wondering if this was too good to be true.

Well, it's about forty-five minutes on the highway. You take I-93 North to Bow and get on I-89 North to exit four Route 202/4. Go past Henniker to downtown Hillbro," he paused.

"But the best thing for you bro is that all the other salesmen just sit on their asses all day, so you won't have any competition with me feeding you," Lucky laughed, knowing it was true.

"Damn Lucky, that sounds wicked. Let me call you when I get off."

"Cool."

TWENTY EIGHT

HE WAS ON his way back to Laura's condo, enjoying the hot Summer evening when he started dwelling on City Corvette, and how he could get even. His mind raced as he thought to himself that there had to be more going on with all these expensive 'Vettes being shipped up monthly from South Florida on car carriers, then other 'Vettes being shipped south on the return trip. Why?

Then it dawned on him from his Coast Guard days in Key West. But instead of boats, it was 'Vettes. What a great way to smuggle drugs up from Florida he grinned to himself, reaching over to crank up Boston's 'More Than a Feelin' on Rock 101.

He was cruising in a brand new, limited edition WS6 six speed Trans Am, fire engine red with both T-Tops out. "Fuck you Big Mike," he screamed excitedly, realizing he was driving the brand new model to Big Mike's old classic.

His A.D.H.D was kicking in and his thought pattern raced back and forth. He was amped. Now he was back on the old man and Ryan. His excitement built and built thinking about spying on his old boss and imagined that just maybe Ryan would know when the next shipments of 'Vettes were arriving. He grinned thinking how easy it could all fall together. "Yup, I bet it does," he mumbled, tapping his left hand to Boston cranked up on the powerful stereo.

His phone rang.

"Hello," he yelled over the music.

"Hey, what are you at, a concert?"

Lucky laughed, turning down the radio. "I wish."

"So Lucky, whas up bro?"

"You my man, you."

"Okay, then I wanna come up 'n' check out this wicked deal, how bout tomorrow after I get off work?"

"Sounds good. But remember I told you they're closed on weekends. It doesn't matter. I can still meet you if you want?"

"Shit, okay. How about five-thirty tomorrow? I hope to get outta here by five p.m., and between us I'm getting really sick of all this shit goin' on around here," Ryan whispered, glancing around City Corvette's showroom. "Hey Lucky, you were serious, three bills a week salary, plus commission?"

"Of course"

"Jesus, that's sweet."

"No shit huh – but hey, keep it to yourself okay. I don't need the old man finding out I'm trying to steal one of his guys," he told him cautiously. *At least not yet.*

"That's for sure...so I'll catch you tomorrow...where you gonna be?"

"Call me on my cell. I'll be in Hooksett at Laura's so we can meet at her place and we'll take my demo up okay?"

"Sounds great...till tomorrow."

"Later Ryan."

*   *   *

The following day, Saturday, Ryan showed up at Laura's condo right after work, all excited. They jumped into the new Trans Am and headed for Hillbro on I-93 North. Lucky pulled off exit one on I-89North and stopped at the Bow Mobil where he gave Ryan a five-spot to buy some Cold Molson Golden.

Back on I-89 they made great time cruising at ninety, while they sipped cold ones. After two beers each, they pulled into Johnson's well lit mega car lot.

"Wow, this place is huge," Ryan said enthusiastically while Lucky slowly cruised the dealership.

"No shit, I told you. Just look at all those vehicles. It's a fuckin goldmine." "And most of them are way over priced," he mumbled.

"Just imagine you and me on a Saturday all alone, and every customer we wait on is all yours." *That's right suck it all in homeboy. I got you now, you'll be workin' for me real soon.*

"You mean that shit?"

"What? Of course I do…shit, I can't make any commissions off my own sales so I may as well give 'em to you," he smiled. "And of course if you want, you can kick back a little love," he laughed waiting for Ryan to finally figure it out. "It's true, I only get a bonus if we sell a certain number, so it only helps me meet my goals if I feed you deals."

"Okay, okay…It's just I got to convince my old lady…cause it's a long fuckin' way from Westborough."

"True – but we do close at 8 p.m., not nine like City Corvette so you'll be home at about the same time," he paused looking at Ryan. "Don't forget weekends are optional, so you'll have a lot more time with your kids, and of course three times their base salary doesn't hurt either."

"Man, oh man." *No wonder you sell so many cars.*

Lucky laughed. "Hey, hopefully you'll want to come in here and make some coin, seriously bro, I can't do this alone, these guys are like zombies." *For real.*

They went inside and he quickly showed him the new fancy showroom and where his desk would be. They left the Country dealership and stopped at a local corner store for four more Molson Goldens for the trip back.

They started back to I-89 on Rt. 202. Ryan was relaxed and in a great mood. He took a swallow of the cold Canadian beer and said, "So three bills a week and a decent demo day one, right?"

Lucky nodded, carefully cuffing his Marlboro Light so he wouldn't put a burn hole in the expensive leather bucket seats.

"Shit, plus your sales on top of mine, that's too good to pass up." *You bet it is.*

Lucky smiled in agreement. "Oh yeah, I'll feed you sales, don't worry, I won't let you down. You, of all people, know I can sell," he grinned at Ryan. *I'm not gonna say anything else except…go for it."*

Ryan thought, God, he used to sell twenty a month plus my twelve, shit, that's thirty-two. Even if we do half that, I'm ahead of the game at sixteen. "God Lucky, I really can't stand those assholes at work. Shit, I could have a nice fresh start, and be a star, Lucky's star," Ryan joked.

Lucky expertly flicked his butt out the T-Top before getting on the highway. In no time they were back at Laura's condo. It was seven fifty-five p.m. He pulled into her reserved spot beside Ryan's beat up demo that City Corvette issued him and shut off the sweet sounding V-8.

"Listen, do me a favor, let me know either way so I can hire someone…but hey. I do hope it's you, cause if I know how to do one thing," he looked at Ryan seriously, "it's making money selling cars and you know that. I will spoon feed your ass. Man, I can't stand any of the sales team so it'll be you and me."

Ryan eagerly listened.

"I got every car on my computer and I know exactly what we own it for, that's a huge advantage…but whatever you decide, don't say shit to anyone but your old lady."

"Okay. I'm not stupid, I know the old man's after your ass."

"Did I say you're stupid?" he joked. "Listen, what are you doin' Monday?"

"I'm off."

"Good. If you want to ride up with me and spend the day, you know, see if you like it and I can probably line up a quick interview," he hesitated before pouncing. "Then if you take the job, I'll let you pick out a killer demo and you could start on Tuesday."

"Shit Lucky, don't you think I ought to give a notice because you know how the old man is?"

"Fuck him," Lucky roared angrily. "They need you, you don't need them. The minute you give a notice, it'll be the worst last week of your life and you know it."

"Shit, I never thought of it like that," Ryan responded eyeing his watch. "You better go dancing and I better get my ass home, but hey, thanks."

"Hey Ryan, before you go, they got any new 'Vettes coming up from Florida?"

Ryan, holding the door open on his used Subaru, turned around thinking. "Yeah, we should have a load coming in tonight or tomorrow. At least I hope so because I sold a ninety-two triple black convertible that's on the carrier and I'd sure like to deliver it tomorrow, it's a pretty good lick and I could use the commission."

That's great news, wonderful news.

TWENTY NINE

H E WENT INSIDE and changed into his dancing duds. While they each were getting ready, he made them tall Captain Morgan and Cokes.

It was a gorgeous night.

In the Trans Am, he left the T-Tops out and when he glanced over, he was extremely pleased at what he saw. Laura looked hot as usual in her red silk dress and matching red pumps. But what really excited him the most was the sheer crotch-less panty-hose she was wearing that he had surprised her with from Victoria Secrets.

He started to grin while he drove. All he could think about was her sexy exotic stockings and the tiny red bikini panties she slid on over the top of her delicious legs, so they could be removed easily.

As usual, the two of them dominated the over thirty crowded dance floor in the music hall. Every Saturday, the old dance club in Concord came alive with old Rock-N-Roll dance classics. Even the owner himself, dressed in a tux,showed his expert skills as a D.J. constantly jamming the dance floor.

The club was hot and they sweated while they continued to drink down Cold Captain and Cokes. Finally, after Laura had a good buzz going, Lucky convinced her to shed her skimpy panties in the ladies room.

Now he was really turned on. They slow-danced to Eric Clapton's "Cocaine." Slowly, he slid his hot hand down her spine, lower and lower his fingers caressed until his palm felt her scantly covered almost naked bottom. Through the thin sheer silk fabric of her red dress, his hand could lustily feel everything.

They moved closer.

Tighter, they danced closer. He responded by rubbing his hardness into her, making sure she could feel his eager manhood.

"Mmm…you're so naughty," she whispered into his ear, obviously turned on by her nakedness.

"Yes I am…but you see what your body does to me," he sighed, heavily kissing her ear again with his tongue, teasing her neck."

After a few more Spiced Rums and fast dirty dancing, Laura was really starting to loosen up. Every time Lucky went up to the oval shaped bar for drinks or to the men's room, the same young stud would move in on the highly intoxicated, sexy Laura.

He barely looked twenty-one, solidly built, and very cocky. Persistently, he continued to demand her to dance flirting and strutting with her as he tugged on her arm lightly.

Smiling, loosely, she kept telling him no. Lucky eyed the young stud lusting after her on two different occasions he tried to make his strike. But Lucky smiled knowing the way she checked him out when he walked away that she thought he was good looking.

When the next fast song started, Lucky encouraged her to go ask her admirer to dance.

Shocked, she didn't know what to say. "What, are you sure?"

"Yes, I'm sure baby…go ahead, tease him for me," he ordered helping her to her feet.

"Well okay, just one dance," she mumbled nervously, walking over to ask him to dance with a sly grin.

He watched them boogie to a couple fast songs, then a nice slow song started and she turned and said thanks and started to leave the dance floor. But the young stud wouldn't give up and before she knew it, she was in his strong arms, slow dancing.

Boldly, the young stud started grinding his crotch into her while he eagerly squeezed her ass with his big hands. He knew the kid must be rock hard and he watched closely to see if he needed to come to her rescue. Laura blushed and smiled sexily as he whispered something into her ear. *God, he's so hard.*

Finally, the slow dance ended and he made his move. Quickly he tried to kiss her but she turned away at the last second.

Stubbornly, she broke free of his paws and worked her way back over to Lucky with weak knees.

"Whew…wow…," she said grinning, taking a sip of her rum and coke. "God Professor, is that part of my schooling?" she sighed, shaking her head. "God, do you know his hard thing was grinding into my nakedness…and…I couldn't pull away," she blushed excitedly.

"I saw, and you loved every minute of it," Lucky replied, giving her a hungry French kiss.

On the way out Laura leaned over and whispered "Guess what he told me?"

"What…tell me?"

"Is that guy your hanging out with bothering you, cause if you want I can take care of him if you want me to?" she joked with a devilish grin.

"Are you sure you want to leave?"

"Yes. Yes, I'm very sure and very horny," she whispered.

He whispered back, "Sure you don't want to bring your young stud along? Maybe he'd like to substitute teach."

She laughed loudly, "You're crazy, ya I bet he would too…come on, let's go before you really corrupt me," she said pulling his hand towards the Trans Am.

All the way back, he caressed her scantily covered legs and eagerly, he teased her bare moist mound while the cool night wind blew in from the roofless T-Tops lifting up her sexy dress exposing her naughty crotchless Victoria Secrets stockings.

They were both so turned on they barely made it inside her condo. Once inside, they slammed the door, fully aroused, they attacked one another.

Hungrily, he dropped her on the bed and quickly slipped a pillow under her ass before devouring her wetness with his mouth.

She was so close to ecstasy that when he started talking dirty to her about her young stud being in the other room, all the while increasing the speed of his tongue and fingers, it was too much for her and she screamed out in delight digging her nails into his shoulders.

Once he finished her off, leaving her moaning and groaning, he spryly shed his sweaty clothes and displayed his hard manhood proudly.

He entered her slowly while she still had her dress, stockings, and heels on and it was driving him into a frenzy. Aggressively, he sucked on her firm exposed nipples holding her legs back with his strong arms. The thought of the young stud turning her on was too much for him.

Wildy, he pounded her faster and faster and faster, seeking relief from all the excitement. Closer and closer the pressure built till they both exploded together.

"God that was great, Honey, whew," she exhaled exhausted, and gently wiped the sweat out of his eyes. "Mmm…Baby, that hit the spot, mmm twice," she giggled.

He tenderly kissed her while he gently undressed her and cleaned up their mess with a warm face cloth. Lightly, he tucked her in bed giving her fifty milligrams of trazadone, his psychotropic sleeping medication.

"Are you sure I'll be okay?"

"Yes baby. You need a good night sleep putting up with me all week and tomorrow's the only day you get to sleep in." *And I need to sneak out so take it and sleep like a baby, cause if you find out, I'm screwed.*

"Oh okay, if you say so…Loverboy." *What, that's Alexis's word.*

Smoothly, he handed her the trazadone and a glass of water. "Nighty night, Angel," he mumbled, cuddling up to her while he waited impatiently for her to pass out.

Twenty minutes later, she was snoring in all her glory. Carefully, he slid out of the bed naked, guarded not to bother Taffy who was curled up in his own doggy bed.

Silently, he grabbed the gym bag out of his closet and tip-toed out to the living room, gently closing the bedroom door.

Rapidly, Lucky slid on a long sleeve black t-shirt and black Levi's jeans, then he tied his black Nike Jordans in double knots. On his way towards the door, he grabbed his backpack and Nike black ball cap. He hesitated, which car? he thought. "Fuck it," he mumbled and grabbed Laura's keys to her Lincoln and shut the door.

THIRTY

Manchester, NH
2:00a.m.

I N HIS BACKPACK, he had his black driving gloves, a mag light, and a pair of expensive night vision binoculars he had permanently borrowed from the Coast Guard.

It was late, the bars were just letting out and the roads were filled with drunks. He pulled Laura's big Lincoln into an all-night Market Basket supermarket, and went inside.

After scouring the meat department, Lucky finally found what he was seeking. Two fat juicy meat bones. In the check out he grabbed a pack of Marlboro Lights and an ice-cold Coca-Cola Classic.

His eyes switched from the dashboard clock to the rows of 'Vettes off in the distance through his night eyes. Impatiently, he waited...and waited.

What the hell am I doing here?
Nothing's going to happen.
Yes it will...Just be patient.
Remember, don't ever forget, he tried to kill you

The dashboard clock said three-nineteen a.m. when finally something happened. He couldn't miss it. A beautiful car carrier cruised by...full of pretty Florida 'Vettes. Excitedly, he slid lower in the seat eyeing the carrier as it carefully backed into the alley beside City Corvette. His heartbeat raced while he watched the driver slowly unload his precious cargo one at a time.

Systematically, the driver drove all seven 'Vettes into the back fenced in lot and then he put lock boxes on each driver's window with the individual 'Vette keys locked inside the box.

Instantly, Lucky rubbed his jean pocket feeling the master lock box key he stole out of the manager's desk on the last day when he got fired from City Corvette.

At last the empty car carrier pulled out and left. A few minutes passed before the old security guard pulled in and unlocked the back lot. Lucky watched through his big eyes as the security guard opened the back of his enclosed truck and two Doberman Pincher attack dogs jumped out. Expertly, he pushed them into the back lot and slammed the heavy gate, locking it.

Oh shit, Lucky thought.

He glanced at the dashboard clock. Five past four. Shit, it's getting really late, he thought. Why the dogs?

His heart began to race, and he pulled on his black Nike driving gloves. He smoked waiting for the security guard to leave before he sat back up and started the Lincoln.

Glancing all around, he pulled out and crossed over to the other side pulling into the 24-hour self-service car wash next door to City Corvette.

Smoothly, he backed the Lincoln into the last stall concealing the license plate. Quickly, he exited the car and crossed the alley. Discretely, he followed the fence line to the back of the dealership clutching his backpack he followed the fence line into the woods.

Lucky could see the two Dobermans prancing around sniffing everything. His adrenaline was racing through his body as he dared himself to climb over the security fence. He prayed they were the same two dogs he met at a party months earlier at the security guard's home.

Please be the same King and Queen.
Man, this is fuckin' crazy.
Don't chicken out now.
Okay, okay, here I go.

He wasn't sure if his idea would work, but it was too late now to back out. Up he climbed, over he went. He touched the ground on the inside of the fence and immediately unzipped his backpack, pulling out the pack of juicy bones.

Both dogs froze at the sound of the fence vibrating, alertly they sniffed the air. Swiftly, both dogs responded silently, stalking towards the noise.

Lucky was breathing rapidly, slowly he shuffled towards the new 'Vettes. *Come on, where are you?*

Nervously he eased forward trembling, clutching a fat juicy bone in his hand. Bravely, he called out, "Here King...here Queen..."

The next thing he heard was a deep vicious growl close by. Terrified, he inched forward very slowly, "Come on boy," he whispered, alertly looking around behind him to see if he was about to get attacked.

When he sensed movement, he spun back around to see King posted up directly in front of him, blocking his way crouched in an attack stance growling and showing his teeth.

Oh shit...Oh shit. He could feel the sweat pour out of his body and he tried not to panic.

Deep breath. "Hey King, hey boy, there you are. Look what I brought you, yeah, good boy," Lucky said, friendly tossing the fat five dollar beef shank to King.

King sat back and eyed the bone, then lifted his head and eyed Lucky. "Go on boy, that's it, take it boy, please," he whispered.

Slowly King shimmied up to the bone with shifty eyes and sniffed the bloody bone.

Oh no... He sensed the attack from behind by Queen, the second Doberman who had snuck up behind him while King distracted him.

Desperately he spun around just in time, stalling the attack. He faced Queen head on, wide-eyed, and trembling. "Hey Queen, remember me girl, huh? Yeah, I brought you a treat just like King," he said desperately holding out the expensive bone, trembling.

Queen, ready to pounce all of a sudden sat back and licked her chops. Surprised, Lucky glanced back at King. He was gone and so was the bone. A sense of overwhelming relief came over him; he turned back towards Queen and tossed her the bone. She didn't hesitate after watching King snag his bone, she grabbed it and disappeared. *Thank God.*

He didn't realize he'd been holding his breath the whole time till he started getting light headed. Then he exhaled deeply taking in a mouthful of fresh oxygen.

I gotta move fast he told himself.

With newborn energy, he walked quickly to the seven 'Vettes and glanced around nervously pulling out his lock box key, he opened up the first 'Vette in line and searched.

There's gotta be something here.

Who the hell puts dogs in right after they get used cars.

I know it, it's here somewhere.

By the fourth 'Vette, he was getting frustrated. "What the fuck am I doing out here," he yelled angrily. I should be back in bed with my goddess…shit this sucks." *I'm so stupid.*

It wasn't till he climbed into the sixth 'Vette that he found something. "Bingo…oh my God…oh shit…oh shit…" he mumbled, as he shined his little mag light across the bag holding ten kilos of cocaine wrapped in Juan Valdez Columbian coffee wrappers.

Crazily, he filled his knapsack with all ten kilos. "Holy shit this is heavy." *Twenty-two pounds of cocaine, holy shit.* Quickly he put the keys back in the lock boxes.

Excited, he glanced around nervously. "Shit," he mumbled, "let's get the hell out of here" With his heart pounding, he started for the fence, praying the dogs would leave him alone.

The last thing he wanted to do was stumble upon King and Queen on his escape. His heart was beating so hard he could hear it pumping with the heavy pack pulling on his chest.

At last he reached the fence, exhaling to catch his breath when he felt it, a cold wet nose on the back of his wrist.

"Shit…"

Don't move, don't move.

Very slowly, he glanced down and back to see King only inches away. Trying not to shake, he said, "Hey King, you comin' to say goodbye? … Good boy."

Taffy's milk bones in my pack's outer pocket, please be there, he thought anxiously.

Smoothly he eased the pack off his shoulders and set it on the ground. Nervously he bent over and unzipped the tiny outside pouch and reached in. "Yes!" He felt four wonderful milk bones in his hand.

King watched every move silently. He had Lucky pinned against the fence. Very slowly, he opened his other empty gloved hand and bravely held it out to King to sniff.

"Come on, do it," he told himself. Steadily, he reached out further and patted King's head gently while Queen stood guard on the opposite side. "Good boy King…here you go boy," Lucky whispered. Nervous as hell, he dropped two of the small milk bones on the ground.

King snatched them both up and disappeared under the closest car. Carefully, Lucky turned and spotted Queen. "Hey Queen, here you go girl," he said very relieved, tossing the last two bones at her. She plucked the bones out of the air and took off.

"Whew," he mumbled, grabbing his pack he climbed the fence.

I'm outta here.

THIRTY ONE

AT FIVE-TWENTY-FIVE A.M., he quietly slid back naked into Laura's warm bed, and was too excited to sleep. Lustily, he glanced over at Laura who was out cold, naked, and in a very desirable position snoring away.

He stroked his manhood until he was ready and then he rolled over carefully on top of Laura, carefully keeping his weight off as he entered her slowly.

She was still nice and wet from all the sex earlier. She was knocked out from the trazadone and spiced rum and before she could really respond consciously to what was happening, he climaxed inside her, collapsing onto his side of the bed spent. "Unbelievable," he muttered.

At noon time, he awoke to a wonderful smell. "Room service sleepy head," she said with a happy smile. Slowly he stretched and yawned while he looked over at the delicious smelling tray of food. Steak, cheese omelet, toast and fried potatoes, and on the night stand was hot coffee and fresh squeezed O.J.

"Man oh man, this looks wicked good, just like you."

"Thank you teacher…I'll be in the shower if you need me."

Wiping the sleepys out of his eyes, he asked, "What did I do to deserve all this?"

You'll see after breakfast. "So eat up, it's getting cold," she smiled as she started to leave the bedroom. "Oh, by the way, I had this wild dream last night that someone made love to me in the middle of the night. I don't know, it must have been that pill you gave me, because my dreams were so vivid that I woke up very excited," she laughed very naughtily with her hands on her hips.

"Did you now, well I guess I'll just have to give the cook a tip for bringing me my favorite breakfast. Won't I?"

"You bet you will," she responded going out the door. "Oh, by the way, you could use a shower," she grinned. *You bet I could.*

Starving he dug into the steak and eggs, thinking about his night escapades, when he turned his head he spotted his black Levi jeans and pull over tee shirt in a pile by the closet. Then it sunk in, he really did pull it off.

"Payback's a motherfucker," he laughed thinking how pissed the old man would be when he found out his precious drugs were missing.

Hungrily, he devoured all the food and carried the empty tray into the kitchen before joining Laura in the steamy shower.

Because she was almost finished, she started helping him wash. She scrubbed his arms and shoulders then concentrated her attentions on his hard firm chest and tight rippled stomach. Slowly she moved lower and lower washing and cleansing his manhood.

"Well now…what's this…is he waking up?" she grinned licking her lips.

He moaned pleasurably, "Yes, he sure is." Slowly he lowered his lips to her erect nipples. A few minutes passed before the teacher took charge. He spun her around and had her lean forward with her arms outstretched on the wall.

Then he adjusted her long flexible legs, putting one up on the side of the tub arching her ass back. Perfect, he thought, as he slowly entered her from behind while the steamy hot water cascaded down on top of them.

He reached around touching her with his left hand in her most sensitive spot, while he continued to thrust in and out. She reacted with moans of pleasure and he could feel her love muscles contract squeezing him tighter and tighter.

She was so close he could sense it. He quickened the pace with his hand while the pressure continued to build. Finally he felt her let go flooding him and caused him to release his seed deep inside her. Both weak kneed with ecstasy, they held on clutching each other while they laughingly washed off the mess they made.

THIRTY TWO

HE COULD HARDLY contain his excitement knowing he really had ten kilos in his backpack stuffed in the trunk of the Trans-Am.

Unsurprisingly, Ryan decided to join him for the day on Monday. Excitedly, Ryan told him, "Yup, I talked it over with my wife and she was like, go see if you like it," he laughed. "Yeah, like I needed a push."

The trip to Hillbro was the slowest one on record. Amazingly Lucky kept right to the posted speed limits the entire way, fully aware of the trunk's precious cargo.

While Ryan met the sales team and interviewed with the two owners Lucky looked through the local classifieds for a small place to rent close by. During lunch, Ryan and Lucky drove out to look at a barn apartment located five miles out in the sticks.

It was perfect.

Lucky didn't hesitate, he handed the burly farmer two one-hundred dollar bills. One for the first weeks rent and the second for a security deposit. Then he handed the farmer who was glaring at the fancy Trans Am his business card. The farmer eyed the card and said, "No parties," handing Lucky a set of keys.

Casually Lucky unlocked the hatchback and grabbed his backpack going up the steep steps to his new apartment. Once inside he went into the small bedroom and hid the backpack. He locked the deadbolt on his way out. Relieved, he took Ryan to lunch. They spent the afternoon going over the large inventory, setting up Ryan's desk and picking Ryan out a nice demo.

Ryan had decided to follow Lucky's advice and not give City Corvette a notice. Thankfully, he had delivered the 'Vette from Florida on Sunday so he was just going to start the following day, Tuesday.

"Thank God I delivered that 'Vette yesterday," Ryan said while he sat in Lucky's office. "Man, there was a lot of shit goin' on yesterday."

This caught Lucky's attention. "What ya mean?"

"I don't know. It was really strange. They wouldn't let anyone near the Florida 'Vettes except the one I delivered. And the old man and his son were wicked pissed off all day," he said shaking his head. "I'll tell ya, I'm glad I'm outta there, this will be a good change…oh yeah, yesterday the old man was screaming at some derelict dude while the guy went through all the 'Vettes. Man oh man it was the strangest sight, fuck 'em all."

"You got that right! Listen, five cars your first week. Whatever it takes okay, because I gotta hit my bonus," he said eyeing his chart on the wall. So you only gotta sell about thirteen cars in seventeen days."

"Sounds good as long as you're helping me!" Ryan laughed. *I can do anything.*

THIRTY THREE

LUCKY CUT OUT of work early and went shopping. After he bought everything he needed, he drove out to his new hideaway.

Once inside he locked the doors and went straight for the backpack hidden under the twin bed. Eagerly, he pulled out one of the kilos and set it on the sturdy kitchen table. The apartment was completely furnished with everything including sheets and dishes. *I just can't believe this.*

Meticulously he pulled out his new triple beam scale he had just purchased at the local Hillbro Hardware store in town. Excited, he took it out of its hard molded case and set it up on the sturdy kitchen table.

Grinning, he zeroed in the scale. Then he set one block of the Juan Valdez coffee wrapped cocaine on the scale. "2.30 lbs..yes sir," he exclaimed, shaking his head in awe. "Now let's see what you look like?"

Carefully he took out his new razor knife and slit open one corner. His heart raced as he sniffed the strong acetone smell. Excited he cut out a large chunk and set it on a dinner plate.

Should I or shouldn't I? I have to try it.

He cut off a smaller chunk so he could crush it with his Bic cigarette lighter into a powder. Then he also removed a single edge razor blade from it's green plastic case that he'd purchased at the same time as the scale.

Drooling he scraped the cocaine off the Bic lighter and expertly chopped up the pile into a fine powder, quickly making a mouth watering fat line across the plate. *Here I go again.*

Before he knew it he had a new Ben Franklin bill in his hand. Automatically he rolled it up. With his heart racing in anticipation he snorted up about a half a gram in one shot.

"Wow," he hollered feeling his nose burn and eyes water. Instantly, he knew it was uncut. He could taste it in the back of his throat as it dripped potently down from his sinus cavity.

Man oh man, this stuff's killer, whew.

Just then he heard a car pull in on the gravel driveway. Scared, he jumped up and eyed Ryan pulling into the driveway with his new demo, a one-year old Ford Taurus.

Panicking, Lucky put the kilo back into the backpack and hid it in the bathroom. Then he hid the triple beam scale inside a kitchen cabinet.

He could hear footsteps coming up the wooden stairs. Nervously he grabbed the dinner plate and stuck it back in the cupboard with the ten gram chunk on it.

Wiping his nose, he opened the door just as Ryan was about to knock.

"Hey dude, whas up? ... I thought I'd bring you a little house warming present," Ryan smiled clutching a twelve pack of Budweiser.

"Great, come on in."

They drank a cold Bud while Lucky was still zooming from the blast he did. On the second beer he broke down and asked Ryan if he wanted to do a line.

Surprised, he replied, "Sure sounds good."

Lucky pulled the dinner plate out of the cupboard and set it on the table.

"Holy shit Lucky, that's a serious chunk."

If only you knew dude, if you only knew. "Yeah shit's killer too – just wait n' see." He cut out four lines and slid the plate over to Ryan who eagerly grabbed the loose hundred dollar bill and tightened it. "Guests first," he grinned.

Ryan clumsily snorted a line up each nostril. Stunned, he sat back with his eyes wide open in shock. "Holy shit, that stuff's wicked…man that's…that's the strongest stuff I ever had, wow."

Lucky laughed, "I know bro, I know," he mumbled while he snorted up his two lines.

They drank a few more beers then Lucky pushed the plate over to Ryan and told him to cut a line for the road for both of them.

"I gotta go back to Manchester anyway, all my clothes are at Laura's."

"Alright, twist my arm."

After they snorted the to-go lines Lucky handed Ryan a packet of cocaine to take with him. "Go ahead, share it with your wife, it's on me!" he said handing Ryan a gram.

"You sure?"

"Sure...go ahead...bro...don't worry, you're gonna make me a lot of money anyway," he snickered slapping Ryan's shoulder as he went out the door.

"Well, I'll see you tomorrow, thanks Lucky."

"No problem, thanks for the beers and drive safe."

THIRTY FOUR

LUCKY'S MIND RACED.
He was high and a little scared. He wanted to make some quick money, but he knew he had to be extra careful because people on the street would be on the lookout for all this missing cocaine.

Systematically he weighed out five ounces and put them in separate plastic sandwich baggies. Then he crushed and chopped up enough to fill two glass vials that held two grams each. Both of them had a little silver spoon attached, and he also grabbed the six gram boulder left on the plate.

Carefully he placed the nine kilos between his mattress and box spring. Then he covered the small twin bed with a huge comforter.

Out in the new Trans Am he pulled out of the gravel driveway with money, lots of money on his mind. After he thought about it, he knew there was only one person who could handle this kind of weight.

Romeo.

It was just past six p.m. when he dialed Romeo's pager and entered in his cell phone number along with his 007 code.

Laura didn't expect him till nine p.m., so he was in good shape time wise.

"Hey gringo, where you been at?"

"Hey Romeo, I've been being good. But I do need to see you."

"What you be needin' bro?"

"I got something for you to look at!"

"Wow, really – that's a first. Well okay, come on up. It's just me and Sasha."

"Good, I'll see you in ten minutes bro, no visitor's okay."

"Loud and clear gringo." *Click.*

*　　*　　*

He pulled into the same corner store and bought a twelve pack of Bud and cigarettes for Sasha. Lucky knew he couldn't trust anyone else with the cocaine except Romeo and Sasha.

He had his nine-millimeter stuck in his shorts while he carried the backpack on his shoulder and the twelve pack in his hand. He climbed the four steep flights of stairs and gave his coded knock. The three deadbolts clicked and the heavy reinforced door opened a crack. Romeo stood there with a glock in his hand.

"Hey gringo," Romeo barked, waving him inside while he eyed the stairs listening before he slammed and bolted the door. "Sasha, your boyfriend's here," he yelled out following Lucky into the old fashioned kitchen.

He set the beer and backpack on the table. Sasha walked in wearing a tiny pink mini skirt and a white thin tee shirt. Looking incredibly sexy, she said, "Hey Lucky," giving him an affectionate hug. "You brought me some beer?'

"Yup."

"You're so bad," she giggled putting the twelve pack in the fridge. When she turned back around, Lucky was holding a pack of Marlboro Lights in his hand. "No way, you're too much," she blushed slightly as he tossed her the new pack of smokes.

"So amigo, why the big secret...what you got to show us huh?" Romeo demanded impatiently sipping a cold brew.

"Here," Lucky responded handing him one of the two gram vials.

"A sample huh? Well you know I don't snort...but I'll sample it and test it. Honey, get me the tester kit okay." While Sasha left the kitchen, Romeo filled the small silver spoon attached to the lid by a silver chain and did a bump in each nostril.

"Muy bueno gringo that shit ain't stepped on at all. Here Sasha, try this." Sasha who loved to snort eagerly grabbed the small vial and did a few spoonfuls. "Mmm, oh Lucky," she beamed, "That's so strong, Romeo, oh my God!"

"Where the hell did you--? Okay, never mind"

"Yup, it sure is. But anyway I thought you two and maybe your cousin might want to buy some of this primo stuff because it's so clean," he paused. "But of course this would have to be strictly between us."

"Damn gringo, that be funny me getting' my shit off you…but I'll be damned if it ain't rocket fuel…you got more?"

Lucky pulled a fat ounce out of his pack and set it in front of Romeo. "Hey baby, grab my scale. Let's see what we got here."

She returned with a top of the line digital scale. And she also handed Lucky a mirror. "Can we do a line Lucky please?"

"Sure, how can I say no." *When you look so hot.*

Romeo set the baggie on his expensive scale. "Right on gringo, 30.2 grams including the baggie weight. Man you be right, this shit straight off a key, it ain't been hit at all." *Shit, I could make this into two ounces easily.*

"Yup, I figured you'd rather buy it clean like that then after it's stepped on."

"Bet your ass I would…so the million dollar question gringo is how much green…and can I get more?"

"What have you been payin' for an o-zee?"

"Shit I pay between twelve to fifteen, but not like this quality."

"So if I give it to you just like that for fifteen per o-zee you'll be happy?"

"Fuck ya gringo, that's straight off a key and you damn well know it."

"Oh, but you're gonna have to do me a favor."

"Name it gringo."

"I need you to cook up an ounce of powder for me because I can't do it myself."

"We can do that."

"So how many you want?" Lucky smiled putting the other four ounces on the table.

They locked eyes, and Romeo shook his head and laughed, "Where the fuck…okay…okay…never mind, I don't wanna know."

Romeo left the room and came back with a huge wad of green bills in his hands. Street drug money. Fives, tens, and twenties he stacked on the table in piles equaling a hundred bucks. Fifty stacks later, Romeo ran out of money. "Five grand gringo. Count it."

Lucky visually counted the piles picking up one or two randomly to count.

"Yup, five gees, so what you wanna do?"

"Shit – I want all four, but I'm light a grand."

Fuck, I hate fronting shit. "Okay listen, I'll give you the four and you can owe me a grand okay! Now cook up that cookie for me so I can get the hell out of here," he glanced at his watch. "I gotta be home by nine p.m."

"Deal gringo, deal."

Romeo disappeared with the four ounces while Lucky picked up the huge wad of small bills and stuffed them into his backpack.

"Hey gringo, you do know this shit is gonna make a monster slab with this shit bein' so pure I bet when I cook it, it'll all come back."

"Go for it, I'm gonna watch."

He watched as Romeo took out an oversized silver kitchen spoon, baking soda and a chunk of cocaine from Sasha's mirror.

Smoothly he put a few drops of tap water into the spoon, then he added equal amounts of baking soda and cocaine.

In one hand he held a piece of coat hanger broken off into the shape of a short poker. And in the other hand he held the spoon over the hot gas burner. In less than a minute, he walked over to the table and poured the excess water onto a paper towel. Then Romeo popped the hard rock loose with the coat hanger and dropped it on the counter in front of Lucky. "There's your sample."

"Shit, I can't get all geeked out – but I'll sample a hit," Lucky said, dropping the whole sample rock onto the glass stem. It only took a second before the bells were ringing and the train was screaming, while his heart beat tripled.

"Holy cow, that took my head off man, whew this shit is wicked potent," he whispered loving the endorphin rush.

"I told you bro, be careful man, you can't smoke that shit like normal shit."

Trembling from the hit he watched while Sasha and Romeo skillfully cooked up his whole ounce at one time in a large round plexiglass like container. They mixed the cocaine water and baking soda till it was thick goo.

"Usually we add other shit, speed, heroin, baby laxative, procaine, vitamin b-12. All sorts of cuts to stretch it out, but I'll keep yours clean for you okay?"

He just nodded and watched in amazement. Within ten minutes of constant mixing they were done cooking it in the microwave, then they stuck the whole container in the freezer.

"About ten minutes it'll be ready," Romeo bragged as he reached over and grabbed the mirror snorting a line.

Ten minutes later Romeo pulled out the container and cautiously drained off the excess water. Then he flipped the container upside down on the cutting board. Carefully he tapped the bottom, suddenly like magic, the monster thick cookie slid out.

"Bingo."

Stunned Lucky smiled.

"Shit let's see what it weighs,' Romeo said placing it on his digital scale. Look at that gringo, forty grams, Holy shit. I put fifteen grams of baking soda on an ounce, that's what, forty-three grams total. Shit man, we can make some serious money on this shit," he declared wrapping up the cookie in plastic wrap for Lucky.

He glanced at his watch. It was already eight p.m. Only one hour before he faced Laura. Anxiously, he dug through his pack until he pulled out his pill case. Impatiently he popped out two fifty milligrams of trazadone to help him come down quickly.

"Listen Lucky, if you can get more like this, count me in, you don't need to go no where else, you know what I'm sayin' gringo? Man I can get the boys together and we can come up with some serious coin."

"That's exactly what I figured anyway Romeo. I really don't want to go nowhere else with this shit…you know what I mean? In other words,

I was never here," he told him point blank packing up all his stuff. *Five grand already, I can't believe it.*

"Oh, by the way Sasha, you can keep the rest of that boulder on the mirror."

"You're too good to me," she smiled giving him a very friendly kiss. *God she is so young, so hot, so...damn I better get out of here before...*

THIRTY FIVE

THIRTY MINUTES LATER he pulled the Trans Am into Laura's a few minutes past nine p.m. Lucky felt pretty good because he hadn't done any drugs in the past hour, and the strong trazadone was helping him come down rapidly. *I can make it.*

He breathed in deeply trying to relax because he was still nervous of getting by Laura's sixth sense. Every time he smoked or snorted, his sexual appetite and wild imagination would soar through the roof, and she could tell a mile away.

"Hi, Honey."

"Hi," she smiled glancing at the clock. "Right on time, lucky for you. I've got a nice dinner once you take your shower," she told him handing him a glass of white Zinfandel.

"It sure smells good," he said smiling. Even *though I'm not hungry, just horny.*

After his shower he slipped into his silk boxers and sat down at the dinner table while she served him a juicy New York sirloin medium rare with sautéed mushrooms and onions, on the side was a loaded baked potato and her delicious Greek salad.

It smelled too good not to make an effort. So slowly he started eating, forcing himself at first, then before long with his favorite A-1 bold steak sauce readily available, he consumed most of it.

After dinner, they retired to the living room where he grabbed Laura and pushed her firmly into the big Lazy Boy recliner. Down on his knees he started slowly kissing her sweet smelling thighs while he slowly undid her lacy expensive robe with his fingers.

His member was throbbing in anticipation, and she gradually responded by parting her long legs as she leaned back in anticipation. Eagerly he teased her, devouring her with his horny tongue. Closer and closer Lucky climbed up to her sweet nectar using wet kisses to work her into frenzy.

Wildly he took her right there in the recliner, burying himself deep inside, her while he pinned her legs back with his arms.

Animal like, he thrusted in and out seeking relief until they both collapsed from powerful orgasms.

"God Lucky, you're going to kill me," she purred. "Oh shit, I still gotta walk Taffy before it get's too late. You wanna come?"

"I already did!" he laughed.

"Stop, not that."

"No baby, I'll hang out here."

"Okay, we'll be back."

"I know, be careful."

"I will," she replied heading out the door.

As soon as the door slammed shut he made his next mistake. Quickly he grabbed the stem out of his suit jacket and stepped out on the ground level patio. Naked he blasted away where anyone walking by could see him.

After he hit the stem a second time his endorphins screamed loudly. Paranoid he rapidly pulled on his Levis and Tee shirt and headed out the door after Laura and Taffy.

Things were moving very fast.

He had this awful feeling that they weren't safe. Carefully he followed them at a safe distance until he ducked behind a big old oak tree and hit the stem again. He was really zooming now. Nervously he inhaled his Marlboro Light to calm down.

"Are you watching us?" she asked with a curious grin as Lucky emerged out of the darkness.

"Yup. The best security is the one you can't see," he said grabbing her extended hand.

"You're still worried about him aren't you?"

"You bet I am." *If you only knew.*

Back in side he was already ready. Hard as a rock. They made love again. This time on her bed, he set a frantic pace with the cocaine running through his veins.

His pleasure was magnified to the max, while he madly flipped her over and entered her from behind watching himself recklessly in the big oversized bedroom mirror until he exploded once again.

By eleven p.m., they both finally lied down for the night. She was exhausted and he was still wired. By midnight he was still wide awake and tuned into her breathing. Impatient, he made his next mistake.

Quietly tip toeing out of bed, he slid into the bathroom where he snuck another hit of crack. Bug eyed he glanced in the bathroom mirror feeling his heart beat race.

Paranoid. *They're coming, they're coming.*

His imagination started running wild. Fearfully he hit the stem again. Now every little noise made him jump. Quietly he listened. Something told him he heard a noise from the bedroom and he panicked, immediately locking the bathroom door and turning on the shower full blast.

Then it happened thirty minutes later with the shower still running, he continued to smoke crack in the steamy bathroom.

"Let me in right now, or I'll call the police," she screamed loudly, pounding on the bathroom door. *Oh fuck.*

Scared he quickly did another blast. *I'm zooming, oh shit oh shit, hide everything, they're coming, quick hide.*

In the mean time Laura had gotten a steak knife from the kitchen and was jimmying the lock outside the bathroom door. Laura came flying into the bathroom like a tornado, knocking Lucky backward through the shower curtain into the tub on his ass soaking him.

"Get the hell out…right now," she raged waving the steak knife angrily. "How dare you smoke that shit in my house," she screamed looking horrified. "I want you outta here right now.'

"But…but…Laura…It's almost two a.m… I can't go nowhere now," he pleaded high as a kite.

"You can and you will! You got three minutes, then I call the cops," she stormed, turning back. "Oh and all your shit will be packed and on the patio in the morning. Now give me my key and get the hell out."

Oh no, hurry up, they're coming. She's pissed, run.

Briskly, he grabbed jeans, sneakers, and a shirt, and a handful of dress clothes on his way out the door. Nervously he pulled her key off his ring and slapped it on the counter. She clutched the phone ready to dial.

It was time to go.

He sprinted to the Trans Am in his boxers and yanked on his jeans throwing the rest of his clothes into the car. Recklessly he tore out of the parking lot and headed for the highway.

Scared…paranoid…he kept glancing back in the rearview expecting to see blue lights. Just as he approached the on ramp his nightmare came true. Blue lights racing towards him off in the distance.

Wildly he cranked the wheel into a hard right turn almost sideswiping a pickup truck. Swiftly he recovered downshifting the powerful new six speed and flooring the accelerator.

Oh shit, dead end.

"Fuck," he screamed.

That's when he spotted the Bates Motel sign still lit one street over. Like a magnet he pulled right up to the manager's office just as the neon sign went dark.

Fuck.

Lucky jumped out of the Trans Am and pushed the buzzer while he pulled on his shirt. Impatiently he waited expecting the cops any second. Then the top half of the door opened and the old man leered at his watch. "You just made it."

"Great, had a fight with the wife, gotta sleep somewhere."

"That's forty bucks…cash…here fill this out," the old man said handing him a clipboard with a registration card.

Lucky filled it out with the first name that came to mind then handed the man two crisp twenties.

"Nice car you got there, brand spankin' new, even still got the window stickers on it," he commented admiringly.

"Yup, sure wish it was mine, but I just sell em."

"Here's your room key, number nine, check out's eleven a.m."

"I'll be long gone by then, gotta work." *I hope.*

THIRTY SIX

LOCKED INSIDE ROOM number nine, he shut the old fashioned curtains and opened his knapsack. Exhaling he broke off a chunk from the cookie with his leatherman tool knife. His hands trembled in anticipation while he jammed a chunk into the brillo end of the glass stem.

It all started again.

Each hit he inhaled, the worse it got.

He strained to listen over the noisy a/c wall unit, while he constantly peeked out the curtains expecting to see the Manchester cops surrounding his car.

There's no one out there.
Yes – I can hear them – ssshh listen.
Man, I know she called the police.
Maybe not.
Shit, I got all this crack and cash.

The faster he smoked the more he hallucinated. Sweating, he stripped down to his boxers leaving his Nikes on in case he had to run. Then he strapped on his leather shoulder holster over his bare chest and chambered a round in his military model baretta.

Breathing deeply he started tip toeing back and forth to the heavy curtains. Paranoia took control. Jittery he shut off the a/c wall unit expecting unwanted visitors any second. Bug eyed he wedged a chair frantically under the door handle.

The silence was driving him insane. Skittish and tense the hallucinations ran wildly through his head. He was really convinced they were now outside, and he continued to sweat and panic.

I can feel it they're coming.

Shit what was that?

Man I gotta hide, but where…

Quickly he turned the a/c back on and grabbed four pillows off the bed. Armed with his back pack, drugs, and pillows, he locked himself in the bathroom.

Two hours later at six a.m., Lucky finally ripped the bathroom door open clutching his gun. He was completely geeked out; his mouth was going a mile a minute, grinding his teeth back and forth. Slowly he stepped out of the bathroom covered in sweat, trembling.

He glanced back into the well lit bathroom and saw the large crack cookie sitting on the toilet seat so he could flush it if they were out there. But the crack rock was so big that he'd have to break it up to flush it.

Then he tried to get his breathing under control.

Deep breaths – exhale slowly he told himself.

He continued to worry about the time, as he glanced at his Casio 'G' Shock for the hundredth time. He knew Laura left for work at seven-thirty a.m. and his clothes would be sitting outside on her patio true to her word. *Man, what am I gonna do?*

THIRTY SEVEN

AFTER A NERVOUS hot shower he still felt light headed, but a little better. He then got dressed in wrinkled work clothes and put his drugs and paraphernalia away. Reality started setting in quick the lighter it got outside. *Shit I gotta leave soon.*

At seven a.m. he left the Bates Motel feeling like shit. Depressed, hungry, and irritated, he drove past a Burger King and pulled into the drive thru. Slowly he gnawed on a bacon, egg, and cheese croissant with hash browns.

He fought the food down knowing he had to eat. Between bites and sips of coffee he used his portable Gilette razor.

By the time he arrived in front of Laura's condo, it was seven-forty-five a.m. and he was finally starting to feel a little better. Her Lincoln was gone so he pulled in her vacant spot next to the convertible Camaro he had given her to use.

Looking around he spotted three large green trash bags sitting on her outside patio. "Bitch," he mumbled feeling his heart ache while he carried the heavy bags to the Trans Am.

Lucky had to hustle to make it to work by nine a.m. When he pulled up at Johnson's Chevy, Ryan was already there waiting.

"Man Lucky, you look like shit bro."

"Thanks, I feel like shit," he responded making his way to his office with Ryan trailing along. "So what did they say at City Corvette?"

"I haven't told them yet," Ryan laughed raising his muscular arms. "I'm gonna call now and tell them that way they can't really do shit over the phone," he snickered. "Fuck em if they can't take a joke."

"Go ahead, call em and then let's go sell your first car," Lucky said exhausted, eyeing the sales board. "Oh shit, we got a sales meeting at eleven a.m. in the break room."

"I'll be there, you know that."

I know, I just hope I will be.

With no sleep, depressed, he continued to hit the coffee pot. "Listen if you can't sell them a car on the spot and they qualify, check with me and we'll talk about over nighting them. It's known as the twenty-four hour sale," he stressed at the sales meeting.

"Why do this? Because you got about an 80% chance of closing the deal when they return. It's simple, it works. They get spoiled with a new car in the driveway, especially when all their family, friends, and neighbors see it and start talking positive about their new car."

He paused, pacing back and forth. "The key is you always keep the customers trade-in here. Make sure before they leave you pull out everything and put it in the new car, you know, like the baby seat, packages, etc. And once they leave, immediately hide their trade-in out back out of sight. It doesn't exist anymore," he told them looking up at the four salesmen and Ryan. *Boy I'm exhausted.*

"Now as Ryan can verify, I sold two-hundred cars in about ten months. How did I do it? People buy from those they like, so first impressions are very important. Also, asking the right questions and pre-qualifying your customer will help you close more deals. No matter how good you are, or what you do if you don't get them on the right vehicle, most likely within seventy-two hours they will be driving off someone else's lot with the right car," he said sipping more coffee.

"If someone likes the color, I love the color, if someone digs the interior, I really dig it," he laughed. "The point is to focus on what the customers get excited about and not what they don't like.

"So say it's used, with a rip in the seat, a scratch on the door and it needs two new tires. All negatives, right? Wrong. 'So Mr. Customer, if we fix the scratch and the seat, plus take care of the tires, you'd take it home today, isn't that true?' That's right, any objection you can overcome if you're on the right car. The one they really want, and can afford. Just write it up. Customer offers x, offer is subject to scratch on door, tires that pass inspection, and rip in driver seat repaired. And I'm sure I don't have to remind any of you that it's not an offer unless you get a deposit. Cash, check, credit card, jewelry, watch, get something. It shows they are serious. Get it?"

Heads nod.

"Good. Oh, one other thing guys you must do is don't let anyone leave without meeting me. Yes, that's right, I want to greet every single customer before they leave," he paused. "Why right? Believe it or not most people who come onto a car lot or take a test drive are ready to buy. But most of them will tell you they're what?...Just looking. And you believe 'em. It's true that 76% of customers who come on a lot or test drive buy a vehicle within seventy-two hours somewhere. Most don't even know they're ready to buy so that's where I come in. If you just introduce me and let me talk to them before you dismiss them, I guarantee you'll each sell one or two cars more each month."

Also while he was on a roll, he told them about Saturdays and Sundays from noon to six were now optional. That Ryan and he would be here this Saturday and anyone who wanted to join them would get free pizza.

Then he went on to explain what he had planned for all of them for the rest of the day.

"I want a detailed list of every car and truck on the lot that won't start, flat tires, needs gas, etc. What ever you think it needs, write it down. Also, every night you guys will now take home a different used demo so you can fill out a sheet on it," he said handing them each a copy of the new form he devised.

"Brakes, tires, pulls to one side, shakes, runs rough, broken radio, whatever it needs, just write it down. What I'm going to try and do is get as many cars sell-able as possible so we can move'm out of here." *In our dreams.*

He sipped his coffee wishing for sleep. "Oh as we all know, people don't buy broken down cars. So I'll either fix 'em or we'll move'm to the back and I'll send 'em to the auction in Concord. One last thing before we move the lot around. A lot of the vehicles are way overpriced and we all know it. Not anymore. I'll be marking new prices aggressively right on the windshields so no matter what anyone offers you, bring all offers to me, now let's ride." *Damn I need a hit.*

Reluctantly they followed him outside in the hot afternoon sun to the huge parking lot clutching three hundred sets of keys. Three hours later and thirty-two jump starts later, they all collapsed exhausted in the cool showroom.

Ryan sold his first car at four p.m. By 6 p.m. Lucky was worn out. Even the nine cups of coffee weren't helping him anymore.

"I'm outta here Ryan. I still gotta move all my stuff in. You want'a help?"

"Sure, let's go."

THIRTY EIGHT

B ACK AT HIS apartment they lugged the green trash bags up
the long outside stairs. He really needed a blast, but he wasn't
sure if Ryan even knew what crack was. He was so damn exhausted
that he just layed out two fat lines and after they each did a rail, Lucky
realized how much he was craving a hit of crack.

"Hey, you ever smoked this shit before?" he asked Ryan while he
pulled two glass stems out of his pack, and dropped a chunk of crack
on the dinner plate.

"Nope, can't say I ever have, but I've heard stories. So what's it like?"

You'll see. "Well my friend, there's only one way to find out," he
chuckled packing both stems with a hit. "Watch," he told him as he
carefully demonstrated how to melt the crack onto the brillo. Slowly
Lucky exhaled then he showed Ryan how to hit the stem. Immediately
his tired brain woke up.

Ryan felt pressure, so he took his first hit of crack. Stunned he
shook his head in awe. "Holy shit, that stuff's wicked," he mumbled.
"No wonder so many people get addicted to this shit. Whew man, oh
man, what a fuckin' rush."

"You can say that again."

"Okay"

"So what did they say when you called?"

"Man Lucky, they were really pissed; especially when I told Tom
I was up here working for you. I guess Junior was in his office and
overheard our conversation," he smiled buzzed. "I could hear him
cussing me out…Hey fuck them…they treated me like shit anyway."

"Yup, been there." *A few times.*

"But uh, I still need to go by and get my last commission check this Friday, hopefully you'll let me take off early?"

"Yeah, you can go. But you be damn sure you don't mention any of this shit to no one," he said seriously pointing at the crack and powder cocaine.

"Fuck, who the hell would I tell?"

Uptight Lucky started unpacking his wrinkled expensive suits. Quickly he got more frustrated and threw the clothes back in the bags.

Fuck this, let's go have a drink and drop all this shit off at a dry cleaners. It'll cost me an arm and leg but…oh well…it's gotta get done and I'm not fuckin' with it." *Not when I got five grand of the old man's money.*

"Shit Lucky, I'm high as a kite, but hey boss man I'll come along for the ride, what the hell."

They dropped off two large trash bags full of suits, pants, dress shirts, and ties at the local dry cleaners.

The man behind the counter about had a heart attack when he counted eighty-six items. "Sir, this is gonna be a lot of money. Are you sure you want to do this all at once?"

Lucky eyed the massive pile, "Just dry clean all the suits and ties. The rest of the pants and shirts, just have them washed and ironed. That'll cut down on the bill," he told the man handing him his sales manager's card. "I will become a very regular customer if the price is reasonable, and of course if you need a vehicle, I'll personally make sure you and your immediate family get a huge discount!" he boasted as they walked out of the cleaners both laughing at Lucky's strong arm tactics.

At the tavern they ordered a pitcher of Michelob Light and the house special. Half pound black angus bacon Swiss sirloin burgers with homemade onion rings.

"Don't get too used to it bro, I can't treat you all the time."

"I know, I know. But hey, I do appreciate it. Hey by the way, what kind of commission did I make today?"

"As soon as they take delivery tomorrow you mean?" Lucky laughed. "Well total gross was eighteen hundred and you get twenty-two percent so you'll get about four bills. Just don't forget about my measly fifty bucks, you'll be glad to give it to me, trust me."

"Hey, I got no problem with that."

"You better not. I treat you like a king and you've only sold one car. But you and me are gonna work this Saturday, and I want us to write at least five deals between us so we can show everybody what they're missing."

"Sounds good…I'm there!"

They stopped at the local grocery store while Ryan pushed the cart, Lucky filled it up with expensive steaks, shrimp, chicken breasts, burgers, and deli sliced roast beef. Fresh corn on the cob, Spanish purple onions, mushrooms, and bell peppers. He grabbed Hunt's ketchup, Gray Pupon, and A-1 Bold. The next aisle, they came away with Pepperidge Farm onion rolls, multi-grain bread, and farm fresh eggs.

Kraft cheese slices, Concord grape jelly, and a pound of butter. The largest bag of Lay's potato chips, Doritos, and a box of deli honey dip donuts. On the way to the beer aisle he grabbed a large container of fresh chopped garlic in olive oil.

A carton of Marlboro Lights and four cases of beer, after all he thought, it's five miles one way to the store. Two cases of Molson Golden and two cases of Michelob Light along with two twelve packs of Coca-Cola classic.

On the way through town, he spotted the tiny New Hampshire Liquor store where he dropped another hundred bucks of Romeo's drug money on the biggest bottle of Absolute Vodka, Kaluha, and Captain Morgan's Spiced Rum.

Finally they were on their way back when he spotted it outside the hardware store. Quickly he did a u-turn right on Main Street. The Ace Hardware manager, a Mr. McGowan recognized him immediately from all his purchases the day before and gave him a good deal on the top of the line Fancy Webber 50,000 B.T.U gas grill that caught Lucky's eye.

The new Trans Am was packed full. There was no way it would fit in the expensive car so Lucky smartly paid the local high school kid who worked for Mr. McGowan twenty bucks to put it in his old Ford

Ranger and deliver it after they closed in a half-hour. Lucky made sure they filled both gas tanks and then they left.

Back at the barn they put all the food away, then relaxed sipping Captain and Cokes.

"Hey you think I could buy a little of that shit from you?" Ryan asked eyeing the large crack rock sitting on the dinner plate.

Oh oh, he's hooked. "Man I don't know bro…you know how expensive that shit is?…man I don't know I hate to get you started on that shit…I'll tell you what, I'll sell you powder…but any rock you gotta smoke here." *If he only knew how much shit I got he'd shit his pants. You can't tell 'em, God if he told anyone I could end up dead.*

"How about fifty bucks worth and I'll pay you on Friday?"

"Are you sure? I hate to be a bad influence," he stopped. "But I guess it's too late for that huh!"

Lucky pulled out a two gram vial of powder and handed it to Ryan. Then he broke off a hit of crack and dropped it on the table.

"That's two grams of coke and a free blast of crack. You owe me a hundred on Friday."

"Wow, thanks," he responded eagerly breaking off a piece of the crack and melted it like an old pro onto the glass stem.

THIRTY NINE

OVER THE WEEK, Ryan sold three more cars and was very pleased with himself. Before he left on Friday afternoon to get his last check at City Corvette, he stuck his head into Lucky's busy office.

"Hey boss, is it alright if I take off now so I can go get my last check? I want to be rested for tomorrow's big day," he grinned happily thinking about all the money he made this past week. "Hey I grossed twelve hundred plus my three hundred dollar salary so my wife will be pleased."

Lucky smiled, "Good and don't forget about me."

"I know, I owe you three bills total. Two for the four cars I delivered and one for the other stuff."

Lucky nodded.

"So what time you want me here tomorrow?"

"We'll start around nine and work till we write five deals for you. Also if you want we can sell five more on Sunday," he told him seriously.

"Damn, you mean it don't you?"

"Damn right Amigo, I want to hit my bonus numbers, otherwise I'm outta here."

"Okay Lucky, I'll be here at nine. Later, and thanks for everything," he said excitedly. "Oh by the way, I really do like it here. This place could be a friggin' goldmine like you said," Ryan whispered as he shot out of the showroom.

FORTY

BACK AT STATE Police Headquarters in Bow, Lt. Frank Brooks continued his investigation of the deadly car chase.

After he reviewed the 7-11 store surveillance video tapes that showed Lucky and an unidentified shapely blonde leaving the all night store at two-fifty eight a.m. He also had interviewed two willing witnesses that saw a green Mustang tear out of the 7-11 around three a.m.

"Too much of a coincidence don't you think Herb?"

"I'd say so Frank. I think it's time for another talk with your boy Lucky Sullivan. He obviously knows more than he's telling. Are you gonna pick him up or what?"

"Well Herb, I gotta find him first. He quit Big Mike's, but it shouldn't be too hard to find since I've got his cell phone and girlfriend's phone number. But what bothers me the most is he seems like a decent guy from a nice family. Why would gang bangers in a stolen car from Roxbury be shooting at him?"

"Maybe drugs."

"Maybe…but I don't know, something's missing…and that's the part I need to figure out," the Lt. paused glancing over the growing file with weary eyes.

The D.A. responded, "You know without a confession there really isn't anything I can charge him with, especially since that hot rod he was driving was cleared of any excess speed on the night in question with you as a witness…" *I might add.*

"True, but before I pull him in I'd really like to find out why those punks tried to shoot him, then maybe I can get some answers."

"Okay Frank, sounds good. If you need any help, I'm available, although what happened to those gang bangers didn't upset too many higher ups," he snickered. "Yes, I know it's still a possible unsolved homicide." *But.*

"True, true I guess I'm after the reason why it went down, and if Sullivan was involved, and it does look that way, then he's damn Lucky to be alive. Get it? Lucky's…lucky," Lt. Brooks chuckled at his own corny joke.

"Ya well maybe he won't be so Lucky next time. Those punks meant business packin' heat. Hopefully for his sake they don't have any more unfinished business."

After Trooper Brooks's conversation with the D.A. he made a few phone calls. His first call was to Big Mike's Muscle Cars where he didn't learn anything new. Then he called City Corvette where he spoke with Tom and learned Lucky was now the sales manager at Johnson's Chevy which really surprised him. "That's way out in Hillbro isn't it?"

"Yup."

"Hey Tom, when Lucky left City Corvette, did he leave on good terms or what?"

Tom laughed, "Well, he got fired for screwing a lawyer's wife. Right before he sold her a $40,000 'Vette which really pissed off her husband because Lucky talked her into trading in his 1968 Classic Mustang," he laughed. "But hey don't get me wrong, Lucky can flat out sell cars like there's no tomorrow."

"Really?"

Tom hesitated looking around the showroom. "I hated to see him go, he was a money maker. But it was out of my hands, I couldn't protect him, not this time. The old man had to fire him immediately or face a lawsuit."

"Wow that's interesting, but Tom tell me when they fired him was there any words or a bad scene or did anything abnormal happen?" Come *on, tell me what really happened.*

"Well Lt., you know people can get upset when they get fired, especially if you're the top gun. Egos get in the way and it wasn't a pretty scene that's for sure Sir." *What's he after?*

"Tom, I'm curious because I'm looking into something that may or may not involve Lucky and I'm just trying to get some background to fill in some spaces." *Like the truth would be nice.*

"Lt. he left here running his mouth, and making threats. He's definitely not welcome here anymore," he said aggravated scanning the showroom. "But sir, between you and me, I didn't blame him. He made the dealership a lot of money and was top salesman every month he was here." *Now my bonuses are gone.*

"Really?"

"Yeah the guy was really likable, a real workaholic. He just sometimes ran his mouth and it got him in trouble." *I miss him.*

"I just hope Lucky didn't upset anyone enough where someone might want to kill him," he paused letting Tom hear the message. "Because one way or another, I'm gonna find out." *So tell me damn it.*

"Sir no disrespect, but I've said all I'm gonna say about Lucky, like I said, I've got no beef with him at all." *But the old man certainly does.*

"Between you and me Tom, I've heard a lot of rumors about your owner and they're not all good. I just hope for your sake there's nothing going on I should know about?"

Abruptly Tom responded coldly, "I told you all I know, now is there anything else?" *Asshole.*

"No Tom, not at this point, I know where to find you when I need you."

Lt. Brooks could sense there was more to the story and Tom was protecting someone. He quickly decided to run a background check on Tom and the old man.

His break came when he checked in with the D.A. and found out surprisingly from Herb that there was an undercover Federal Narcotics Task Force investigating City Corvette and was now working in conjunction with the New Hampshire Drug Interdiction Team, better known as (N.H. D.I.T.)

According to the fax he just received it said a very reliable confidential informant (C.I.), overheard that City Corvette is moving cocaine inside 'Vettes delivered from the huge dealer auctions in Orlando, Florida up the Northern Corridor to New Hampshire hidden in 'Vettes that are on car carriers.

The latest tip received a day late for the Narcotics Task Force to put a surveillance team in place for the last shipment of 'Vettes they just received. So now everyone was waiting for a phone call from an undercover federal officer working at the auto auction with the C.I.

Lt. Brooks continued to read on and smiled. There was interesting intelligence on the old man and a known accomplice, a Hector Santiago who was a known gang leader of the Northern Kings and was wanted on drug and gun charges and questioning on other suspected related crimes.

The level one secure fax had two blurry pictures of the old man and Hector. Also enclosed was a picture of the old man with a huge king fish taken in front of his expensive yacht, a sixty-foot Hatteras named the "Fast Lady"

"Bingo."

The following day, Saturday, he decided to pay Lucky a surprise visit at Johnson's in his unmarked Ford Crown Vic. dressed in his black swat team fatigues which he was obviously a member of.

Lucky showed up at work at eight-forty five a.m. and opened up the showroom for business. Finally he had gotten a good night sleep after breaking up more cocaine and taking two-hundred milligrams of Trazadone he passed out by nine p.m.

After he fired up the showroom coffee pot, he sat down a dozen donuts next to the coffee machine that he had picked up on his way in at Dunkin' Donuts. He had already devoured the three honeydips he ordered for himself on the ride over.

Lucky saw Ryan pull up and park, so he went outside. Ryan jumped out of his Ford Taurus all excited. He couldn't wait to tell Lucky all about him picking up his check.

"Hey Lucky, now I know how you felt. Shit I got the third degree, then the old man went into a wicked rage. He screamed 'Who do you think you are quitting on me! No one quits on me. Now get your damn check and get your ugly ass off my property!'", Ryan giggled holding his chest. "Can you believe that shit? Oh…oh…and on my way out someone yelled 'I heard you're workin' for Lucky…good luck.' I guess the old man didn't know, you should have seen the look on his face, I was outta there," he laughed.

"Who said that?"

"Your buddy Mark. He's such an asshole sometimes," Ryan told him handing him three one hundred dollar bills he owed him.

"Hey thanks. Sure wish I could have seen the look on the old man's face, I really would have enjoyed that."

Shortly thereafter, the lot was extremely busy and both Ryan and Lucky were waiting on two or three customers at once. They managed it rather well by sending people out on test drives by themselves, something Lucky was taught not to do by Joe Verdi, the professional automobile sales expert.

By three p.m. they had written six deals, taken six deposits, and overnighted four other couples. They ran out of spare dealer plates and never got to stop for lunch, so Lucky ordered three large pizzas delivered to share with the customers still lingering.

By three-thirty p.m. Lt. Frank Brooks pulled onto the lot in his unmarked state cruiser where he parked and watched Lucky send a couple out on a test drive in a new Chevy Silverado pickup.

Quietly he hopped out of his car, "Hey Lucky, what you doin' way up here?" he asked loudly.

Stunned, Lucky lit a smoke giving him a few seconds to recover, "Hey Lt. I didn't recognize you in that get up," he replied eyeing his swat fatigues and matching nine millimeter shoulder holster.

"You gotta minute, we need to talk?"

"Yeah I guess, that's about all I've got. We've been slammed all day. But come on inside for a minute and we'll grab a slice of pizza, my treat."

They sat in Lucky's small office for some privacy. Lt. Brooks got right to the point. He proceeded to tell him about the 7-11 surveillance tapes with his picture in it, at two-fifty eight a.m. early Saturday morning with an unidentified attractive blonde.

Then he continued on while he finished his free slice of pizza and told him about the two Northern King gang bangers who survived the crash weren't playing ball, and that the more he looked into it the more the old man appeared to be somehow involved with the kings.

"So what you think Lucky, am I getting warm?" he asked with a big shit eating grin looking all around to see if anyone was listening in.

Then he leaned in closer. "Honestly I really don't give a shit if that was you out on the highway driving the mystery car," he said seriously. "What I want to know is why those punks were way up north on my highway discharging firearms at you, but most of all I want the asshole who ordered it." *And so do I.*

He paused trying to keep his temper under control keeping his eyes locked on Lucky. "So Mr. Smarty-pants you can either help me or when the shit hits the fan you can go down with it," he said standing up glancing at the 1953 Corvette picture on Lucky's wall. "It's your choice."

Lucky didn't know what to say. Thank God, he thought when he spotted the new Silverado returning from their test drive. "I gotta go Trooper, but I'll think about what you said and I'll let you know if I can help you", he told him unconsciously shaking his head as he started towards the showroom exit.

Trooper Brooks grabbed Lucky's arm and stopped him. "Just tell me one thing. You think the old man put a hit on you because you ran your mouth? Hey I mean help me out here, the guy tried to seriously hurt you."

Lucky looked up and hesitated, eyeing the hand holding his suit jacket he pulled free, "Look Lt., I think you already know what I think and I'd say you're a lot smarter than I thought," he told him throwing a quick salute before he hustled back outside. *I'll take care of the old man myself.*

Lucky welcomed the nice couple who were going over the new truck's interior very carefully. He watched while the Lt. climbed into his unmarked and started to pull away. "Excuse me," Lucky said quickly to the couple before he turned towards the Lt. catching his eye. "Hey Lt. The answer is yes, I definitely think so."

Lt. Brooks nodded, pleased and drove off.

FORTY ONE

O N THE WAY back to headquarters he glanced at his pocket notebook and put another asterisk beside the old man's name. He knew Lucky wasn't going to tell on himself, and in a way he didn't blame him.

Without a confession after being Mirandized, everything he had on Lucky was circumstantial evidence. But he was pleased that he'd given him an answer to his questions. Now he definitely knew he was getting much warmer.

His next move was to go lean on the two punk gang members still in his custody at the Merrimack County Jail Medical Ward. He hoped to get one of them to confess in exchange for a lighter sentence.

After reading the two gang members files he decided to focus on the younger of the two whose prints were found on one of the discharged illegal handguns found out on the highway. He knew with his past record he'd be facing fifteen to twenty years. Armed with that knowledge he called the D.A. and told him what he'd like to do so he could confirm who the man was who ordered the shooting.

The D.A. liked Lt. Brooks. They had a history. Lt. Brooks had intervened at a D.W.I. roadblock when the D.A.'s wild seventeen year old daughter was stopped and almost arrested. Brooks had stepped in and put her in his cruiser, and drove her home to the wrath of her embarrassed father.

"Well Lt. if you think it would help move your investigation along, go for it. I was going to push for maximum. But I could live with five years mandatory if you can get the bastard to talk," the D.A. responded.

"Hey thanks Herb, I think that might get one of them to open up. Could you fax me over an offer with your signature so I can put it in front of this kid's face?"

"Sure Frank, I can do that for you, but no deals unless this scumbag sings. Get everything you can," he paused thinking. "So what's your angle on all this?"

He told him how he now believed Sullivan was driving the other car, but without an actual confession there really wasn't much to go on, with the speedo-meter verifying that he wasn't speeding. Then he told him what he really thought was going on. That according to 7-11 witnesses', four punks in the Mustang deliberately scratched Sullivan's Trans Am.

Which he said caused Sullivan to give chase and once out on the interstate the Trans Am caught up with the Mustang. Apparently Sullivan must have passed the Mustang, when they fired on him discharging three separate rounds before the driver of the Mustang lost control and flipped.

Lt. now frustrated said, "But what I want to know is why they were way up here in a stolen ride shooting at Sullivan who just happened to have been fired from City Corvette a week earlier. Apparently he really ruffled some one's feathers on his way out the door."

"I guess you know Frank who owns City Corvette. The guy's on the federal hot sheet for possible narcotics trafficking."

"Yup and on top of that I really believe he put the hit out on Sullivan and somehow he went out of state to arrange it, and that's what I'm trying to prove." *I'll get 'em somehow.*

And leave out his trip up to Hillbro to see Lucky at his new job and how he reacted when he told him about the 7-11 surveillance tapes and witnesses who put him at the 7-11 at three a.m. so he had demanded his cooperation in nailing the asshole who had ordered the shooting.

"What did he say?"

"It's not what he said, but what he didn't say that told me I was on the right track…the old man."

"Is this the same Sullivan whose parents live in Bow whose father works for the governor?"

"Exactly. But he seems like a decent guy, just a little scared and I don't blame him," the Lt. laughed nervously. "But he did steer me in the right direction so-."

"Hey Frank, do me a big favor, don't move on the Sullivan boy without letting me know. His old man's well connected and if you decide you need to take him down I need to make sure we got all our ducks in a row."

"Don't worry from what I hear he's small time. Does a little recreational cocaine and pot, and sells a hell of a lot of cars. But I do need his help to take down the old man. He knows more than he's telling me."

"Sounds good Frank, just be careful. I got your back, so watch out for the feds, you know how they get when you step on their big toes. Just clear it through me before you make a move."

"Count on it Herb. Hey, how's your daughter doing?"

"Much better thanks," the D.A. answered. "Look Frank, I owe you one, so I uh really appreciate what you did. Shit with elections only a few months away you really saved my ass from a lot of public embarrassment." *To say the least.*

"Hey don't worry about it."

"Well I'll never forget it. Oh by the way, I got box seats to Fenway next weekend, and I can't use em. Why don't you take your boy and go watch Pedro Martinez beat the Yankees."

"Geez Herb that would be great." *My kid will love it.*

"Good. Oh stand by your fax and I'll send you over a signed offer okay. And Frank, stay in touch."

"Yes sir."

FORTY TWO

LUCKY WROTE UP one more deal making a total of seven. They high fived as the last couple left the showroom.

Then proudly Lucky took all seven deals with deposits inside the folders and lined them up on the finance manager's desk.

They grinned. "That ought to keep him busy Monday morning," Lucky laughed with a shit-eating grin looking at Ryan. "Now we can take tomorrow off, I told the four overnight test drives to stop by Monday after work."

Ryan shook his head amazed. "Wow Lucky, seven fuckin deals all in my name...damn...I don't...I don't...know what to say but thanks," he giggled excitedly.

He slapped Ryan's broad shoulders, "No problem bro, just help me break those sales records so I can hit my bonuses and I'll be a happy camper."

"Sounds real good."

"Yup, that's just what I need." *Thirty-five hundred used car bonus and twenty-two hundred new car bonus.*

Ryan was amped up munching on the last slice of cold pizza. "Hey you want to stop by or you got plans?"

"No – no, I'll come by for a while and the beer's on me," Ryan beamed eagerly jumping into his latest demo, a one year old Pontiac Grand Am.

"About time you paid," Lucky climbing into a brand new sky blue Chevy Hightop conversion van, loaded with all the extras. Four captain's chairs, a fold down bed, built-in T.V/VCR and fridge.

He stopped again at the New Hampshire Liquor store and bought another bottle of Absolute Vodka and 100 proof Rumplemintz

Peppermint Schnapps. On the way out to his barn apartment to meet Ryan he impulsively called Alexis on his Nextel phone.

"Hello?"

"Hey there stranger."

"My God what the hell are you doin' calling me on a Saturday night? Don't tell me the super salesman can't get a date?" Alexis snickered teasing him.

"Damn, busted again, how'd you know?" he chuckled.

"Shit Lucky, I thought you got lost or killed by now. You just never know with you," she replied seriously.

"Man I got so much to tell you. It's been a wicked week. Laura and I finally broke up and to top it off today that fuckin trooper came by to see me at my new sales manager's job way up in Hillbro. Can you believe that shit?"

"Oh no, is everything all right?" *Do they know about me?*

"Don't worry hot mamma they ain't too worried about the unidentified good looking blonde, with the beautiful tits on the 7-11 surveillance video."

"What!...I'm gonna kill you...Do they really have us on tape?"

"That's what he says, but he's not worried about us. He's going after the old man."

"Who the hell's that?" she demanded.

"The guy who ordered those punks to take us out. But anyway I got a new job and a new crib, and I'd really love to see you tonight," he pleaded admiring the plush van. "Wait till you see what I'm driving, you'll love it." *Sex palace on wheels.*

"Ya well, it better not be another race car, because I won't get in. That was fast enough to last me a lifetime."

"Nope, just the opposite."

"Oh really," she pouted looking at herself in the bedroom mirror fresh out of the shower. "Good surprise me then, 'cause my fuckin' musclehead boyfriend went out of town fishing with his homeboys. Something about male bonding! Can you believe that crap!"

Good timing. "Great that's my girl, I'll see you around nine okay? I'm an hour away and I gotta shower, eat and get sexy." *Because you're in trouble girlfriend.*

"Sure you do, you're hot enough just the way you are lover boy," she purred sexily.

"Look who's talkin'," he smiled listening to her breathe. "Well I guess I'm glad someone thinks so." *Laura kicked my ass out.*

"Hey baby, do me a fava. Dress really sexy for me okay? Maybe we'll go dancing. I know just the place." *To stir up trouble.*

She sighed, "Don't I always?"

"Yes."

"Bye lover boy, don't be late. I'll be waiting."

FORTY THREE

A S SOON AS he hung up his phone, it rang making him jump. "Hello?"

"Hey gringo, whas up wit you dude, you know who this be shoutin at ya?"

"Geez let me guess," Lucky laughed. "What's up Romeo?"

"You da man, I need you to stop by wit two full hands if you can pull it off. I got bidness."

Lucky glanced at his watch. Five-fifteen p.m. Listen I'm coming into the city around eight-thirty or so but I made plans, so it's gotta be real quick when I come by."

"No problem gringo. I gotch you. Just make sure they're the same."

"They will be. I'll call you when I get close okay?"

"Okay gringo, adios."

Ryan was waiting by the fence watching the farmer's cows drinking a Bud.

"So Ryan when's the last time you wrote seven deals in one day huh?" Lucky kidded. "Now we just gotta get that lazy finance manager off his ass and get 'em bought by the bank." *So I can get my bonus!*

"No shit. Unfuckin believable," he shouted excited. "I called my old lady she's shocked! I even told her I was coming over for a while and she didn't even get mad," he grinned. "Now that's a change I can live with."

"Well I got to leave here by seven-thirty at the latest, I got myself a hot date, so why don't you fire up the Webber while I grab a shower."

Ryan cranked up Lucky's new J.V.C. oversized boom box tuning in Pink Floyd's 'Dark Side of the Moon' rattling the apartment.

They ate thick Delmonicos and fresh New Hampshire Silver Queen corn on the cob while they passed a joint back and forth across the table. They washed it all down with Ryan's frosty cold Budweisers stored in the freezer.

Lucky laid out a couple of fat lines for the road and while he changed into a pair of Guess Jeans and a Ralph Loren white tank top. Ryan eagerly cleaned up the small kitchen.

Together they bagged up a hundred and twenty, twenty dollar rocks putting them in individual tiny blue baggies. Afterwards he cut Ryan a hundred dollar slab of crack and a vial with two grams of powder for only a single Ben Franklin.

Grateful Ryan helped load the van up with blankets, pillows and sheets, while Lucky filled the van fridge with various liquors and mixes. Carefully Lucky hid his backpack containing ten ounces of powder for Romeo, a hundred and twenty rocks, his triple beam scale and 9mm Baretta under all the blankets.

"Hey Lucky, thanks man you didn't have to give me all that!"

"I know. Just don't let your old lady catch you smoking that shit, and hey make sure you buy me another stem."

Once he got out on I-89 South bound, he set the cruise control at seventy and tried to relax driving the big van. Casually he sipped his large Absolute Screwdriver with a fresh wedge of lime. *What a life!*

He tuned the upgraded stereo into Rock 101 just in time for a block of Van Halen. His mind wandered, the last thing he needed was to get pulled over with all these drugs on him. Then his mind switched back to Alexis, she really turned him on and he couldn't wait to take out his frustrations on her willing hard body.

By eight p.m. on the outskirts of Manchester he dialed Romeo's pager. When he called back five minutes later, Lucky told him to meet him at the Donavan's country club parking lot. Just look for the sweetest van in the lot with a dealer plate. Oh it's midnight blue."

Ten minutes later, Romeo pulled up in his lowered caddy sporting oversized gawdy gold twenty-inch rims. Once inside the van, Lucky motioned Romeo into the back where all the custom curtains were already drawn. Smoothly Lucky slid the privacy divider from behind the front two captains chairs across the opening sealing them in.

"Gringo boy, this ride's sweet. Why don't you be sellin' me one?" he grinned looking all around drooling.

"Sure you got forty-five grand," Lucky laughed watching his face. "Anyway," he said pulling out his triple beam and weighing out one of the ten ounces.

"Nice Gringo, nice," Romeo commented after he weighed each one quickly stuffing them in his leather Tommy Hilfiger bag. "Here gringo, sixteen large. That takes care of the one I owed you. Oh sorry about all the small bills," he laughed sarcastically. "Later gringo."

Lucky hated to take the expensive custom van down into Romeo's neighborhood, but he had one more stop to make before Alexis's.

He hopped out of the van and set the remote alarm. Nervously he felt his Baretta stuffed behind his back in his waist band underneath his tee shirt. Anxiously, he hustled up three flights of stairs. Exhaling heavily he rapped hard on the reinforced door. All of a sudden it went quiet inside. "Welcome to my crack house," Lucky mumbled.

"Who is it?" a deep voice demanded.

"Lucky." *Your worst nightmare.*

"Who?"

"Lucky," he yelled louder.

"Hold on," a deep voice said as Lucky listened to a bar being removed inside the door, then two dead bolts were undone.

"Let em in Kickstand…let em in," a voice hidden from view barked out.

Lucky felt like bitch slapping the big asshole to teach him some manners, but he held back biting his tongue.

"Hey hombre, whas up?" Julio the den leader asked all friendly knowing Lucky always had bread on him.

Lucky glanced around and saw twelve or so crack addicts sprawled around the room smoking crumbs and trying to push their valuable stems for one more hit. He shook his head at the sad sight and pointed to Julio's bedroom where they could talk. There was no way he was pulling out two grand worth of rocks in front of all these desperate jonesing addicts.

Once inside the dingy bedroom he noticed a crack whore passed out naked on Julio's dirty looking bed spread-eagled.

"Fuckin skank," Lucky mumbled under his breath. "Here try this shit Julio," he said breaking off a hit, knowing how he'd react.

A few seconds passed then Julio whispered, "Man oh man, this stuff's wicked. There ain't no shit on the streets like this."

No shit. "Listen, before you get all geeked out I got a deal for you," he said pulling out a sandwich baggie with a hundred and twenty rocks, worth twenty bucks a piece. He then set his Baretta on top of Julio's bureau making sure he saw it.

Julio's eyes lit up. "What kind a deal?" *Man look it all that crack.*

"A hundred and twenty fat twentys for only eleven-hundred bucks, that's only ten bucks each. Shit a lot of them are twice the size you normally sell, so you can cut em down and still sell 'em for twentys. Man you can easily double your money and get high for free."

"Shit Lucky," Julio mumbled going into a corner of the room and pulling up a small board, he reached down and pulled out a lunch paper bag. "Man I only got two-hundred, what you givin up for dat?"

Lucky got dead serious. "Okay Julio give me the two bills. I'll have to trust you. If you fuck me, I'll beat you down myself and that ox you got out there can't stop me."

"Okay then what's the deal?"

"You get twenty rocks for your two bills. The other hundred rocks I'll front you for twelve each. So you'll owe me twelve hundred when I come back. Julio I know you can still make a killing because you will cut these down to street size so don't give me any fuckin excuses when I show up for my money." *Maybe I shouldn't do this?*

"Okay, okay," Julio responded in disbelief.

"Now put this shit up, don't tell no one you got this much weight and you didn't get it from me, you understand? I'll stop by tomorrow to pick up what cash you got. Be smart Julio and don't fuck with me, and I'll bring you more crack. This shit's grade A, everyone will want it once the word gets out, so don't go gettin all fucked up till later. Take care of business or else," he said picking up his gun and aiming it in Julio's direction. "Bang bang, you're dead."

"Deal Lucky, I'll see you tomorrow. I'll have your bread don't worry." *Oh boy look at all this butter.*

"Don't fuck up Julio, I'm givin you a chance."

"I know." *Boy are you ever!*

FORTY FOUR

A T EIGHT-FIFTY-FIVE P.M. he pulled the van up to Alexis's parents' large apartment complex. Once inside he couldn't help but get excited. Alexis was all dolled up in a very sexy black leather zipper mini skirt with black stiletto fuck me heels and cute ruffle ankle socks.

Instantly he was turned on when he noticed the see through lace top that proudly exposed her Victoria Secret's lacy white half bra and luscious breasts.

He could smell her Estee Lauder perfume and feel her firm after market breasts poke him in the chest when he gave her a warm friendly hug.

"God baby you smell good enough to eat…mmm and you look so delicious," he whispered sniffing her hair and neck.

She giggled enjoying his undivided attention. "Well I'm glad someone thinks so. My fuckin boyfriend is off fishing! Imagine that," she stated grabbing her overnight bag. "Okay lover boy, I'm ready." *I hope you are.*

Outside she eyed the van. "Is this it?"

"Yup."

"Jesus Lucky what's this, a love pad on wheels?" she giggled excitedly ogling the bed with the pillows and blankets Lucky had made up earlier.

"Check it out, T.V., VCR, fridge, thing's loaded. Christ it's only got eighty miles on it," he exclaimed drooling over Alexis's toned tanned legs. "Oh and no high speed chases in this baby, just cruisin."

"Let's hope not, once in a lifetime is enough for me, you almost gave me a heart attack last time."

"Come on," he ordered pulling her into the back where he mixed two absolute screwdrivers with fresh limes. Then he also handed her a two gram vial of cocaine with a little silver spoon attached. "Go ahead do a couple of bumps."

Alexis sipped her cocktail shaking her gorgeous long blond sexy hair. "You sure are full of surprises aren't you," she grinned licking her red lips. "I just never know what to expect with you," she said as she daintily filled the tiny spoon full of potent cocaine and sniffed.

"Whew! Mmm that's wicked strong. God, good coke like this makes me so horny, ooops…," she laughed covering her mouth with her drink. "But I guess you already knew that you naughty boy."

Lucky joined in and did a couple of bumps then leaned over and gave Alexis a deep French kiss. He was instantly hard. Slowly he eased Alexis back onto the bed. Still kissing her, he worked his hand up her short sexy skirt until he felt her silky crotchless panties.

She knew what he was up to and she felt his manhood grinding against her knee while he aggressively kissed and pawed her.

"Stop it Lucky," she moaned removing his paw out of her crotch. "God we haven't even got out of my driveway for Christ's sakes…come on let me up."

"Okay – okay." *Damn I'm horny.*

"Just wait till later, I haven't even finished my first drink yet, you horny toad," she snickered.

"Alright then how bout we go dancing?"

"Sure that sounds safe."

"Don't bet on it," he laughed. "I know a great place up in Concord."

After a thirty-minute ride north on Interstate 93 they pulled up outside Laura and Lucky's favorite Boogin place, the 'Take Five Music Hall.'

They moved into the back two captain's chairs and enjoyed another screwdriver while he gave her the vial, and she helped herself to a couple more spoonfuls. She tried to hand it back.

"No…no hold on to it. I got another one," he grinned. "Hey baby grab that pack over there and open it."

She opened up his backpack confused. "Oh my God," she exclaimed pulling out a handful of cash. "Shit Lucky, this is a lot of money…what the hell have you been up to?"

He gave her a look like 'you don't want to know.'

"Okay never mind you bad boy," she said raising her hand in defense.

"You pay tonight," he told her pointing at the pack.

She nodded stuffing a couple hundred in small bills into her purse along with the two gram vial.

"Hey let's do a shot of ice cold Rumplemintz."

"What the hell is that?"

He laughed at her facial expression. "It's imported expensive peppermint Schnapps. The good stuff!"

"Okay, lova boy let's have a Peppermint pawty!"

They toasted with Dixie cups shooting down the ice cold 100 proof Schnapps. "Oh by the way Laura might show up with her girlfriends so I want you all over me okay?"

She giggled almost spilling her drink. "Shit Lover boy, I'll do it anyway. I just hope she doesn't start any trouble with me," she said seriously. "I'd hate to have to deck her in public, but she threw you out, so you're all mine…at least for tonight."

"Hey."

FORTY FIVE

INSIDE THE MUSIC hall they were getting wired off the strong cocaine and potent absolute screwdrivers. Wildly they danced up a storm until they were both sweaty. He knew about half the crowd and they were all eyeing Alexis in shock, because everyone was so used to seeing Laura with Lucky that they whispered back and forth.

Alexis hung all over Lucky and flirted endlessly. She strutted back and forth to the bar buying them sixteen ounce absolute screwdrivers. Her fetching bleached blonde hair, large thirty-six double dees and rock hard tanned legs in sexy stiletto heels acted like a magnet for every man's eyes.

"Hey Lucky who the hell's that?" one of Lucky's bar friends asked eyeing Alexis with lust as she strutted to the bar looking wicked hot.

"Oh just a friend," Lucky laughed.

"Damn bro she's smoking hot, dude you lucky dog!" he drooled watching her lean over the bar and flirt with the hunky bartender. "Hey what happened to Laura?"

"She's around," he replied eyeballing Alexis as she returned with fresh drinks.

He smiled knowing she was enjoying all the attention. "Hey my friend thinks you're smoking hot," he teased.

"Does he," she grinned. "Well as long as you think I am then I'm okay," she teased back leaning over giving him a deep French kiss.

"Well honey I'm goin to the little girls' room and I'm taking the bumper okay?" she asked snatching her tiny purse with a sly grin she teasingly licked her red upper lip. *I'm so bad.*

He laughed at all the attention they were getting, "Sure baby have fun," he smiled.

A few minutes passed as he lit up a smoke, a cute married hot brunette walked up and grabbed his arm pulling him to the dance floor. She gave him an affectionate hug and peck. She was a great dancer. He knew her from many Saturday nights and she always came alone.

"Come on playboy, you're the best dancer in here and you're hot girlfriend's busy, so let's do it."

"Sure Debbie, I'd love to."

They dirty danced together, teasing and playing with each other, grabbing one another's bodies. He always fantasized about making it with Debbie, their bodies fit together perfectly and the way they moved so smoothly together he knew she'd be awesome in bed, but his exotic thoughts were short lived when he glanced over towards the bathrooms looking for Alexis, and spotted Laura and her cast of girlfriends coming in the door.

"Oh shit."

"What?"

"Look who's here," he said jerking his head towards the entrance.

"Oh, oh and here comes your blonde bomb shell," Debbie kidded covering her mouth.

Not believing his eyes, he watched Alexis walk right past Laura and her friends unknowingly on her way back to their empty table. Laura and her three girlfriends grabbed four free bar stools and ordered cocktails. Before long one of Laura's friends pointed at the dance floor right at Debbie and Lucky.

Debbie and Laura were already friends. After the third fast song ended they hugged and said goodbye as both Alexis and Laura casually watched.

"Good luck, you're gonna need it," Debbie whispered.

"Thanks a lot," he muttered heading back to Alexis.

"Can't leave you alone for a minute," Alexis smiled jokingly.

Nervously he sat down and drank his screwdriver. "We got company at the bar."

"Oh really?" she said casually eyeing the busy bar. "Which one is the wicked vixen anyway?"

"The dark haired Greek looking goddess with the tight white jeans on."

"Damn lover boy she's pretty. What the hell did she ever see in you," she snickered. "I know, don't tell me it's because you're so good in the sack!"

"No way, it must've been my wonderful personality," he laughed. *It certainly wasn't my drug habit that's for sure.* "Come on Alexis, let's dance…time for you to earn your pay."

Out on the busy dance floor Lucky could feel eyes burning into his back as they continued to dance for three songs straight ending it with a long slow song. Alexis willingly flirted recklessly while he pulled her in closer crushing her big breasts into his chest.

On the way back to the table he whispered to her, "We're under heavy surveillance you better watch out."

"Oh yeah, she said pulling him into a hot French kiss.

"Mmmm Jesus you're something else," he said shaking his head. "Go on big spender make yourself useful and get us some fresh drinks." *Boy this could get very interesting.*

"Sure lover boy, don't go anywhere, I'll be right back."

Relieved she was gone, he watched her strut up to the bar right in the midst of Laura's friends. He surveyed the scene waiting for some type of explosion.

Oh shit Alexis's crazy.

Laura never gets jealous.

Maybe this wasn't such a good idea.

Damn it I still love the bitch.

She's so…so…perfect.

Quickly Laura's friends surrounded little Alexis while she flirted shamelessly with the big Italian stud behind the bar totally ignoring the four girls trashing her and laughing,

Boldly Alexis turned towards Laura with two sixteen ounce plastic red cups full of absolute and o.j. For a second he saw her smile and say something to Laura.

Oh shit.

Don't throw the drink Alexis.

She's gonna do it. Fuck.

No she won't I'll kill her.

Finally, she returned to the table with a shit eating grin while Lucky nervously huffed on another Marlboro light.

"Here you go honey," she said nicely sliding her chair towards him and kissing him affectionately.

"Jesus girlfriend you sure got a big set of balls," he laughed shaking his head. "For a second I thought you were gonna give them all a vodka and oj bath," he asked her seriously.

She set her drink down shocked. "Who little ol' me?" she smirked. "They were whispering up a storm about how big my tits were and the color of my hair, imagine that."

"So what did you do?"

"Oh first I just kind of elbowed my way up to the hunk behind the bar, but after listening to all their rude comments I just had to say something."

"What?"

"Oh, just girl talk," she teased grinning while they both enjoyed a smoke and sipped on their potent cocktails. After they danced again he casually glanced over towards the bar and noticed Laura and the girls were gone.

Doubting his eyes he started looking all around for the evil foursome, just to make sure. After a good scan he leaned into Alexis and said, "Hey I think they left."

"Doesn't matter you're taken anyway – come on let's get out of here, I'm getting awfully horny," she teased touching her juicy red lips with her hot tongue.

She didn't need to say anymore. He was horny the minute he laid eyes on her, eager and ready they left the music hall at one a.m. pretty damn buzzed. The outside cool fresh air felt wonderfully refreshing to their hot sweaty bodies. He had to be extra careful driving the big van the long mile back to the interstate. It was one of the reasons they were leaving at one a.m. instead of two a.m. because at closing time the Concord police would be out in full force, and even though it was just a mile, they were in the capital and he knew from first hand experience that they would be watching from somewhere.

Once he made it back on I-93 South bound towards the Hooksett Toll Plaza he let out a big sigh of relief, and set the cruise control cranking Lynyrd Skynyrd on Rock 101. Shortly they were back in the Queen City, Manchester, the biggest city in New Hampshire.

After talking it over, they decided to splurge and rent the penthouse suite at the Airport Hilton instead of trashing the expensive van. Four hundred bucks later they were ushered into a plush penthouse suite called Paris.

Excitedly she took it all in. "Oh Lucky, it's beautiful," she cooed walking over to the gorgeous heart shaped Jacuzzi in the center of the room. Then she examined the gigantic king size bed surrounded by mirrors on the walls and ceiling while Lucky grabbed the remote and turned on the 50 inch Phillips stereo T.V. that was hanging nicely on the wall. Quickly he found MTV music videos.

"Nice room huh? Must be why they call it Paris, after his gorgeous blonde daughter, I think she designed the layout, yup I definitely like her taste don't you?" he kidded mixing them White Russians.

"Yes! Let's party!" she bellowed undoing her tiny buttons on her skimpy blouse while she turned on the hot water to fill the big heart Jacuzzi. He ogled her superb hard body from across the room, and instantly felt the blood rush to his crotch.

Then they snorted some more coke almost finishing off the first two gram vial, before Lucky lit up a joint of green bud to set the mood.

Once they were in the tub they hungrily attacked one another. After lots of foreplay, touching and teasing he couldn't stand it any longer and he ended up carrying her wet glistening body to the huge bed where they had sex over and over and over till even the cocaine couldn't help them continue.

FORTY SIX

AT THREE A.M. he called Romeo and waited for a call back. "Who you calling Lucky, you bored with me already?" she purred next to him like a satisfied kitty cat, caressing his body with her long red nails sending shivers up his spine.

He grinned in delight, his mind still zinging from all the stimulants he had ingested. "No baby I'm not bored with you. That's the hottest sex I've had in a long time," he chuckled turning towards her. "I love being with you, you know that."

Flushed she beamed, "Hey what can I say, I'm a high maintenance chick," she replied wiggling her cute ass on the way to the shower.

He sat there admiring her body realizing how toned her arms and legs were from teaching aerobics. Then his phone rang startling him back to reality. "Hey Romeo what are you and Sasha doing?"

"Shit gringo, we just got in from running around all night making money bro. I swear this whole city's high," he boasted. "So where you be at?" *Crazy white boy.*

"The Airport Hilton up in the penthouse. Why don't you two come by and also bring me an o-zee cookie of hard plus baggies."

"You for real?"

"Yup, I'll square with you later, listen I have plenty of good liquor, killer weed, and my gorgeous lady friend is with me so…"

"Hold on a sec…yup Sasha's psyched. She's dying to get out of our castle. Fuckin' people keep banging on the door," he said disgusted. "See you in a few, what room?"

"Paris Penthouse, top floor." *Can't wait, this could get exciting.*

Sasha and Romeo showed up thirty minutes later and were very impressed with the expensive suite. While Romeo and Lucky were busy whipping up four White Russians, the girls chatted. They looked perfect together, two hot blondes, one natural, one not.

Romeo gawked at Alexis sexually and joked with Lucky about how big and firm her ripe melons were. Lucky's ego was growing by the minute.

"God Alexis that tub looks heavenly," Sasha said smiling. "Can we go in?" she asked innocently passing the joint back to Alexis while she sampled the expensive White Russian cocktail.

"Sure we can go in if you want to," Alexis answered exhaling the powerful dirty joint laced with cocaine. Alexis reached over and dimmed the recessed lights around the tub before she dropped her black silk robe to the plush carpet.

Both hot blondes were naked in the Jacuzzi with the jets and air bubbles running full bore. Alexis's waterproof vibrator was still setting on the side of the tub when both girls noticed it and they both giggled with embarrassment. *Ooops.*

They were all stoned and Lucky gave the lovely girls a fresh two gram vial of coke while he and Romeo got down to business. Together the guys broke up the ounce of crack. Romeo the expert, cut up the rocks, while Lucky stuffed the little blue ziplock baggies with twenty dollar rocks.

They finished in record time both wanting to join the girls. Immediately Romeo aggressively stripped off his Tommy Hilfiger clothes eagerly ready to join the girls.

"Mind if I come in?" he told them not waiting for a reply, the girls just giggled. "I guess not," he said dropping his Hilfiger boxers exposing his very muscular twenty year old dark skinned Columbian body. Both Sasha and Romeo were five years younger than Alexis and Lucky who were in their mid twenties.

Lucky put away the hundred and twenty rocks and glanced over to see Romeo kissing Alexis while playing with Sasha. Slowly he watched Sasha and Romeo seduce Alexis as he stripped naked and reached for his stem.

Man I gotta check the quality.

Just one hit.
Don't get too high or you'll ruin it.
God Sasha looks so young, so edible.
I can't believe this is actually happening.

Sasha gently kissed Alexis's perky breasts while Romeo grabbed the vibrator and turned it on. Smiling his hand disappeared below the waterline. A few minutes passed until Romeo sat up on the edge of the tub while Alexis devoured his young hard manhood. Sasha totally turned on had Alexis's legs spread from behind and was willingly working the waterproof vibrator toy, rapidly thrusting it inside Alexis.

Is this really happening, he thought, obviously turned on and very buzzed. He decided he'd seen enough. It was time to join the fun.

Quietly he walked over to the Jacuzzi and sat down smoking another joint laced with cocaine he stroked himself.

Sasha gently reached over and took his hand away, licking her lips. Slowly. He held the joint up to her lips ogling her sweet hard nipples, she exhaled and smiled. Next thing he knew she took him deep inside her warm mouth. His eyes shut wanting more he reached out and tenderly squeezed Sasha's firm ripe breasts.

He opened his eyes moaning in lust, he watched Romeo pull Alexis up onto his lap. She willingly straddled him using her hand to guide him. Romeo hungrily kissed Alexis's erect nipples while she rode him expertly.

Lucky copied his move and lifted Sasha on top of him. Eric Clapton's 'Cocaine' song wailed on the surround sound system as both couples worked themselves into a frenzy. Everyone was moaning, groaning, and grunting. Within seconds of each other both guys exploded in ecstasy.

A few seconds of silence filled the air before they all started giggling as they all realized what they had done. "Damn gringo," Romeo chuckled trying to break the strangeness, "This sure is great, you sure know how to treat your friends Amigo." *Don't I though?*

They partied some more completely naked ending up on the huge bed for another naughty session of swapping partners. Alexis was the first to pass out, sexually exhausted around six a.m.

When Lucky and Alexis came to around noon, Romeo and Sasha were long gone. Their first stop was into the Hilton's dining room for a first class brunch. Afterwards he drove Alexis back to her apartment where they kissed and said good-bye.

He glanced at the dashboard clock. One p.m. Sunday. Free of Alexis, he drove directly to Julio's crack den. Before he climbed out he grabbed his Baretta and the baggy full of rocks he'd broken up with Romeo's help late last night from what he could recall.

When Julio finally opened the door, there were crack heads passed out all over the place. A few were still using which surprised Lucky considering it was Sunday, he figured they'd all be broke by now, but then he remembered what someone had told him. Don't ever underestimate how much power crack has over someone. They will go to any extreme to come up with the money for the next hit, lie, steal, cheat, and con.

He shut his eyes disgusted. Man I hope I never get this bad, he thought going into Julio's pigsty bedroom. On the bed were two naked crack whores passed out, dead to the world. *Nasty.*

"You got my money?" Lucky irritated snapped.

"Yup, sure do Lucky. Just like you said," Julio mumbled proudly going to his stash spot. Anxiously he pulled out a fat wad of wrinkled bills.

"Shit you've been busy!" *Crackhead.*

"Told you Lucky, this shit's the best." Together they counted out twelve hundred dollars. "You want more?"

"Fuckin right, I did real good with that shit, everybody wants more."

"How much green you got?"

"I don't know let's see," he mumbled obviously burnt out from partying all night. They counted the rest of his stash. "How much is it Lucky?"

"Looks like you got seven hundred and twenty-six so that'll get you seventy-three rocks. That leaves forty-six rocks I'll front you at twelve bucks so you'll owe me five hundred and sixty bucks okay?"

"Okay." *Fuckers good in math ain't he.*

"You sure now, listen in a few weeks you'll be rich. Just keep it real," he barked at Julio. As he dumped out the packets. "Count 'em, go ahead."

Then he pulled out his business card and told Julio to call his cell phone when he was ready for more. "Listen call me okay, but don't you dare give my number out to anyone," he said firmly jabbing Julio in the chest.

FORTY SEVEN

T HE FOLLOWING WEEK was Lucky's fourth week of the month at Johnson's. His detailed chart on his office wall showed he had seventeen new and thirty used delivered.

That meant he had seven more days to deliver five more new and four more used to hit his double bonus. Labor day was only a week away. Unlike most dealerships who held a huge blowout sale on Labor Day weekend, Johnson's would be closed Saturday, Sunday, and Monday. So he made plans to go down to Westin, Massachusetts to his brother-in-law's younger brother's annual party.

During the week he managed to sell another wholesale piece to Dirty Shirt Dick earning himself another two-hundred yard tip. By Friday the sales board read twenty-one new and thirty-three used. He only needed one more new and one more used to hit his double bonus.

Saturday Ryan and Lucky worked the lot aggressively. They wrote up three new and three used. Delivering one of each on the spot to hit the bonus numbers. His cell phone rang just as they finished up for the day.

"Hey Lucky, it's Julio, stop by I got your flow."

"Okay dude, I'll be by in an hour or so with more."

After he returned from Julio's he made a chart up in his notebook.

WHO	SALE	PAID	OWE	TOTAL
Romeo	6K	5K	1K	5K
R	15K	16K	0	21K
Julio	1.4K	200	1.2K	23.126

| J | 1.28 | 1.926 | 56.0 | 23,126 |
| J | 0 | 560 | 0 | 23,686 |

He spent Saturday night in his barn apartment hiding his money underneath the living room rug so there were no lumps. There was a total of twenty-four thousand in small bills spread out evenly under the large throw rug.

The depression hit him like a punch. He couldn't stop thinking about the look Laura gave him at the music hall when he was dancing with Alexis. His bipolar mood swings were controlling his thought patterns. Usually he was on a manic swing, but instead his mood had swung completely in the opposite realm, leaving him feeling lifeless. The fact he had stopped taking his psychotropic medications the day Laura threw him out never entered his mind.

Even with all the cash and cocaine it wasn't enough to help him out of his funk. He sat quietly in the kitchen doing shots of Rumplemintz Schnapps that he kept nice and cold in the freezer.

After a few hours of depressing suicidal thoughts he eyed his loaded baretta sitting on the table. Not trusting himself he took his eyes off the gun and downed two Xanex with his next shot. An hour later he passed out on the uncomfortable couch.

Sunday morning he awoke fully dressed in all his clothes and he had a vicious throbbing headache. Disgusted he took a long hot shower. Feeling a little better, he threw a filet mignon on his gas grill. He poured a cold glass of chocolate milk and downed a handful of Advil. *Man I feel like shit. I hate it when I get like this.*

After he shaved and dressed he was glad he was headed out of town. Back at the abandoned dealership he dropped off the conversion van and grabbed the keys to the 1972 Mercedes Benz Roadster. First thing he did was drop the top. It was one of the owner's personal cars that Lucky was allowed to use.

Smoking a cherry Tijuana small cigar, he cruised over to his sister's house in Keene where Lucky took his oldest nephew with him while they followed his brother-in-law's Chevy Astro van down to Weston, Massachusetts.

Sam, his brother-in-law's brother was the one holding the big party and Lucky was feeling his mood change for the better the farther away they got.

By Sunday afternoon, Sam who ran a successful auto body shop and Lucky were in a heated horseshoe match. They both had been drinking draft beer heavily. Between the beer and the potent weed they were both so buzzed that they were evenly matched.

Slurring Sam asked Lucky just as he was about to toss his shoes, "Hey you still sellin' cars like crazy?"

Lucky nodded knowing he was trying to break his drunken concentration on his last turn. Come on, you can do it he told himself.

"Alright ringer, that's game, you lose! Let's see that makes twenty bucks," Lucky laughed rubbing it in. *I love winning.*

"Fuck you, you beat me at my own damn game, sheet. Hey how are you at pool?"

"Shit Sam old buddy, let me go get my cue stick out of my trunk and we'll rack a few games, where's your table at?" *Gotcha.*

"Fuck you asshole," he grinned knowing he'd met another hustler. "Hey you ever come across anything you want to unload, just let me know," he paused. "Nothin like a quick paint job and a new set of numbers to go along with a clean title," Sam said with an evil shit eating grin. *What the hell is he talking about?*

"Yup, I heard you're some big shot at a Chevy dealership," he slurred. "Shit bro, I'll give you three grand for somethin' sweet." *Oh now I get it, chop shop.*

Immediately Lucky thought about the lock box key he had taped to the bottom of his couch. He was smiling thinking pay back time. "You're really serious aren't you?"

"Damn straight. How else you think I made all this bread, paintin' fuckin' cars, get real," he said raising his arms to the expensive Cape Cod house, sitting on a lake.

"Let's take a ride around the block," Lucky said.

"Sure time to burn one anyway, away from the kids."

They climbed in the old Mercedes Roadster and took a mellow ride to smoke a joint and talk. Lucky drove very slow checking out the nice houses on the large lake. He pulled out a vial of coke and handed it to a wasted Sam. Immediately his eyes lit up.

"Don't mind if I do."

While Sam blasted away on the strong powder, Lucky thought about stealing the old man's 'Vettes. The cocaine woke him up from his drunken stupor, "Shit man, this is premo stuff. We could make some serious coin with this – so, tell me about these 'Vettes again."

"Okay, well I want five grand a 'Vette and we could probably get I don't know say ten of them worth about twenty to twenty five grand a piece," he boasted with excitement.

"Man oh man, that's fifty gees on your end," Sam whistled shaking his head. "Man I couldn't come up with that kind of bread up front, so you got any other bright ideas?"

"Yup sure do, pay me a week after you get em," he said as they approached Sam's house. "Listen bro it'll be so fuckin' easy…cause I got the lock box key to a hundred 'Vettes."

He laughed thinking about paying back the old man once again. "All you gotta do is drive em off the lot late at night…shit I could even get you a few paper tags," he said thinking.

"Shit Lucky, that sounds too fuckin' easy, you sure about the set up?"

"Never been so sure, I used to work there. Trust me, no security, no cameras, easy pickins. Christ you could have an empty car carrier down the street and you could fill it up," he giggled thinking about the old man's expression when he found out he got ripped off again.

The following afternoon, Labor Day, when he pulled out of Sam's they both agreed to talk by phone the following week.

FORTY EIGHT

THE NEXT DAY, Tuesday, Lucky was back at work. He wanted to deliver one more new and one more used from the other four cars they took deposits on Saturday. The deal was that any vehicle delivered by the close of business Tuesday, counted towards last month's numbers increasing his bonuses to twenty-three hundred on new and thirty-five hundred on used for a total monthly bonus of fifty-eight hundred.

When he finally left at seven pm, he was very excited and pleased because both deliveries had just driven off the lot.

Sam called and said he was due in Manchester at nine pm. They planned to meet at Applebee's, just down the street from City Corvette.

Lucky grabbed a new trade-in, a 1992 low mileage Mustang GT with a Paxton super charger and after market headers with a Borla performance exhaust system. The car was supposed to be pushing four hundred plus horsepower. His manic mood swing was back. He raced towards Manchester pushing the powerful Mustang at speeds between a hundred and one-fifty making it in record time.

They enjoyed a couple Captain Morgan and Cokes at Applebee's Bar and Grill while they waited for City Corvette to close. By ten o'clock they pulled out in Lucky's Mustang. He pulled right into an empty City Corvette. Casually they cruised between the five rows of twenty sexy 'vettes.

"Shit Lucky, this is a 'Vette lover's dream," he raged twisting his head back and forth like a kid in a candy store. "And…and you got a key to all those little boxes?"

Lucky grinned gripping the master key in his palm, "Yup sure do, here. Take the key, you hold it cause I'm gonna be far away when this shit goes down."

Yup, I'll be in Bow with my parents.
Shit this is fuckin' crazy.
But the bastard tried to kill me.
And paybacks a motherfucker.

He pulled back out on the main drag and headed back to Applebee's parking lot where they both did a couple of bumps while they hashed out everything.

"Man it's too easy havin' this magic key. It's gonna be what I do with the 'Vettes afterwards that matters," he stammered. "Okay dude, let's plan on next Tuesday night."

Sam commented, "Oh and what's up with all this rocket-fuel you keep havin'?"

"Why you like it?"

"Fuckin-a I do…how much?"

"Fifteen bills an o-zeee, cash and carry. Uncut."

Sam whipped out his biker wallet chained to his jean belt loop and yanked out a wad of bills. Lucky smiled watching him count out his money, then he reached into the backseat and grabbed his trusty backpack. Carefully he dug through it and pulled out a fat ounce of uncut cocaine. The good stuff.

Excitedly Sam slapped fifteen Ben Franklins into Lucky's open palm and snatched the ounce out of his other open hand.

"Wicked nice," Sam squealed fingering the large boulder in the baggie. Stashing it in his dungaree vest. "Later Lucky, wish me luck," he grinned slamming the door.

FORTY NINE

L UCKY SWUNG BY Julio's for another pick up and drop off on his way back north to Hillbro. He moved the couch and peeled the carpet back exposing the twenty-four grand.

Then he added Sam's $1500 and Julio's $500 to the pile on the floor. Inside his notebook he wrote down:

WHO	SALE	PAID	OWE	TOTAL
Romeo	6K	5K	1K	5K
R	15K	16K	0	21K
Julio	1.4	200	1.2	21.2
J	1.28	1.926	560	23,126
J	0	560	0	23,686
Sam	1.5	1.5	0	25,186
J	500	500	0	25,686

All week, Lucky was in an upbeat mood anticipating getting his dealership bonus money on Friday, totaling fifty-eight hundred. That along with the 'Vette heist was enough to bring him out of his depressed state and kick in the manic roller coaster cycle once again.

On Friday things didn't go as planned.

After lunch, he was called into one of the owner's offices. "Hey Lucky – hell of a month, you almost broke both sales records on your first month. Incredible," the owner smirked glancing at the printout in his hands.

Stunned, Lucky scowled shocked. "What are you talking about sir? ...Almost...you must have miscounted or something," he snapped back anxiously pulling out his own copy from his suit jacket pocket.

They went over it one by one agreeing till they reached numbers eighteen and nineteen new and numbers thirteen and fourteen used. "What you mean, they don't count?" Lucky fumed trying to control his temper. *Not this shit again.*

"Well Lucky, Bob sold two new vans and two used vans to the Hillbro school district at below wholesale, you know as a community service with our dealership logo painted on the side. So of course those four vans don't count towards your totals."

Lucky's pulse raced. His heart beat faster and faster. He paced back and forth. His brain was in overdrive. Angrily he spun around, "Sir that's bullshit and you know it," he raged. "You never told me that and to pull this shit now is down right dirty and you know it!" *Easy does it.*

The owner with his legs propped up just smirked and casually responded, "Well son, not everything in life is always fair, but like I said in the beginning, no wholesale pieces count period." *So you're not getting shit wise ass.*

Impulsively, Lucky almost smashed the owner's expensive cowboy boots off the desk. Instead, he just glared at him with hatred, spun around and stormed out of the office muttering to himself thinking.

First the old man.
Then Big Mike.
Now this.
What the hell's next?
I'll pay 'em all back if it's the last thing I do.

After he collected his measly six hundred dollar gross salary pay check he walked straight to the souped up Mustang and was gone in a cloud of smoke and dust.

Back in his apartment still hot, he started drinking like a mad man while he weighed out more ounces of cocaine.

I have to get even.
Think of somethin' really good.
Nobody does this shit to me.
And gets away with it.
But shit this is the third fuckin' time.

FIFTY

H E BARELY SLEPT all weekend snorting powder till his nose bled, then he switched to crack, which he continued to smoke till he was so paranoid he began hallucinating and seeing things that weren't there. Quietly he tip toed around in his dress socks clutching his nine millimeter while he peeked out the windows. *They're out there.*

Back at work on Monday, he acted like nothing was wrong, and that's just how he planned it to look. On different deals, he pulled each customer aside and cut the price enough so they both benefited. The grateful customer saved an additional five-hundred after paying Lucky five bills cash on the side. All he had to do was lower the sale price by a thousand dollars.

"Fuck them," he mumbled quietly after he pocketed the second five bills raising his slush fund to a grand. I'll make my own damn bonus," he giggled knowing he was working on borrowed time.

After inviting his parents out to dinner for the following night, the same night Sam planned to hit City Corvette, he decided to go back to his apartment and crash so he could try and look half way respectable the next evening.

He traded demos and chose a late model Cadillac Coupe Deville to take to his parent's. On the way he dropped by Lungs farm house which sat on eighty acres, and dropped by with a present. Lung was no where to be found so Lucky snuck into the old barn, and parked inside one of the empty horse stalls, was Lung's bad ass Ninja 900 motorcycle. Lucky wrapped up his present in a brown paper lunch bag and set it on top of the ninja's sleek seat.

On his way out, he dialed Lung's number and left a message for him to check his bike out. He laughed knowing Lung would flip out when he found his little present a free ounce of uncut cocaine. *Hey what're friends for.*

That evening, the Sullivan's dined at the popular Makris Lobster Pool Restaurant in Loudon on Rt. 106 where you could pick out your favorite Maine lobster from a live tank before they served it to you twenty minutes later. The homemade New England clam chowder and whole belly fried clams were to die for.

After a delightful meal he spent the night as planned with his parents, sleeping in his old bedroom. In the mean time, Sam and company were reviewing the game plan for the night, ten golden 'Vettes.

They would transport two 'Vettes in three different enclosed trailers while the last four 'Vettes would be driven ninety minutes south to a warehouse in Westin, Massachusetts wearing stolen Mass. tags. Seven guys total, three to drive the trucks pulling the three different car haulers and four guys to drive the single 'Vettes to the hidden warehouse. Sam promised them each a grand up front and a grand after the 'Vettes were sold. They all had been up to City Corvette at least one time over the past week to scope out the layout.

The three enclosed car trailers belonged to a shady wholesaler who Sam knew from Boston. The trailers were painted black and very non-descript. The wholesaler who Sam knew wasn't always legit and let it be known that he wanted first dibbs on the stolen 'Vettes.

At midnight, while Lucky slept soundly, Sam's guys made their move with walkie-talkie Nextel phones. Smoothly and quietly they moved into action. The first 'Vette left the lot and two minutes passed exactly when the second 'Vette followed.

The trailers were set up in a wooded vacant lot quarter of a mile away. Once the first two 'Vettes were loaded the old Chevy dually pick-up truck pulled out and headed for the highway observing the posted speed limits.

Within fifteen minutes all six 'Vettes were trailered and heading south on I-93 approximately ten miles apart. Twenty minutes later, Sam in the last 'Vette, a mint limited edition 1991 ZR1 worth all the money, listened over the roar of the powerful motor for any warnings coming over his Nextel walkie talkie. He couldn't help himself he was so pumped up that while he drove down I-93 towards Boston, he pulled out his vial of coke and did a few bumps to keep the adrenaline surge going. He was still amazed at how easy it had been. *Damn Lucky you were right.*

He grinned excitedly when he pulled up behind the spread out caravan. By three am, he had all ten 'Vettes secured in his motorcycle gang's warehouse. Smiling, he paid all six guys a grand a piece making sure to give them each a half gram of blow as a bonus.

*   *   *

The next morning, Lucky enjoyed a nice breakfast with his father before they both had to go their separate ways to work. Dad, a retired marine officer and vice president of a large national phone company was now officially retired. Unofficially he worked as a problem solver for the governor and drove an official looking state vehicle.

They feasted on mom's homemade scrumptious thick French toast served with real New Hampshire maple syrup. "Thanks mom," he told her gratefully. "Boy do I miss your great cooking," he smiled giving her a hug and kiss good-bye.

Once he got on Interstate 89 heading north towards Hillbro, he eagerly dialed Sam's private number.

"Hey cuz, how's everything with you this fine day?" Lucky asked curiously.

Sam was still wide awake zooming on cocaine. The rush of stealing a quarter million dollars worth of adult play toys so easily kept him excited. "Good…very good…Lucky dog…In fact extremely good," he snickered high as a kite. "Man I got you this weekend bro."

"Great, I'm just checkin bro, I'll touch base this weekend." *Yes he did it.*

"Later dog."

*   *   *

With everything else going on, Lucky didn't realize that Julio actually lived in the Northern King's turf, and that Hector the old man's henchman served Julio dope on a regular basis. Hector, the leader of the New Hampshire Northern Kings chapter ran most of the weight in Manchestser other than Romeo and his Columbian hombres.

Hector stopped by Julio's to make a drop, and when Julio told him he was straight and didn't need any product, Hector smelled a rat. Immediately he became extremely hostile.

Violently he beat on poor Julio till he begged him to stop. Then Hector squeezed him for the information he was after: who was supplying product on his home turf.

"Lucky," Julio whispered wiping away the blood from his nose and mouth. Reluctantly Julio showed Hector a twenty piece of Lucky's crack. Hector immediately spotted the quality and even though he was an uneducated hood, he was street smart knowing the crack was too pure not to be tied to the missing cocaine shipment. "Mother fucker's dead," he screamed leaving Julio bloody and cowering on the floor.

On his way back to his hideout it dawned on him where he'd heard the name Lucky. He shook his fat head feeling stupid. It's gotta be the same fuckin' guy the old man's after, he thought. Feeling silly he started to laugh because he's the one who made the call for the old man to the Roxbury Mass. Northern King chapter.

"Fuck," he yelled dialing as fast as possible he called the old man on his private number to give him the latest news on Lucky. But Hector was stunned before he could get a word in he learned quickly from a very angry owner about ten stolen 'Vettes. *Too many things are starting to go wrong.*

FIFTY ONE

L T. BROOKS RECEIVED a courtesy call from the Manchester P.D. in regards to the ten stolen 'Vettes from City Corvette. He listened carefully while the Sgt. read the police report over the phone. The Sgt. told him how the 'Vettes were stolen after midnight and currently there were no suspects. He asked the Sgt. to fax him a copy of the report and inwardly he smiled to himself realizing how things were starting to get very interesting.

He had already leaned on the younger of the two gang members armed with the D.A.'s offer. After a few hours, two cokes and a half pack of Marlboros the young kid finally decided five years sounded a lot better than twenty.

The street smart punk told the Lt. to call in his mouth piece so he wouldn't get screwed in the deal. Once his public defender arrived he spilled his guts on tape. He described how the gang deliberately scratched Lucky's Trans Am at the 7-11 and got him to chase them out onto the highway where they were paid to shoot out his tires at a high speed causing him to crash and burn.

Once he started to sing, he rambled on giving up more valuable information. He admitted that it was another Northern King chapter that ordered the hit. Reluctantly he gave up Hector's name and gang association but he had never heard of the old man or City Corvette.

After his public mouth piece whispered into his ear, the punk responded saying there was no way he would testify against Hector unless he walked away clean, no time served. Otherwise he'd be a dead man inside the joint.

Lt. Brooks told his lawyer that once he could verify the information he would sign off on the five year deal. And if they needed him to testify against Hector they would consider the get out of jail free offer.

Later on the Lt. called the D.A. and also touched base with the New Hampshire Narcotics Task Force who were working in conjunction with the feds.

They agreed to put a twenty-four hour tail on Hector's last known address, because he was already wanted on outstanding warrants for parole violations regarding gang and drug activity. Either way, they all agreed Hector was going down.

Lt. Brooks reviewed the Manchester P.D.'s reports filed by the old man to his insurance company on the ten stolen 'Vettes. He wondered if it was an inside job to scam the insurance company out of a hefty claim. All this focus on City Corvette made him decide to let Lucky walk on the aggravated fleeing and alluding and drag racing resulting in multiple deaths a second degree felony punishable by up to fifteen years. Instead he'd use him to set up the old man, just the thought of it made him smile.

He could easily justify it because the punks had instigated the chase and tried unsuccessfully to run him off the road. Any felony charges against Lucky could possibly tip the old man off. Lt. Brooks had a sixth sense that things between Sullivan and the old man were just starting to heat up.

I'll use Sullivan as bait.
Get the old man to make a mistake.
Maybe Sullivan's more involved than I think.
Is he that revengeful? I doubt it.
How the hell could he steal ten 'Vettes?

FIFTY TWO

DURING THE NEXT week, Lucky did as little as possible at work feeding Ryan a few deals. He was uptight and very agitated, and his mood swings were more extreme and closer together.

It was like a fast train going through a mountain pass. The higher elevations were higher and the steep valleys came up quicker. He tried to compensate with cocaine. It really didn't matter powder or crack, they both fed his natural endorphins keeping the train from stalling in a valley too long.

Friday, after he picked up his measly pay check for six hundred, Lucky hopped into his new favorite ride, the gas guzzling super charged Mustang. He hauled ass heading south on I-89 towards Bow Junction.

His destination, Weston,Mass. He pulled off exit one in Bow and filled up with premium famous Bow Mobil station. The four hundred plus horsepower Mustang sucked fuel like Lucky drank vodka.

Now southbound on I-93 towards Hooksett toll plaza, he did a couple bumps off the tutor while he listened to Rock 101 and "Bad Company till the Day I Die" blasting out of the amplified stereo.

Automatically he increased his speed feeling all the raw horsepower under his foot. The endorphins raced in his brain while he unconsciously accelerated. Glancing down he was surprised to see he was pushing one-forty-five.

The next thing he saw when he looked up was a state trooper sliding sideways across the grass median with his blue lights on.

"Oh shit," he screamed glancing back he floored the Mustang 150…153…155 mph. "Come on baby, give me all you got." *Shit. I got my gun and coke in the car. Not good.*

Things were coming up rapidly and he swerved into another lane to avoid colliding with a car that nonchalantly pulled out directly in front of him.

Adrenaline shot through his veins. 160…163…165…167 mph. He was flying now and begging for more, 168…169…171 mph. Suddenly he saw motion, and jerked his head to the right. Shocked to see a black 911 Porsche Turbo right beside him. The driver casually glanced over at Lucky and grinned like he was on a county back road. A few seconds later he was gone. Amazed Lucky watched the distinct taillights rapidly pull away. "Holy shit," he growled eyeing the speedometer. 175 mph.

That guy must be doing 190, 195. Unbelievable.
Now what the hell do I do?
Toll plaza two miles. They'll be waiting.
Shit no off ramps…except.

The New Hampshire State Liquor store and rest area 1/4 mile ahead. "Please Don't Drink and Drive!" the big green sign stated.

"Yes," he beamed quickly slowing and cutting over four lanes to the right, he barely made the exit. Suddenly he couldn't get out of the car fast enough and went inside to make it look legit.

Impulsively he bought a bottle of Cuervo 1800 Tequilla. Back outside he glanced around the busy parking lot. There were no state trooper cars thankfully, so he climbed back into the Mustang.

Now what he thought. Only one way to exit. That was back onto I-93 southbound towards the Hooksett Toll Plaza. Cautiously he drove back onto the highway sweating bullets. *Where are they?*

Toll plaza dead ahead. He dug three tokens out of the center console, and tried to veer left away from the manned toll lanes. "Holy shit," he muttered when he spotted the black Porsche surrounded by mean green state trooper cruisers.

The poor guy was handcuffed and looking right at the Mustang when Lucky lowered the window to toss the tokens they locked eyes for a few seconds. The guy shrugged his shoulders and grinned. Then he jerked his head as if to say, 'Hey they already got me, go on get the hell out of here…' Still shaking Lucky pulled off and set the cruise control at seventy-five. Five miles an hour over the posted limit till he crossed the border from New Hampshire into Massachusetts, known for the worst drivers in North America.

Automatically he increased his speed to eighty-five, because the flow of traffic started to pass him by. Forty-five minutes later he pulled into Sam's peaceful Cape Cod home and was met instantly by George, Sam's mean ass German Shepherd attack dog.

He lowered his window down a little. "Hey George, don't bite me," he teased, backing away from the window as George lunged up on the car door barking ferociously.

Wish I had a fat juicy bone,
No I don't, he'd probably bite me anyway.
Shit, I'm not movin' till somebody puts him up.

A few minutes later Sam came out of his house all smiles tossing a treat to George, he climbed in the passenger's side. "Hey Lucky I see you met George," he joked. "Mean son of a bitch ain't he," he roared slapping Lucky's shoulder full of himself.

He handed Lucky a dark green trash bag. "Open it bro," he pestered. "Fifty large my good friend. Very, very sweet doing bidness with my new family."

Amazed he thumbed through a few of the fifty bands of money. Suddenly he realized how sweet revenge could be, smiling he tied the bag shut and handed Sam a copy of the Manchester Union Leader with the City Corvette stolen 'Vettes on the front page. "Here you made the front page."

Sam eyed it for a few seconds. "Man we both made out. I wholesaled all ten 'Vettes for fourteen grand a piece so we did real good."

"You got my key?" Lucky asked holding his palm out.

"Right here bro," he responded slapping the shiny master lock box key into his open hand. "So you got any more of that white lightning for sale, say in quantity?"

"I just might know where I can get some, why what ya lookin' for?"

"Shit that stuff was wicked. Best shit anyone's ever seen around here. I'd buy a whole kilo of that shit if the price was right," he laughed evily.

"Let me see, best I could do," Lucky hesitated trying to calculate knowing Sam had a pile of cash. "Shit say twenty-five solid o-zees for twenty five gees, uncut of course, same shit as before and best of all you'd save twelve grand off my usual price of thirty-seven grand. But hey your family, you get a better deal."

Promptly Sam barked, "I call that! …When?"

"How about now? Go get your money and follow me back up, but just you and me bro."

"Five minutes," he responded excitedly hopping out of the car to a vigilant George.

About five minutes later true to his word the garage door opened and he pulled out in a bad ass 1971 Chevelle SS 454 big block motor in mint condition.

Boy this ought to be fun Lucky thought when they hit the highway. Little did Sam know Lucky wasn't driving a stock Mustang. They played catch me if you can and took turns passing each other at ninety or better. It was almost nine pm when the two noisy cars pulled into the farm. "Shit nice place Lucky," Sam said looking all around.

"Yup if you like the country, peace and quiet this is the place, come on."

"Don't you mean the sticks," he kidded. "The boonies."

Upstairs Lucky pulled two frosty Molson Goldens out of his icebox and then realizing he hadn't eaten any dinner he grabbed two thick choice black-angus sirloins and set 'em on the counter. "I'm fuckin' starving Sam, you up for a juicy steak and some premo New Hampshire silver queen corn on the cob?"

He eyed the two inch thick steaks. "Damn straight." They shared a joint while Lucky the chef quickly marinated the choice sirloins in Italian dressing from Ken's Steak House, adding freshly chopped garlic in olive oil, Worcestershire sauce and A-1 bold. Expertly he used a dinner fork to tenderize the steaks stabbing both sides with lots of tiny holes.

Twenty minutes later with six ears of freshly shucked native corn, a pot of lightly salted water boiling and the Webber grill on high. Now that they were stoned it was time to munch out. The strong reefer and cold Canadian beer just enhanced their taste buds for sizzling medium rare steaks and perfectly boiled six minute buttery corn on the cob.

Very little was said during the simple delicious prepared meal. They both grinned satisfied. "Man oh man that was wicked good Lucky, appreciate it."

"No problem, it sure did hit the spot."

After they cleaned up Lucky came out of his bedroom with the same green trash bag that had the fifty bundles of cash, but now it was filled with twenty-six ounces.

He pulled out his scales and set up the triple beam handing the garbage bag to Sam. "Here count 'em and weigh each one," he demanded setting the scale weights on thirty grams. Twenty-eight grams of cocaine and two grams for the glad sandwich bag.

Methodically, Sam set each baggy on the scale till he got to number twenty-six. "Uh – what's this? You gave me one too many," he mumbled double checking his count.

Lucky smiled watching. "Boy I do love honesty," he said slurping his Molson stoned. "Go ahead keep it. That's why I put it in there, but now I know what you're all about, and I like it." *Reward honesty my Dad always said.*

Sam counted out twenty-five grand and set the stacks on the kitchen table packing up the cocaine. "Thanks Lucky."

"Hey we can do that same deal again, but don't wait to long," he warned him. "Oh I'd stick to the speed limit at least till you get to the Mass border, New Hampshire cops love loud fast cars, so watch your ass."

FIFTY THREE

AFTER SAM SPLIT, he pushed the couch back and pulled the big throw rug back until he had to move the T.V. so he could spread out more cash evenly on the floor making sure he took his time so there were no lumps detectable when you walked across the rug.

In his small black notebook he added on to his list.

C-Sales

WHO	SALE	PAID	OWE	TOTAL
Romeo	6K	5K	1K	5K
R	15K	16K	0	21K
Julio	1.4K	200	1.2K	21.2K
J	1.28K	1.926	560	23,126
J	0	560	0	23,686
Sam	1.5K	1.5K	0	25,186
J	500	500	0	25,686
Sam	50K	50K	0	75,686
Sam	25K	25K	0	100,686,

After he spread the twenty-five grand on the floor, he realized the rug had reached it's limit. Quietly he snuck down to the old barn below and eased inside careful not to spook any of the animals. He grabbed an old shovel out of the corner and worked his way across the dirt floor to a far corner.

Swiftly he dug a deep and wide enough hole for the double wrapped garbage bag holding four kilos and the fifty-grand Sam gave him for the 'Vettes. Ten minutes later he was back upstairs, busy weighing out more ounces out of the second open kilo while he waited for Romeo to call back.

Romeo now wanted fifteen more ounces but only wanted to pay fourteen hundred an ounce, plus he wanted him to bring the ounce he owed him for the ounce of crack he brought to the Hilton penthouse party.

It only took Lucky a second to agree to the hundred dollar an ounce discount. On his way out to the Mustang he slid a crisp new hundred dollar bill into an envelope the landlord provided and slid it under the landlord's door for his next week's rent. He climbed into his Mustang strapped with his Baretta, crack, and seventeen ounces of powder.

By midnight, he was at Romeo and Sasha's pad very excited and horny because this was the first night he'd laid eyes on the young blonde vixen since the wild night they had swapped partners.

"Hey gringo, come on in."

"Hey Romeo, hey Sasha," Lucky replied.

Sasha crossed the room and came right up and gave him a friendly hug and peck on the cheek taking the twelve pack he'd brought her. *God she looks good.*

"How's Alexis doing?"

"Good I guess, I haven't talked to her all week. She's probably with her muscle head boyfriend knowing my luck," he said with a shrug.

"Is he really that big?" she asked wondering.

"Shit yeah, he used to play for the Patriots before he blew out his knee. The guy benches like six hundred pounds."

"Jeez poor Alexis," she joked.

They got right down to business. Romeo weighed his sixteen ounces and paid Lucky twenty-one grand all in small bills collected off every street corner in Manchester.

They had a quick beer then he left twenty minutes later with a freshly cooked up crack cookie and all his cash. Nervously, he kept everything in his pack on his back keeping his hands free, because there was a lot of drug traffic coming and going up the long flight of stairs around Romeo's that he was ready to throw down with his baretta if anyone tried him.

Back in the Mustang he stashed the knapsack and drove a few blocks to Julio's passing a grove of drug addicts wandering aimlessly in the known drug zone, jonesing for one more hit of the devil's poison. He parked a block away from Julio's building armed with sixty rocks in one pocket, forty in the other and his Nextel flip phone. He then got out and stuck his gun securely behind his back in his waistband.

It was two am. Prime time on a payday, Friday night. The Manchester cops were cruising hard. Blue lights were flashing brightly down the street. Another unlucky crack head on his way out of town with a mouthful of rocks.

Lucky set the car alarm on the key remote and started walking rapidly before he suddenly halted. Every hair on his neck stood up. He glanced around. Something wasn't right, it was very, very strange the feeling that came over him as he tried to identify the source. *What the hell?*

Nothing.

His adrenaline was really flowing and all of a sudden something told him he needed to move so he shook off the bad feeling. Maybe I'm just paranoid he thought. He accelerated his pace determined to make it into Julio's building which he knew would be loaded down with money grubbing addicts looking to score some good shit.

He loitered letting a slow cruising shit box pass by before he crossed the street to Julio's side.

"Hey man you gotta light?" a dude asked harmlessly clutching an unlit cigarette between his lips.

Lucky hesitated then pulled out his bic lighter. Just as he lit the guy's smoke he sensed it. Movement behind him. He started to swing around when someone smashed him solidly in the back of the head with some type of pipe knocking him forward awkwardly into the cigarette guy who suddenly drilled Lucky in the face with a pair of brass knuckles breaking his nose and mouth.

They were on him like flys on shit. Five crazied drug addicts closed in for the kill. Dazed and confused Lucky tried to frantically block the blows using the eight point blocking system he had studied over and over in martial arts training at Body Works in Concord.

The wooden Louisville slugger smashed him in the ribs crippling him while another thug spun a bicycle chain wildly hitting him in the back and arms.

Falling hard he met the sidewalk angrily spraining his wrist. The bat struck again bashing his left knee cap driving him into a wild frenzy. Again they moved in for the kill. "Fuck," he swore spitting out a mouthful of blood.

Furiously he sat up on the sidewalk and fired off a vicious punch into the closest creep's family jewels instantly disabling him. *Take that asshole.*

The gorilla with the Louisville slugger took a home run swing broadcasting it, Lucky rolled out of the way and eyed an opening out of his one good eye, timing it perfectly he snapped out a powerful side blade karate kick into the gorilla's knee sending him crawling away, howling in pain he dropped the bat clutching his shattered knee cap. *Bastard.*

As Lucky turned on the ground a bicycle chain struck him hard across the ear and face ripping him wide open slamming him onto his back. Stunned he somehow knew he needed to move or he was going to die. That's when he felt it digging into his lower back. A sudden surge of hope raced through him as he whipped out his gun still on the ground screaming wildly, "Come on mother fucker, come on," he yelled waving his gun trying to focus.

One punk with a long metal pipe made a jerky motion from the side and tried to knock the pistol free. At the last second Lucky turned and fired blasting the pipe wielding punk in the thigh freezing everyone.

"Get the fuck outta here now," Lucky demanded ready to shoot the next one who made a move towards him. "Go on, get the fuck out of here, right now," he said again. Hesitating, hearing the sirens they dropped their weapons (and grabbed their shot amigo, and disappeared down an alleyway.

FIFTY FOUR

HIS ADRENALINE WAS maxed out. He started to shake violently knowing he was about to go into shock. That's when he realized how badly he was injured.

The loud siren getting closer forced him to his feet. Clumsily he stumbled in pain towards Julio's crib as fast as humanly possible with his shattered knee. Inside running on empty, he limped up the three long flights of stairs dripping a steady stream of blood still clutching his gun in a death grip with both hands.

Dizzy, winded, and very confused, he pounded on the solid door with his gun, listening to the sirens getting closer and closer. "Open the fuck up," he yelled desperately.

Julio's thug Kickstand who also went by Pitbull opened the door and saw the gun then eyed Lucky's battered and desperate looking face and threw up his arms as if to say don't shoot man!

"Oh my God, what the hell happened Lucky? Shit man you're really fucked up man," Julio whined, helping Lucky to the battered sofa.

Lucky delirious whispered, "Hey you need some rocks?"

"Jesus Lucky you don't quit, who the fuck did this shit, you recognize 'em?"

He shook his head no. "There was five of them, I think," he whispered still clutching his gun. Awkwardly he pulled out his Nextel phone and hit speed dial surprised it still worked after getting whacked with the bat.

The house was full of crack addicts who all looked on in horror till Julio yelled, "Get me a damn towel man, get me a fuckin' towel." Nervously he held it on Lucky's face to try and stop the bleeding. "Man you need to go to a hospital Lucky. This is bad, real bad."

Lucky turned his head looking around with his one good eye and saw everyone was gawking at him. "Mother fucking' good for nothin' junkies," he wailed. "Get the fuck back," he screamed waving his gun violently.

"Easy…easy…bro…these guys didn't do nothin'…hey Pitbull watch the back will ya…no one comes or goes," Julio cried out scared.

Lucky was losing it, the room was spinning just as the police sirens stopped right out front. His phone vibrated against his leg and Romeo asked him what the hell was up with the 911 page.

"Man you gotta come get me, I'm…I'm…really…fucked up bro," he sighed.

"What happened?"

"I got jumped outside Julio's place by five armed dudes and I uh shot one of them."

"Shit – what the fuck are you doin' over there gringo with them low lifes bro? You know you're on King's turf man and the pigs are cruisin' hard over that gun shot, shit sit tight, we're coming." *Damn you Lucky.*

"Hurry Romeo."

"Hey Julio, you got any green?" he asked slapping down a baggie full of sixty twenty-dollar rocks.

The room went silent. All the crack heads stared at the big baggy of crack drooling." Fill me a hit Julio," Lucky demanded still clutching his gun in defense as he pointed at someone's stem left on the table.

Julio hesitated shaking his head. "Man, are you sure?"

"Just do it."

Lucky took a big hit of crack in his bloody mouth then exhaled a large cloud of the devil's smoke. His head spun out of control while Julio lit him a Marlboro light and stuck it in between his bloody lips trembling.

"Five minute crack sale to pay my fuckin' hospital bill," Lucky cried out crazily, "Only five fuckin dollars a rock, line up and pay Julio."

Julio pissed realizing all the money he was losing collected the drug money and doled out rocks till they were all gone and he had three hundred in fives and tens.

Lucky pulled out the second baggie with forty rocks. There was still a handful of jonesing addicts who were so broke they couldn't get in on the sale. For some reason Lucky felt sorry for them because everyone else was busy packing their stems. "Call them all over here," he mumbled to Pitbull pointing at the have not's.

They all scuttled over nervously ogling the loaded baggy and eyeing the gun. "Take one each," he ordered watching them. Then he gave Pitbull two. "There's thirty-two left Julio, you got a buck-fifty?"

Julio snatched the baggy and disappeared into his bedroom. Seconds later he handed Lucky the money.

Romeo only lived a few blocks away. He showed up with his giant Columbian cousin known as Baby Boy. Both were packing heat and looking seriously pissed off. Julio looked up skittishly while Pitbull backed off nervously. Romeo slammed the reinforced door shut with his large ten millimeter glock.

"What the fuck," he bellowed staring at Lucky's face very concerned. "Jesus Christ gringo, you got it good."

Angrily he looked around. "Who the fuck did this shit?" he screamed waving the big gun recklessly. "Five hundred dollar rock for a name...only need one fuckin' name and it's all yours," he stated firmly holding up a big boulder of crack.

Everybody froze eyeballing the boulder wishing they had the name he wanted. "Julio knows how to get a hold of me," Romeo told everyone taking Lucky's gun from him and sticking it in his waistband. "Come on gringo, let's go get you fixed up." *Man you're really fucked up.*

Romeo nodded at Baby Boy who lifted Lucky carefully off the blood stained couch. "You're fuckin' welcome," Lucky added. "And I'll double that reward," he challenged as he went out the door, delirious.

Baby Boy, a 6 foot 5 inch, 270lb behemoth carried Lucky easily down the three flights of stairs while Romeo led the way with his glock in plain view, very aware they were trespassing on Northern King's turf.

"Shit you sure did shoot the motherfucker," Romeo pointed out when they passed all the blood on the sidewalk. Even Lucky tried to grin nodding hoping the asshole was in a lot of pain.

They drove him to Manchester General Emergency Room where Lucky was immediately escorted into a wheelchair and taken straight to the back. They stitched up his face, his lips, his ear, and the back of his hand. The doctor was very concerned about the swollen welts to the back of his head and ordered x-rays to check for internal bleeding. After a resident sewed up his elbow and bandaged his damaged left hand, the doctor came back in clutching some x-rays. He told him he had a concussion and they would be admitting him for the night.

When the doctor started asking him detailed questions about the obvious assault, Lucky just waved him off in too much pain to listen. Minutes later Lucky heard him on the phone talking to the police about his assault. He didn't like what he was hearing and he knew it was time to go. Slowly he pulled on his bloody shirt.

Cautiously he weaved his way towards the exit clutching the doctor's clipboard. He stopped at the check out desk and dropped three hundred dollars in drug money on top of his chart that he yanked off the end of his bed. "Bill me if it's more," he muttered limping out of the emergency room door.

Romeo and Baby Boy were still sitting in their caddy arguing about something as Lucky very painfully climbed into the back seat and collapsed in agony. "Let's go man," he growled. "The fuckin' doctor called the cops – can you believe that shit?"

They pulled out of the big parking lot just as a cruiser passed by up to the emergency room entrance.

"Damn that was cutting it too close," Lucky groaned knowing they would have his name within a few minutes. *I'm screwed.*

FIFTY FIVE

THEY TOOK HIM back to Romeo's. While Big Boy carried him up the four flights of steep stairs, Romeo drove the Mustang back onto his turf.

"Oh my God Lucky, what the hell happened?" Sasha cried out shocked. "Who did this to you? Romeo, my God Romeo, you gotta find out who did this shit."

Romeo eyed her, never seeing her this mad, he continued to rap with Baby Boy. "Me and Baby Boy are gonna walk the hood," he told them setting Lucky's nine on the coffee table. "You sit tight with Sasha...and don't answer the door for nobody but us...I got eyes watching."

"I ain't goin' nowhere," he moaned. "Hey Romeo get my backpack out of the Mustang, it's got all my shit in it...and I don't need it ripped off." *Man this sucks.*

"Already got it bro...chill," he said pointing at his pack.

* * *

Once they left, Sasha fussed all over him giving him a cold beer with a flexi straw because his mouth was so swollen. He washed down two Darvocets she gave him to help ease the pain.

She wanted him to explain everything while she tried to soothe him. Confused, he tried to recall what the hell happened, and even beat up and extremely sore he couldn't help think about the wild sex he shared with the beautiful, oh so close young Sasha. She looked so hot even through one blurry eye. I'm *dreaming again.*

"Jesus Lucky, I can't believe that gun fire was you – what the hell were you doing with scum like Julio?"

"He didn't do it, it was some other punks."

"Poor baby. Don't worry, if they're still around, they'll find 'em. Especially since you shot one of them, news travels fast around here," she laughed trying to cheer him up.

He nodded off on the couch trying to forget the nightmare. The next thing his brain registered was far far away. A tiny voice called out to him, "Wake up…Hey Lucky, wake up gringo." His mind panicked but his body wouldn't move. He felt tied down. Cautiously he opened his one good eye and tried to focus on the pillow. Confused he tried to sit up and figure out where the hell he was.

"Don't get up gringo…relax," a familiar voice said.

"Okay," he whispered back. *"I can't fuckin move anyway."*

Painfully he turned his bandaged face towards the voice. Baby Boy had a crack head in a full nelson whose face had obviously suffered some serious blows.

"Is this one of the scumbags who jumped you?" Romeo asked him.

Lucky knew right away that it was the guy who asked him for a light and punched him in the face with brass knuckles shattering his nose and mouth. He nodded, "Yup, he punched me in my shit with brass knuckles."

Baby Boy tightened his deathly grip lifting the punk a foot off the floor while he struggled to break free. Romeo turned and struck a vicious blow into the scumbags gut knocking the wind out of him.

Baby Boy stood him up again while Romeo hammered him in the face with leather gloves that had small steel spikes covering his knuckles. His face ripped and spurted blood as Romeo threw jab after jab into his splattered face.

Then Romeo patted down the punk's many pockets and found what he was looking for. His brass knuckles. "Look what I found," Romeo smirked sliding them on his right fingers, he rapidly drilled him in his exposed rib cage causing him to cry out.

Romeo repeatedly bitch slapped him in the face. "Now motherfucker you're gonna talk or I'll break every finger you got one at a time," he scowled grabbing the punk's hand and one finger with his other hand.

"Who are your partners huh?" he demanded.

"Oh man," he cried out pouting, "if I tell you I'm a dead man."

"If you don't, you're a dead man anyway scumbag," Romeo growled bending his middle finger back till it made an awful crunching, snapping sound.

"Stop, stop please," he begged as tears flowed down his bloody face. "Okay – okay, it was me, Blacky, Razor Red, and the twins," he spit out all at once hoping they'd let him go.

But not a chance. Romeo grabbed the wrenched middle finger and squeezed. "Why amigo – why? And don't spin no bullshit, give it to me straight."

He began mumbling with his eyes clenched shut in distress. "Man, some dude gave us each a fifty piece of crack to jump that dude and another fifty when we found him. We been waitin' three days."

"Who?" he yelled. "Who paid you motha fucka?"

"Man no way, no way dude I can't tell, please," he begged.

Romeo grinned at Lucky. "No problemo fuckboy," Romeo laughed evily grabbing his pinky, he snapped it like a popsicle stick. The hood howled and started to pass out so Romeo grabbed Lucky's ice water and dumped it over his head.

"Wake the fuck up shit for brains," he challenged slamming him in the ribs again and again.

"Name the bitch, I want the name. Don't fuck with me," he said stepping back angrily so he could kick him hard in the balls. After the wicked steel toed boot landed, Baby Boy slammed him powerfully onto the hardwood floor laughing.

He curled up in a ball holding his testicles screaming in pain. "Shut da fuck up," Big Boy demanded kicking him hard in the back with his size fifteen steel toed Army Ranger boots.

"Get the fuck up."

"No…no…no…let me be," he belly ached. "Please."

"Last chance – what's the name?" Romeo ordered, nodding at Baby Boy who looked like he was winding up to kick a soccer ball on a sandlot in his native Columbia. Instead, it landed solidly into his mouth, breaking teeth, which instantly got the punk's attention away from his swollen testicles, blood went everywhere.

"Hector man, Hector," he mumbled sobbing.

"That's what I thought," Romeo said satisfied. "Tie em and gag em and put his sorry ass in the back room so we can go check out this piece of shit's story."

Baby Boy hog tied him with Home Depot duct tape and stuffed an old smelly sock in his bloody mouth using more duct tape to secure it. He also taped his eyes shut, then smiled at his handiwork dropping him on the back bedroom floor with a wicked thud.

"Keep an eye on him Sasha, me and Baby Boy got some people to check out. We be back."

*   *   *

Thirty minutes later, they showed back up with a third Columbian and two familiar scumbags in tow.

Baby Boy had his luger stuck to the side of one of the evil twin's heads. Lucky and Sasha had done a small bump while they were gone, so now he was more awake for the entertainment.

The twins eye was swollen totally shut. Romeo looked at him for the confirmation nod holding the two battered riff-raff out in front of him.

Through his swollen mouth and puffy lips he angrily responded wishing he could get off the couch. "Yup, these two fuckers beat me with a bat and chain."

"Oh really...well now, payback's a bitch," Romeo said sarcastically nodding to his cousin who immediately smashed his luger into the twin's head knocking him out cold. With a solid thud, he tumbled to the hard floor making no attempt to break his fall.

The other twin threw a wild punch grazing Romeo's ear. Bad mistake. A trickle of blood ran down from Romeo's ear from the twin's razor sharp nails. Romeo lost all control and quickly slid on his new toy, brass knuckles. "Fuck boy, now you're really gonna pay," he hollered wildly as all three Columbians moved in for the kill.

The two Columbians grabbed his arms while Romeo crushed his nose in with the deadly brass knuckles. His second punch broke off three front teeth while the third and fourth cracked ribs.

They switched places . Baby Boy hit him with sledgehammer sized fists so hard Lucky swore he heard the guy's jaw bone break in two. Just warming up, he threw a wicked combination of crushing punches blooding both eyes and flattening his nose like a pancake. Even animal Mike Tyson would have been proud of his last punch, a vicious upper cut lifting him a foot off the floor, knocking him out cold.

Romeo in a frenzy started in on the other twin kicking him solidly in his unconscious face, then into his ribs. "Motha fuckin' street scum," he yelled continuing to really hurt the unresponding punk.

Sasha screamed breaking his trance. "That's enough Romeo. Don't kill 'em, we don't need that shit."

Romeo took a deep breath and spit in the punk's face. "Hog tie 'em, put 'em in the back," he ordered.

An hour later, the Columbians found Razor Red at Julio's smoking lovely. They dragged Julio and Razor Red along against their will. Razor Red was severely beaten by the time they returned to Lucky and Sasha.

"Julio's got somethin' to say Lucky…Don't you Julio…you piece of shit," Romeo shouted, slamming him in the gut while Baby Boy easily held him off the floor in a full nelson.

Once Julio got his breath back he talked willingly. He told Lucky about Hector's visit the week before, and how Hector beat him up till he told him where he was getting the grade A crack from.

But he adamantly denied knowing anything about Lucky getting jumped. Then Razor Red who was lying on the floor in pain muttered "No man, he didn't know nothin."

Razor Red told them that Blacky, the fifth scumbag Lucky shot in the leg went to some hospital so they let him be. Razor Red had no problem selling out. "Yup, I helped Hector set up the jump on Lucky, but I don't know why he wanted it done," he shrugged covered in dried blood.

Stunned, Lucky looked on. They dragged both of them into the back bedroom to join the others.

The three Columbians sat down with beers bringing one for Lucky with a straw. "Well that's all of 'em Lucky. I told you we'd take care of it," Romeo grinned satisfied, eyeing Baby Boy, who hardly ever showed any emotion.

Painfully Lucky raised his beer in a job well done toast. "Thanks guys, that meant a lot," he told them opening his pack and pulling out a wad of green money.

He gingerly counted out three stacks of a grand a piece and tried to give it to them. "Here bro, thanks man," he said sincerely pushing a pile towards Baby Boy.

"No man, you be Romeo's homeboy. No money," the big brute replied shaking his head holding up his enormous hand in refusal.

But Lucky refused to take no for an answer. "Take it please. Believe me it was well worth it," he grinned awkwardly out the side of his mouth.

The two Columbians looked to Romeo their obvious leader who eyed Lucky, then nodded yes. They scooped up the cash immediately and smiled at Lucky. *Never hurt to have friends in this neighborhood.*

FIFTY SIX

THE MANCHESTER POLICE had got Sullivan's name and information from the doctor at Manchester General Emergency Room. Willingly, the cops decided to find out how Mr. Sullivan was assaulted, and why he snuck out of the hospital against the doctor's advice.

They also noted a Spanish male was treated for a gunshot wound at Manchester General's sister hospital, Brown Hill Hospital and also disappeared under similar circumstances at about the same time as Sullivan vanished.

The following morning the oncoming shift Sgt. spotted Sullivan's file flagged in red. Meaning it needed to be reviewed by a supervisor. Once he read the doctor's report, he immediately picked up the phone. "Hey Lt. Brooks, I got something interesting for you on your boy, Lucky Sullivan. Last night, he paid Manchester General a visit. Listen to this, apparently he was assaulted by multiple suspects and had numerous injuries. The doctor tried to keep him overnight, but he vanished when the doctor called the police."

"Oh really?"

"Also over at Brown Hill Hospital, some punk was dumped off with a gunshot wound to the thigh at about the same time. I don't know if they're related, but they could be, and he also disappeared."

"Can you fax everything over to me?"

"Sure, no problem sir."

"Hey Sgt., I appreciate the heads up."

"If I find out anything else, I'll make sure you get it okay."

"Thanks, I won't forget it." *Now Lucky, what've you been up to?*

*   *   *

When he finally stirred on Romeo's old divan he was so battered and bruised he couldn't get up to relieve himself.

Now he knew he had to get up or he was going to piss his pants. But when he went to stand up his left leg collapsed. Angry and frustrated, he looked down and saw his left knee was four times the size of his right knee. "Shit," he muttered irritated knowing his bladder was about to explode. He balanced himself on his right leg and clumsily hopped to the bathroom clutching his cracked ribs in pain.

The toilet never looked so good. He finished relieving himself, and when he looked at himself in the bathroom mirror, he didn't recognize himself. His left eye was completely swollen shut and was turning black and blue. His swollen nose was caked with dried blood. "Man oh man, they really fucked me up," he mumbled eyeing the bloody gauze bandage the hospital nurse used to wrap up his head and face to cover the stitches and wounds making him look like a war victim.

"Holy shit," he whispered seeing all the blood stains on his shirt. On his way back he couldn't resist taking a peek into the back bedroom and leer at the five bodies still hog tied miserably sprawled all over the floor. The room smelled like urine and bad body odor. A couple of the uninvited occupants squirmed hearing the squeaky door open. Someone tried to speak.

"Huh…I can't understand you…speak up," he giggled slamming the door heading back to the couch.

"Fuckin' assholes," he muttered.

He sat there miserable, thinking what the hell had he got himself involved in. He really wanted to leave right away but he knew he couldn't drive a stick shift. Especially the Mustang with the heavy duty after market clutch plate. So he called Ryan and told him to come trade demos with him.

Thirty minutes later, Baby Boy literally carried Lucky down the dangerous steep four flights of stairs to the street where he helped him climb into Ryan's Bonneville. Lucky asked the Columbians what they were gonna do with all the trash in the back room.

"Oh well, we're gonna let 'em go after each go one more round with Clubber Lang," Romeo said smiling as he put his arm on Baby Boy's shoulder. "They need to feel your pain bro, hey you gonna be okay to drive? Cause we'll take you."

"I think I can make it, thanks guys, you've done enough."

"Hey get some rest, I'll look into this Hector shit, but he's real bad news, so we gotta move slow."

"Good, appreciate it, just don't get fucked up over it." *Like me.*

"Nope, not us. But we're gonna find out why. Cause it's more than you servin' dope to Julio in his turf." I know why Lucky wanted to say.

Ryan was horrified and barely recognized him. But he was a bit intimidated around the Columbians so he didn't ask. Lucky told him he'd tell him everything later.

His first stop was Maribeth's Apothecary shop. He pulled the big Bonneville right up on the sidewalk stopping directly in the front of the main doors. The owner inside leered out the window and once she saw his battered bandaged face, she quickly came outside to help.

The owner, Maribeth, a registered nurse, told him to stay in the car while she wrote down everything he needed, and went back inside to fit him for crutches, plus fill the prescription he swiped off the doctor's clipboard, Tylenol fours with codeine. While he watched the pleasant looking owner go back inside, he moved the big car back into a parking space.

Ten minutes passed before Maribeth came back outside with adjustable metal crutches and a large bag full of bandages, gauze tape, medical tape, two types of antiseptic, and most importantly, his prescription. He thanked her immensely giving her a big tip, and wondered why he could never meet a good looking brainy chick like Maribeth.

He drove over to Laura's condo and very, very slowly he crutched his way to her door clutching the apothecary shopping bag and his backpack loaded with money.

"Who is it?" Laura asked as Taffy barked ferociously.

"Lucky?"

Unsure, she opened the door a crack and was shocked by what she saw. "Oh my God, what happened? ...come in...come in," she sighed heavily helping him to the couch. "Okay now what the hell happened?"

"I got attacked last night by five dudes."

"Are you okay? You look awful. Damn you, I've been so worried about you even though I'm mad as hell...I still love you, you know," she said very concerned.

He felt like crying, "I know – I just fuck everything up, don't I?"

"Yes, yes you do. So tell me who did this, some guys trying to rob you?"

"Who knows," he whined. "It seems like it's connected somehow to the car chase. Payback I guess, I just don't know anymore." *I'm in over my head.*

"Ssshh, it's okay, you're still alive, calm down," she said trying to get him to relax a little.

"I guess I just wanted to say I'm sorry in case I don't get another chance, you know? I guess if it's okay with you I'd like to stay here today because I can barely drive and I'm pretty messed up." *Inside and out.*

She eyed him compassionately. "Yes you can stay but no drugs Lucky or I'll blacken your other eye. Now let's get you cleaned up and somewhat comfortable," she said taking charge, cutting off his bloody shirt with scissors. Carefully she gave him a nice sponge bath and then filled the two ice packs conveniently provided in the apothecary bag. She then brought in pillows and sheets. "You poor thing, your face looks just awful."

He went over his injuries with her while she made him one of his favorite lunches, grilled cheese and Lay's potato chips. He swallowed two Tylenol fours with an ice cold Coca-Cola Classic through another straw.

While they watched an old John Wayne western on her VCR, he nodded off until his cell phone rang waking him up. Irritably he answered it, "Hello?"

It was the last person he wanted to talk to, Lt. Tom Brooks.

FIFTY SEVEN

"LUCKY I NEED to see you today," he demanded firmly. "I know what happened to you last night. You and I need to talk now, so where are you?"

"Lt. can't this wait; I'm in no condition to go anywhere."

"I'll come to you, where are you?"

"Hold on," he said covering the phone with his hand he asked Laura if it was okay if Lt. Brooks stopped by.

"Of course it is."

Thirty minutes later New Hampshire State Trooper Lt. Tom Brooks knocked on her door.

"Come in sir," Laura offered nicely.

"Jesus Lucky, my God they really got you this time," he said shaking his head disgusted. "You should've stayed in the hospital like the doctor wanted."

Laura heard what he said and looked over at Lucky with daggers. "We're going for a walk," she declared as Taffy came in the room with his leash.

"Have a seat Lt., you wanna coke?"

"Sure."

"There in the fridge, help yourself and grab me one if you don't mind."

They watched the Red Sox and Yankees battle it out on the TV. Bottom of the ninth, two strikes, two outs, everyone was on their feet when Manny Ramirez hit a towering home run over the green monster in glorious Fenway Park. The crowd went ballistic, the TV flashed Red Sox 7 Yankees 6 Final.

He sipped through his flexi-straw and waited for him to start with his accusations.

"Listen Lucky, I know it was you driving the Trans Am in the deadly car chase and I can prove it," he said raising his hand to cut off any reply.

"Before you respond you better hear me out. At this point I could charge you with felony fleeing and alluding and possibly vehicular manslaughter…but I'm not."

Lucky listened carefully and waited for the bomb to drop. *And why is that Lt.?*

"Now I talked with the D.A. who agreed with me that if you decide to cooperate with us he will overlook hundred and eighty mile an hour reckless driving habit because there's a lot more at stake," he said evenly watching Lucky light up a Marlboro Light.

"So I don't know what you know about stolen 'Vettes or Florida cocaine shipments, but what I'm going to tell you is strictly between us," he said seriously. "Because people's lives are at stake including your own and if I think for a second you're not being straight with me I'll lock you up for your own protection. Now I need you to tell me the truth about last night. What the hell happened?"

Fat chance, man this sucks the big one.
Shit my gun is in the bedroom with all that cash.
Smart move, idiot.
Man get rid of it, ASAP.

"So tell me what happened and I want to know who was behind it Lucky and listen, I already know about your cocaine habit so be straight with me. Don't play games Lucky, things are getting violent."

That's for sure. "Well I got jumped by five guys late last night. I got a few licks in, but they had weapons, a bat, chain, pipes, and stuff so I got the worst end of it." *At least the first round.*

"You think it was robbery motivated?"

Unsure how to answer Lucky hesitated. "Yeah, I thought it was at first, but then I also found out early this morning that they were paid to jump me."

"Really. That's what I suspected, but I needed to hear it from you. So who paid 'em?" *Come on you can tell me.*

The moment of truth, should I tell him?

Fuck it. "The guy's name is Hector. I guess he's a real bad ass Northern King gang leader, who deals a lot of drugs to half of Manchester, and somehow he's tied in with the old man," Lucky said quickly, glad to get it off his chest, hoping he didn't say too much.

Lt. Brooks nodded pleased. "Lucky, this scumbag Hector is seriously bad news, and he is connected to the old man," he said. "First I think the car chase was a set-up to seriously hurt you and secondly I think last night was a stronger message by the looks of you."

He listened carefully to what the Lt. was telling him and he realized his life was falling apart. "Yes, you're probably right sir, but there isn't much I can do about it in my sorry condition," he pouted depressed.

"We don't want you to do anything. Just be straight with me because we're in the process of building a strong case against Hector and the old man."

"What a fuckin' mess Lt."

"So you heard that ten 'Vettes were stolen last week at City Corvette?"

"Yup, I heard about it," he replied nonchalantly.

"He put in an insurance claim for a quarter of a million; you know anything I should know?"

No I don't know shit, he thought feeling guilty, then he tried not to respond defensively. "No sir. I can't say I'm not glad about it, but I've got over three-hundred cars and trucks to use, besides I don't steal cars, I only sell 'em," he joked sarcastically.

"Right, okay, but just for the record where were you last Tuesday evening?"

Hiding at my parents… "Um let's see, last Tuesday…oh yeah, I think um it was Tuesday night that I took my parents out to dinner at the Lobster Pool in Loudon and then I spent the night in Bow with my parents," he replied smoothly. "But you can always check with them, I'm sure they'd be thrilled to verify my alibi."

He was jotting information down in his notebook. "No I don't think that'll be necessary at this point, mainly because I don't think you'd be stupid enough to steal ten corvettes." *You're right!*

Lucky nodded in agreement.

"Now about Hector Santiago. You sure he ordered this assault?"

"Damn straight sir, that much I do know, I just hope I get the pleasure to pay him back in person once I'm feeling a little better." *I'll kick his Northern King ass.*

"No you don't, we'll do all the paying back, understand?" He wanted to ask him about the gun shot victim that arrived at the other hospital within minutes of Lucky's arrival across town. But he didn't want him to clam up now that he had him talking.

"Okay Lucky, one last question," he asked sternly draining his Coke can. "What do you know about cocaine shipments?"

Lucky shook his head no.
Oh sure I got seven kilos buried in my barn.
And fifty grand cash under my rug.
Lt., my dirty gun and eighteen grand are in the bedroom.

"Nothing sir."

"Well, the word on the streets from our snitches is someone ripped off a ten kilo shipment that came up from Florida inside a 'Vette on a car carrier. And supposedly Hector, Mr. Big Shot himself moves all the dope so the old man keeps his hands clean. According to my snitches, some of this high test cocaine is now hitting the streets here in Manchester and Hector is going crazy trying to find the source." *Boy oh boy this guy's sharp, too sharp.*

Lucky nodded. "Yup that makes sense. I know the old man's got his two million dollar yacht, the FAST LADY down in Palm Beach somewhere, and I know he buys a lot of 'Vettes at the auto auction in Orlando and ships them up regularly. So it would be easy enough to throw a few keys in the back of a 'Vette and ship it up on a loaded car carrier." *So bust his ass.*

"Yes Lucky, what you said make a lot of sense doesn't it? When you put it like that I think that's exactly what's going on!" *Now what else do you know?*

"They're expecting another shipment of 'Vettes anytime so we're gonna nail their asses," he said strongly standing up to pace. "So what I need from you is for you to lay low and stay the hell out of the way," he ordered, concerned hoping he was making the right decision. "There's a lot more people involved in all this than I can tell you, but you need to call me right away if you hear anything, anything at all. Your life might depend on it."

"I can do that." *Yes, bust his ass.*

He stopped concerned. "Are you staying here?"

"No – no I have my own place up on a farm in Hillbro and only two people have been there, so I should be pretty safe, besides I can shoot lights out," he grinned.

The Lt. almost asked but didn't. "Yeah well, just be careful whose lights you're shooting out," he warned.

"Besides I don't think I'll be going to work for awhile," he said eyeing his swollen knee cap.

"No…no…you can't work like that. You need me to call work and let them know you were assaulted, would that help?"

"Sure if you'll call the dealership tomorrow morning."

"I'll do that. All I ask is you play it straight with me the rest of the way. This is no longer a game Lucky, these guys mean business." *Yeah, no shit, just look at me.*

The Lt. threw his empty Coke can away. "We're gonna take Hector down hard, but we're waiting for the next shipment so we can catch him dirty, so just lay low, stay alive, and get better okay? Whatever the hell you do, stay out of Westborough."

He started for the door. "Hey do you still have my number?"

Lucky nodded waiting for him to finally leave.

"Hey Lucky get off that shit, really if you need any help just ask. You come from a very nice family and your parents would be highly pissed if they knew what the hell you've been up to, and you know it."

Ain't that the truth. "Okay Lt. I'll stay in touch," he responded sincerely.

FIFTY EIGHT

JUST WHEN HE started to nod out again his phone rang. It was Ryan who had to know what happened. Lucky stuck to the truth as much as possible. "Dude I got mugged by five crazy guys. They had a bat, a chain, and clubs so that's why I look so fuckin' bad."

"Shit man, you're lucky they didn't kill you. You gonna be able to work?"

"Fuck no…you saaw me…I'm on crutches and my face looks like shit. I'd probably scare away all the customers," he chuckled lightly downing another pain pill.

"If you need anything at all just call. I'll stop by after work tomorrow and cook you dinner okay?"

"Okay. Thanks Ryan. Later."

*   *   *

He spent the night with Laura and she willingly changed the gauze bandage on his head and face before she left for work.

He drove up slowly to Hillbro and decided to swing by the dealership before heading out to the farm. Thankfully one of the brothers was getting out of his old Chevy pick up when Lucky pulled up beside him.

"Holy cow Lucky, you alright?" he asked, stepping up to the driver's window concerned. "What the hell happened?"

"I got mugged late Friday night by five guys in Manchester. They had a bunch of crude weapons, but I'll be okay sir, I just need some time off to rest. I look and feel like shit."

"What did they do, rob you?"

Lucky nodded looking down at his swollen knee.

"You take care, as long as you need. We'll be okay, and don't you worry, we take care of our own, you'll still draw your full salary."

Oh boy... "Thank you sir. Maybe I'll be able to walk later in the week. Oh and a Lt. Frank Brooks from the state police will be calling you this morning about my assault. He's the one investigating it. But since I was on my way home from Manchester, I wanted to see you face to face so you'd know."

"I'm glad you did. Now, go get some rest and that's an order. Ryan's got your cell number if we need to reach you, right?"

"Yes sir."

Lucky eased the big Bonneville through the back rutted cow field entrance scraping the underbelly repeatedly on the uneven two tire track path. He knew he didn't want to struggle up the demanding two flights of wooden stairs to get to his apartment from the farmer's main driveway. So he creeped up very slowly to the back of the barn level with his Webber grill and sliding glass door leading to his living room.

Painfully he threw his backpack over one shoulder and also grabbed the apothecary shop bag in the other hand ineptly crutching his way to the back door. Once inside he dropped his cumbersome packages on the couch. Without any hesitations the first thing he did was call his best friend Lung who just happened to be taking the day off from work to finish a few projects around the old carriage house his dad left him. After listening to Lucky's sad story, he hopped on his bad ass black Ninja 900 and flew up to Hillbro.

Lucky and Lung were still very tight even though they didn't hang out like they use to in high school playing football, chasing women, and doing drugs.

He heard the bike's modified racing pipe long before it arrived. It sounded like he was pushing it, which he probably was. Lung pulled the glossy black bike up to the back porch with no helmet or shirt on.

His hair was obviously spiked back from all the excessive speed and his muscles were ripped and glistening with suntan oil. Seven years out of high school and he still looked like he could bench 400lbs.all day.

Lucky sat on the couch and waited feeling a little better already knowing his buddy was there. When Lung stuck his head in the slider he shook his head silently at what he saw. Lucky was propped up on the couch, a daytime soap, his mother's favorite "Days of Our Lives" intro song blasted from the TV. How appropriate, feeling like shit he was drinking a potent absolute screwdriver.

"Man oh man you don't look so hot. What husband caught you in bed with his old lady?" Lung asked seriously eyeing the baretta on the coffee table and the shotgun close by.

"Is that the piece you shot the dude with?"

"Nope that one's in the Merrimack River," he grinned proudly, glad he'd been smart enough to toss the evidence. Quickly he popped two more pills, this time opting for percocets that Sasha had also provided.

Lung hated crack with a passion, but finally agreed to help Lucky bag up three hundred twenty dollar rocks so he could unload them. Halfway through they stopped to smoke a joint and cook up two twenty ounce T-Bones on the Webber. They bullshitted while the baked potatoes, specially prepared roasted in the pre-heated oven. Both talented cooks, Lung washed the two choice Russett bakers and rolled them in light vegetable oil. Slick with oil, he rolled the potatoes in a mixture of salt, crushed black pepper, and garlic salt. With the oven preheated to 350°. Lung set the taters right on the middle rack setting the timer for twenty minutes. You couldn't help but devour the skin it was so crunchy and delicious.

"Man you're fuckin' crazy rippin' off those dudes, what the hell were you thinking?" Lung said after Lucky told him everything else he'd forgotten on the phone. He trusted Lung with his life and it felt really good to finally tell somebody everything. No matter what, he knew Lung would never ever give him up.

"You know Tats if you really need me, all you gotta do is call, and oh by the way, thanks for the unexpected present on my bike seat," he laughed heartily. "You were right that shit's deadly. You okay now?"

"Yup. Hey you haven't used that nickname in years, Tats. Boy oh by talk about a lot of memories," he mumbled reminiscing about the good old days in his first car with him and Lung cruising Hampton Beach in his 1972 Red Triumph TR4 convertible.

Three hours later at two pm, Lung had finished breaking up three kilos into twenty-eight gram ounces for a total of a hundred and five ounces.

There was a hundred neatly packed ounces in an old YMCA gym bag beside Lucky's bed. The other five ounces Lucky gave to Lung for all his hard work.

Then Lung pulled the living room throw rug back as Lucky instructed and whistled. "Holy shit Tats, you have been busy!"

"Fifty grand in rug padding," Lucky joshed. "Hey Lung there's eighteen grand in my backpack, do me one more favor and spread it out for me."

Lucky watched Lung tediously spread the small bills out thinking about getting rid of all the cocaine and taking a long vacation. He reached over and pulled his black notebook out of his pack, then he was ready to bring it up to date.

After Lung finally split, Lucky reluctantly called Romeo to find out the latest. "Hey Romeo, it's me."

"You okay gringo?"

"Not really, but I'll make it, you got your ears on?"

"I'm listening gringo."

"Things are heating up on my end, you feel me?"

"Ya I hear you."

"And since you and your boys showed me some love I got a deal you can't pass up."

"I'm listening."

"Are you sitting down? A hundred large pizzas with all the same quality toppings at only seven fifty each."

"What! Shit Lucky you got that much weight?"

"Ssshhh of course not. The guy told me it's a going out of business sale."

"Oh now I understand, okay man you got to give me some time, I gotta make some calls to raise that much flow."

"Even better, the guy says twenty-five down and the rest in a week."

"You sure?"

"I just put my face on it, you haven't fucked me yet and I'm giving you a raw deal; I'll take your word."

"True that gringo."

"What's the word on our mutual friend?"

"I'm glad you brought it up. I met with one of his turf dogs, you already know he runs the N-K's around the city?"

"Yeah I heard the same shit on my end, what the hell is that exactly?"

"It's a blood lifer gang gringo. They're a small sister chapter of the Southern Kings out of Daytona Beach, Florida. Anyway once you earn your colors, you're a brother for life. Before all this shit, we had an understandin' until you came along. The deal was they don't fuck with us Columbians and our designated turf, and in return we don't fuck with them or their turf," Romeo paused. "But the word is all deals are off. They know we beat up those punks they paid to beat your ass, but what's got 'em really hot is they now know we got a bee line to a new main source. So now some blood's gonna spill and we be outnumbered six to one."

"Interesting shit." *Time for me to leave town.*

"No just business as usual. And gringo the word is out on the street that you're the bee line to the pure honey and now you're really, really hot."

"How hot?" *Shit they know.*

:Ten grand green and get this, a used 'Vette thrown in."

Lucky exhaled heavily interpreting the street lingo. "Wow I didn't realize I'd become so damn popular."

"Hey don't blame me man, I knew what time it was. A little birdie been signin' excitedly that you been movin' grade A honey on their turf…that you use to be the hot mouthpiece at a place where all the pizzas came up burnt."

Shit time for me to haul ass, I'm in way over my head. "Anything else?"

Romeo continued, "So gringo, we both be stirrin' the pot. You be sellin' premo grade pizzas and me and my boys triplin' deliveries, grabbin' new customers right and left."

He really didn't like what he was hearing, especially being so handicapped. But he really felt Romeo wouldn't sell him out. Not as long as he kept supplying him grade A honey. They were both along for the ride.

"Listen up. Even though they think you be the beekeeper they still don't know where the hive is, so you 'n me need to change things up. No more routine stops, we do everythin' like they be watchin' every second. No slip ups, you feel me?"

"Loud and clear. No more room service deliveries, we meet somewhere else, I'll come up with a place."

"Cool. I'll ring you back as soon as I got my hands on twenty-five large okay? Just stay low and stay away. Adios."

FIFTY NINE

H E LEANED BACK glad his handgun was so close by. It was the same exact Baretta as the one he tossed in the Merrimack River in Bow. He bought them the same time on sale at Riley's Gun Shop in Hooksett. It didn't hurt to flash his Coast Guard petty officer I.D. to get an extra discount. Lucky loved the seventeen shot military model Baretta, the exact same gun he earned his expert service ribbon at the Coast Guard Gun Range on Trumbo Point, Key West Florida.

No way I'm bringing Romeo here, no way no how, he thought trying to digest all he had just heard. An hour later at three pm, Romeo called back.

"Hey gringo, that's a go. Twenty-five on the pizzas. Where we gonna hook-up?"

"Exit one off I-89 Bow exit. Directly across from the Bow Mobil station and Hampton Inn there's a restaurant called the Bow Tavern. Meet me in the parking lot in forty minutes, say three-forty-five."

"Where the fuck's that?"

"Ask Sasha, better yet bring her, she's from Bow," he told him. "I'm driving the same car I left your crib in yesterday."

"Later gringo, I'll be there."

Five minutes later he left his apartment wearing his Oakley sunglasses and his autographed Roger Clemens Red Sox ball cap.

The car was only a few feet away. Carefully he glanced around and spotted his landlord riding his John Deere tractor through the back pasture.

He lugged the six pound bag of cocaine with his good hand, balancing on the crutches. Cautiously he tucked the hollow point loaded

Baretta under the front seat arm rest just as the farmer who saw the crutches pulled up in his tractor and eyed him.

Quickly he shut off the powerful tractor. "Jesus Lucky, what the hell happened to you? You get in a car accident or something?"

"I got mugged in the great city of Manchester, but I'll be okay. Oh sir, by the way, can I get the key to that bad ass lock you got on the slider so I can park here for a while, it would sure make it a lot easier so I don't have to climb those stairs with my crutches?"

"Sure Lucky, I'll leave a key in your mailbox. Just keep using the pasture road in from street. That'll bring you straight up here. In fact I'll knock down that center rut so you don't ruin all your nice cars."

"Thank you sir, I appreciate it, see you later, I gotta run."

"Okay, you need anything just let me know. I see you been eating some of the silver queen corn I grow. What do you think?" he asked firing up his green and yellow pride and joy.

"That corn is the best. Delicious," he yelled waving as the owner pulled off in his expensive tractor.

Lucky drove exactly the speed limit knowing he had enough cocaine to get a long stretch in Concord at the New Hampshire State Prison. Uneventfully, he pulled off exit one, the Bow exit. Nervously he glanced straight ahead only a quarter mile up.

Shit. Right up the street, he thought as he turned left down Logging Hill Road past Jerry's Auto Clinic underneath the interstate where he passed by the on ramp for I-89 North and turned left into the Bow Tavern right on time. He spotted Romeo's Cadillac with its twenty inch gold rims and fat gangsta white walls. Sasha and Romeo watched him pull in without a tail and dressed incognito.

He parked the Bonneville next to the caddy and waited while Romeo got out and came over with a brown paper grocery bag and climbed in.

"Hey Gringo, you still lookin' like shit," he grinned.

"Thanks Romeo, I feel like shit."

"That for me?" he asked pointing at the old YMCA bag Lucky had owned since sixth grade day camp.

Lucky nodded, and Romeo quickly unzipped it and discovered the hidden treasure. Enthusiastically he whistled. "Man oh man, no wonder they want your ass," he kidded closing the bag back up. "There's twenty five large in new big bills in here and I owe you fifty more within a week right?"

"Right," Lucky nodded. They banged fists and Sasha smiled and waved when Romeo climbed back into his caddy.

Forty-five minutes later back at the farm he fished the key left by the landlord in his mailbox and drove back around to a freshly groomed pasture road.

The last thing he remembered before he passed out on his small twin bed was Romeo warning him to watch his ass cause the kings were out for blood.

Exhausted he slept soundly. Dreaming he was back in Key West on a forty-one foot Coast Guard Cutter watching a huge Panamanian registered freighter anchor a half mile off shore from the famous Duval Street. It was late, very late, like two am in the morning.

The Coast Guard boarding team waited impatiently in dark black swat fatigues for the word from the Station Miami Beach who controlled the southeast hotbed known as sector seven for drug intervention. Miami was waiting on word from Washington D.C. who was still waiting on the go ahead from the Panamanian government for permission to board the suspect freighter that was obviously unloading drugs over the side to small boats.

Lucky watched anxiously through the expensive night vision goggles that made the sea calm as small black go-fast cigarettes pulled up rapidly beside the freighter and waterproof packages were quickly lowered over the side by funny looking tiny men who all looked green through the heat sensitive binoculars. It really pissed Lucky off, here they were all eye witnessing the hostile offloading of cocaine and they were the law of the sea, yet they were powerless to stop it.

Boldly the small go-fasts raced off with the devil's powder knowing they could probably catch one of the small boats with customs and Florida marine patrol's help, but all the rest would get away. The idea was to bust the mother ship before too much was offloaded and confiscate the ship.

Suddenly the secure scrambled radio frequency barked, "Hostile boarding approved, go in hot, the Regional Commander in Miami declared also frustrated by the long delay.

The boarding officer, a first class petty officer pointed at Lucky who was immediately ordered F.O.B. (first on board). All six members' M-16As were locked and loaded for three round bursts as the skilled cockswain, a second class boson mate pushed the twin screws to full throttle and at a maximum speed of 28 knots the 41 foot cutter cut ahead on collision course with the big mother ships side. At the last possible second the skilled petty officer swung the cutter sideways jamming both throttles to full reverse.

Quickly the cutter skipped sideways in a nifty maneuver up against the hostile freighter. Full of pent up frustration, Lucky with an adrenaline surge reached out over the dark ocean and latched on to the heavy rope ladder hanging over the side that the tiny green men had used to offload their precious cargo only minutes before.

He never recalled the wild four story night climb up the side of rusted steel hull. It was a moonless night, and up on deck he realized it was totally pitch black. Immediately he dropped to one knee and pulled down his one eye night vision scope over his left eye. Nervously he scanned the dark lifeless catwalks, ladders, and passage ways looking for the tiny green men hiding. His M16A was aimed and ready, he anxiously held point till all six boarding members were on deck. The take down leader pointed at Lucky soundlessly who followed his finger to the first open hatch directly in front of them. Boldly he thought, time to move.

They worked in a standard two man search and secure method taught by many law enforcement agencies worldwide.

It's just that many of the smart tactics implemented weren't feasible for shipboard maneuvers.

The next few minutes were etched in Lucky's memory forever. Moving to the open hatch followed by another boarding team member, he aimed his machine gun down the dark hole. Nothing. Unable to go down the steep steel ladder holding his machine gun he strapped it tightly over his shoulder so it wouldn't bang against anything giving his location away. He mounted the ladder and started down undoing the safety strap on his military issued 9mm Baretta snuggly in it's holster on his police belt. He continued down on the longest journey of his life.

Step after step, deeper and deeper into the evil belly he descended silently, trying to listen for his backup above him and any noise below him. It took every ounce of control not to turn on his six D police battery mag light hanging from his gun belt and shine it into the scary blackness below. But training took over and he knew he'd be a sitting duck unable to fire back with both hands gripped securely on the vertical ladder.

The lower he went, the worse it became.

The feeling of an endless hell with no beginning and no ending. Lower and lower he stepped, thirty feet he thought anxiously...forty feet, he counted the steps. Come on he told himself, you can do it, you're a coasty, fifty feet...sixty feet he estimated. Feeling less and less confident he froze listening for foot falls above him.

Nothing.

The deeper he went the more lonely he became. Seventy feet... eighty feet, shit that's eight stories; I'm four stories below water level he told himself amazed. The only sound was his heartbeat thumping.

*Shit...*He froze knowing he heard movement. What the hell was that? Don't move, find the sound his brain screamed. Close by he could smell a foul odor of saltwater, bilge oil, and body odor.

Fresh, smelly human body odor.

Exhaling slowly he took the next step down landing in ankle deep brackish water. Automatically he crouched down and yanked out his only friend, his 9mm Barettta. Frantically he swung it side to side trying to find a hostile target in the black belly of hell.

Fear of the unknown screamed through his amped up body. Fight it wait for your backup, where the hell is he? Come on hurry the hell up, he impatiently heeded. His night vision was no good, it was too black, then he remembered his night eye still strapped to his head and he pulled it down over his left eye. He scanned back and forth wildly leering at the bay hales and wall of fifty-gallon drums lined up in rows against the bulkhead.

Still nobody came down the ladder.

Movement first to the right. Then he heard it before he saw it, all at once the creepy silence exploded loudly as five fifty-gallon drum lids flew through the air and echoed earsplitting off the steel deck. Rapidly he came to his feet in a combat stance without thinking he watched five tiny green Martians through the one eye night scope pop up out of the lidless drums and start firing little Uzis wildly in every direction.

Scared shitless, Lucky automatically fired back with deadly accuracy, splattering all the tiny green Martian heads. The next memory is a blur. It's like somebody paused the tape. The four bullet holes in his second chance vest sent him crashing backwards into the steel ladder smashing his head, knocking him out cold almost drowning him in four inches of water. The other team member twenty feet above pulled Lucky's face out of the nasty bilge water while he called for help over his radio.

He was back there sweating heavily, then the sound returned louder and louder in his brain. They're coming, they're here he heard his mind scream, wildly he jumped up grabbing his Baretta off the night stand and fired all seventeen rounds into the walk-in closet emptying the clip. Shocked that their were no tiny green men, just a thousand dollars worth of bullet riddled clothes.

Then realizing it was just another bad dream, he was sweating like a pig when he registered the sound was real and it was coming from the front door. Shaking in disbelief he hobbled over to the door to face the tiny green men with another full clip locked and loaded.

"Ryan, Jesus Christ!" *I could've killed you, whew.*

"Holy shit, what the hell are you doing?" he asked scared at what he saw in Lucky's battered eyes. "Who are you shooting at, are you okay?"

Lucky nodded. "Just an old nightmare," he mumbled worn out.

"I'll say, Jesus! Hey I got cold beer and your favorite Micky D's quarter pounder with cheese, extra onion and pickle. Just the way you like it."

Still trembling from his deepest nightmare surfacing, he rinsed his face over and over in the kitchen sink careful to keep his bandages dry.

They ate very quietly. Ryan was very concerned. He'd never seen Lucky so depressed and distraught.

Shit, I got all this fuckin' money and premo coke and I'm still fuckin' miserable, he thought chewing aimlessly eyeing the farmer's cows chewing their cud out in the back pasture.

Ryan interrupted his drifting thoughts. "Hey did you hear about City Corvette getting ripped off?" he asked laughing hysterically.

Lucky grinned thinking about the old man, he took a big swallow of the frosty Budweiser Ryan brought, washing down two more pain killers.

"Oh yeah, I also wrote one deal and got another be-back set up for tomorrow," he bragged proudly. "But shit Lucky, it ain't the same without you around. Pretty damn boring actually."

His gaze and thoughts came back to reality and he narrowed his good eye on Ryan's face. "Good, I'm glad you're doing okay, but it'll be like this for awhile, I'm afraid." *Maybe forever.*

*   *   *

Hector scowled with rage while he listened to his blood brothers tell him how the Columbians were stealing all their customers with grade A white.

"You son of a bitch," Hector screamed violently punching the closest gang member in the face, splitting his lip wide open. Hector turned and leered at Lucky's picture pinned on the clubhouse wall from an old City Corvette advertisement.

"I want that fucker dead, better yet bring his ass to me and I'll personally show you what we do to people who steal our shit," he paused working up a head of steam. "Ten grand cash from the boss, plus a used 'Vette, after we take care of this scumbag, we'll deal with those greasy Columbians. Now go find him and bring him to me."

SIXTY

H E COULDN'T STAND it.
Living in the now, dealing with reality was making him miserable, much more depressed than he had a right to be. His desire to escape the heavy feeling overwhelmed him and he did what only came natural, breaking out a chunk of crack for dessert. They both indulged smoking the demon's drug. After they each did a couple of blasts, Ryan's friendly concerned nature was wearing thin. Lucky threw a chunk at Ryan and told him to hit the road, he needed to rest.

He told Ryan to trade cars leaving him a late model Lincoln Town Car and told him he'd check in at work later on in the week. His rapidly cycling mood swings from super manic to suicidal were increasing in frequency. Lucky's mind ran full steam ahead while his tired broken down body felt lifeless.

Some recent thought triggered it and now all he could think about was his innocent sweet virgin ex-wife that he corrupted into a cocaine loving sex nympho. God did he miss her and he hated himself for what he'd done. Then his mind raced forward like the wind blowing over meadows of tall grass he tried to block out the reality of his beautiful, highly intelligent, second wife and adorable baby girl living down in Palm Beach waiting for him to get his shit together. Knowing that wasn't going to happen any time soon just made his desperation worse.

They had separated a year before because of his inability to deal with reality, straight. Screwing up both life partners really made him feel worthless and very lonely. He did the only thing he had conditioned himself to do when he felt useless. He reached for his favorite girl, the one who never let him down. His crack pipe.

The higher he got, the farther from reality he was, and the worse he felt inside.

He only stopped to chain smoke Marlboro Lights and wipe the sweat off his battered puffy face. By two am, he was afraid to lie down. The little green men were creeping back into his mind seeking revenge, but this time he was still wide awake.

Like clockwork, he started doing it all over again. Peeking out the dark windows waiting for someone to come. His mind told him so, someone was coming. The police, the Northern Kings, or the little green men, it didn't matter, they were all enemies. The more his mind dwelled on it, the more sure he was that someone was out there watching and just waiting for him to slip, because his vivid hallucinations started to convince his over stimulated mind that what he was imagining was real.

His one eye and two ears were on hyper-alert status. They kept playing little tricks on him. Paranoid, his altered mind kept reassuring him that someone was definitely out there while the other sane part tried to tell him he was only imagining the staring eyeballs outside in the darkness.

Panicking, he loaded up all the on hand cocaine, crack, and loose cash that wasn't hidden under the living room rug and stuffed it into his American Tourister Suitcase which he recklessly put into the bathroom tub. Then he rapidly grabbed pillows and blankets and tossed them onto the bathroom floor.

Once locked inside the small bathroom he sat on a pillow using the blankets to wedge his back up firmly against the toilet bowl. Situated comfortably, he pushed his one good leg up securely against the inward opening bathroom door. I'm safe in here he told himself.

His Remington 12 gauge pump shot gun sat on the floor facing the door packed full of shells while his trusty Baretta with the safety off, sat uncomfortably on top of his family jewels with a full clip of sixteen black Talons and one in the chamber.

With chunks of crack lined up all the way around the toilet seat, so he could quickly flush them when they came for him, he hit those stems again and again. Silently between blasts he listened for any stray noises. The over stimulated endorphins raced faster and faster in his brain as the train he boarded a few hours ago was now at full speed and racing down a steep mountainside out of control. The swifter he inhaled the devil's smoke, the crazier his ride. Fear, phobia, anxiety boarded the manic train laughing in the face of sanity.

They're coming, they're coming.
Don't worry you got your gun.
They're gonna kill me and steal all my stuff.
No they're gonna put me in a padded cell and lose the key.
Stop shaking. Oh my God I can feel the damn door.
It's happening, they're here inside – now.

The pressure on the door increased. He glared at the brass door knob as it started to turn. The harder he pushed with his one good leg the harder it was to jam another rock into the hot glass stem. Not realizing he was burning himself.

The evil smoke filled his stoned lungs. Greedily he inhaled a monster hit of insanity. Feeding the tiny green men.

More fear, more craziness, more paranoia, surged throughout his sweating body causing his brain to overload. Too much stimulation all at once. The sweat stung his eyes, but he still clutched his Baretta shaking. Bug eyed he listened and watched intensely.

There it was again. That noise.
Shit they're definitely inside, I can smell them.
Man I can't get caught with all this crack.
Okay think, who is it? The cops, Hector…little green men?
No…no I killed all of 'em…didn't I?

Faster and faster he smoked the door started changing shapes. His good leg ached from pushing so hard so long. Every little sound made him jump. By three am they were out in the kitchen searching for his stash.

Now they entered his small bedroom just outside the bathroom. Jittery he shut off the bathroom light and sat in the dark. Then the pressure increased on the door as the handle rattled. Frantic he pushed back harder. His gun hand shook, his arms ached. The full moon shined brightly outside the bathroom window reflecting strange shadows off the brass door handle showing faces laughing at him.

No…don't let them in.

Push harder.

Oh my God, there's two of them.

He was almost hyperventilating. *Oh shit.* This was no dream, they were really pushing now. *Panicking he pushed with all his might. No…no…I can't let*, they were picking the cheap lock. Clutching the gun he took his last hit of crack.

Then the door bowed, creaked. "Oh no…oh no," Lucky mumbled. His body shook with fear, he was so afraid, so defenseless with his battered and bruised body he hysterically started flushing all the crack down the toilet twisting his body awkwardly.

It happened all at once.

Lucky's good leg, his right foot pushed through the hollow press wood cheap paneled door crushing the inside panel and pushing his sock covered foot all the way through into the bedroom. Shocked he jerked his right leg back leaving his sock stuck inside the hole. Instinctively he reached up and hit the overhead light. Scared, he flung himself backwards towards the tub landing on top of his American Tourister suitcase.

The gun never left his right hand. He knew they were right outside the door. Hector's henchmen had found him. Minutes passed, a slight noise…tick…tock…tick…tock.

"Fuck it," he muttered bravely grabbing one crutch he hobbled to the bowed door and couldn't stand the waiting anymore. Quickly he twisted the cheap lock and pulled the door inward ready to shoot.

His heart beat raced. Nothing happened. He stared wildly into the dark bedroom. Grinding his teeth he slowly edged forward expecting an attack.

It never came.

Slowly, cautiously, he moved towards the living room. Shit my cash, sixty-eight grand is under the rug he thought, hoping it wasn't already gone. Madly he swung his shooter to and fro looking for a moving target.

He edged into the small kitchen. Empty. The noise, there it was again. He reacted so fast he lost his only crutch when he spun around. It was the last thing on his mind when he saw movement across the room by the sliding glass door.

The curtain moved.

He froze in place in a two-fisted grip he learned on the Coast Guard range in Cape May, New Jersey. Wait for a target he told himself. Now he was wide awake and running on adrenaline.

Seconds passed. More movement. Carefully he reached down and snagged his crutch never taking his eye off the moving curtain.

Boldly he moved closer facing his fears. Me or them, me or them, he thought as he yanked the heavy curtain back pulling it off it's rod exposing the glass doors.

Nothing. "What the…fuck…?"

But the slider was wide open. He moved closer in shock. On the top step was the farmer's tomcat 'felix' lying there looking up at him.

"Meow…meow."

Unbelievable. He shook his head to break his hypnotic trance. Anxiously he reached for the switch on the wall flooding the backyard with spot lights.

Nothing.

"Unfuckin' believable." The turkeys gobbled, and Felix blinked, but he didn't see Hector, the police, or any green men. Slowly, he exhaled and lowered his Baretta trying to catch his breath.

Felix wrapped himself between Lucky's legs and purred for a treat. "Whew…what a fuckin' rush…I swear there was somebody here," he mumbled. He couldn't believe it. *Did I leave the damn slider door wide open? When? Jesus I'm losing my mind.* He was too high to remember. Angry at himself for being such a fool, he slammed the slider shut and turned off the outside spotlights.

Together he and Felix worked their way over to the refrigerator where Lucky grabbed a chunk of Vermont cheddar cheese and a slice of expensive smoked turkey for Felix and a cold Molson for himself.

He collapsed heavily into a kitchen chair with a big sigh. He fed the hungry cat. "Jesus I'm really losing it," he told Felix wiping the sweat off his face with a kitchen towel. Eyeing the pills on the table he downed two trazadones, two darvocets, and two Tylenol with codeine. "Maybe I'll sleep right through this nightmare."

Minutes passed by and the pills started kicking in. He put Felix on his lap and rubbed his ears the same way he used to rub his own cat Key West. "My only friend," Lucky moaned feeling sorry for himself, as Felix purred licking his paws.

Then he exploded like an ocean wave crashing against the rocks. Tears poured down his face, he sobbed heavily disgusted with himself. His buzz was slowing rapidly from zooming to dragging the runaway train had hit it's brakes hard.

Depression and sorrow set in swiftly. After a few long minutes he wiped his eyes a final time and put Felix back outside. A few minutes later he was passed out completely naked on his twin bed as the pill cocktail shut down his over stimulated mind.

SIXTY ONE

UT HE STILL dreamed. It seemed like hours later he was running really fast through the woods. Slowly they were gaining, making him run faster than he ever had, he was trying to break free, almost…a little more…no they were still gaining on him… somehow…someway.

Closer and closer.
Then they surrounded him.
And he tripped falling hard.

Stumbling,he got up and ran to his left but he saw them block him so he bolted to the right only to see more Northern Kings stalking him. Laughing.

Carefully he backed up against the big pine tree. Helpless, he screamed out, "Leave me alone." The circle of thugs got smaller and smaller as they laughed at him smacking their big clubs and sharp knives banging them in a death chant. Closer and closer and closer till he couldn't breath. Get away.

Desperate for air, any air, he exploded at them full of wild rage screaming, but the tree limbs were alive and held him captive. Frantic he broke free. Flying through the air, he landed very hard on the on the bedroom floor.

"Ouch," he moaned in agony. Then he looked up at his bed and realized it was just another bad dream. An omen. Jesus, that was so fuckin' real man, he told himself, feeling the pain shoot through his cracked ribs and swollen knee.

It was well past noon when he climbed out of the shower remembering to remove his suitcase before turning on the water. After drying off, he saw the bathroom door. "Sure fucked that up Lucky," he laughed at his own stupidity.

His poor attitude and outlook weren't any better, just dwelling on what a lousy husband and father he was depressed him further when he eyed his beautiful daughter's picture on his bureau.

He pan fried a black angus filet mignon in butter and fresh chopped garlic and ate it with scrambled eggs and Kraft American cheese. Thirsty he washed his late breakfast down with an absolute screwdriver.

Lucky was funny when he went shopping. He'd buy any product that said Gillette or Kraft because Mr. Kraft owned the New England Patriots and they played at Gillette Stadium. He was a loyal fan and he liked the products anyway.

While he was daydreaming about Kraft cheese, it dawned on him right away. He didn't feel safe anymore and it really bothered him that he couldn't remember leaving the slider wide open. But there was nothing missing. Maybe Ryan did it, who knows, he contemplated shaking his head disgusted with himself. *Could all that noise have been the cat or did I imagine it all?* "Fuck if I know anymore," he mumbled.

On his crutches looking out for his landlord he took the bag of cash Romeo gave him out of his suitcase and hobbled down the dangerous stairs to the barn to bury the twenty-five grand with the other stash of fifty grand and four kilos.

Finally back upstairs pooped and winded, but pleased he rewarded himself with a fat line to clear his head. Immediately he pulled his notebook out of his backpack and added the deal.

WHO	SALE	PAID	OWE	TOTAL
Romeo	6K	5K	1K	5K
R	15K	16K	0	21K
Julio	1.4K	200	1.2K	21.2K
J	1.28K	1.96K	560	23,126K
J	0	560	0	23,686K

Sam	1.5K	1.5K	0	25,186K
J	500	500	0	25,686K
Sam	10	50K	0	75,686K
Sam	25K	25K	0	100,686K
R	21K	21K	0	121,686K
J	450	450	0	122,136K
R	75K	25K	50K	147,636K,

Hours later, Ryan stopped by after work on Wednesday. Lucky was very high once again and Ryan saw another side of Lucky he'd never seen.

When he started whispering to Ryan telling him to be quiet and turn down the Red Sox versus the Oakland A's so he could listen while he peeked out the windows.

"Jesus Lucky, you're high as a kite man…Relax bro, there's no one out there," he told him handing him another Molson.

"Go ahead help yourself."

"Don't mind if I do," Ryan grinned grabbing the dinner plate full of coke and crack.

Four hours later at midnight, Ryan was still there. He was geeking out worse than Lucky. "See I told you dude," Lucky whispered. "You hear it too!"

"No shit, now I know what you mean. I'm so glad I called my wife earlier and told her I was staying over to look after you," he sighed bug-eyed grinding his teeth. "She'd kill me if she saw me like this."

"Ain't that the truth," Lucky added realizing he could almost see out of his swollen left eye finally.

They alternated between lines and rocks. Lucky was beyond caring. They had already snorted and smoked a grand worth of product in just over five hours. His loaded Baretta sat ready for duty on the coffee table while they polluted themselves and eyed the old movie on the silent TV. Quietly they whispered back and forth but both weren't listening.

Lt. Brooks popped in Lucky's mind; suddenly he knew what he needed to ask. "Hey Ryan do me a favor. First thing tomorrow morning call City Corvette and find out when the next shipment of southern 'vettes is due in okay?"

"Okay."

"I met a dude with cash money lookin' for a Florida 'Vette. Don't worry, you'll make something off the deal." *Yup sure you will, like a gram of coke maybe.*

"Sure I'll call first thing, then I'll let you know on your cell phone answering service, okay?"

"Yup."

"Man I'm wicked high…when…hey you okay?"

Lucky hesitated. "Just fuckin' tweaked bro, but I'll live."

I hope.

At three AM, Lucky gave Ryan a trazadone, while he swallowed his own pill cocktail. Then he hid all the contraband because he knew neither one of them could get any higher, and the nature of the drug was to keep chasing that first hit. It was time to quit for the night.

SIXTY TWO

WHEN HE FINALLY stirred sometime around noon, he followed his usual routine of late. A long hot shower and a delicious breakfast of three grade A large brown farm eggs over medium, a half pound of thick sliced hickory smoked bacon, grilled Thomas English muffins, and Concord grape jelly.

After breakfast, he grabbed a full box of 9mm Black Talon hollow points sold only to law enforcement officers, which were better known on the street as cop killers, because body armor was not immune to the high velocity exploding tips.

He grabbed a garbage bag full of empty green Molson bottles and limped slowly without his crutches out to the duck pond behind the barn.

Carefully he set up six empty Molson bottles on top of the dock pilings. Painfully he paced off twenty-five yards with sixteen in the clip and one in the chamber he slid his spare clip into the back pocket of his dungaree shorts.

Exhaling, he fired his first shot and missed badly. "Shit, I need practice." Concentrating, he fired again spraying green glass into the pond, startling the turkeys who gobbled relentlessly with fright, as the field full of cows stared with wide eyes.

Five paces back he squeezed the trigger with a standard two handed police grip and missed. "Control your breathing, squeeze easy," he mumbled trying to recall everything the gunner's mate who was a world class shooter taught him.

Concentrating he fired once again drilling the second bottle, then swiftly he took aim and squeezed gently shattering the third bottle.

He grinned excitedly, "I still got it." Backing up a couple of steps he fired again, and missed. "Exhale slowly, aim and squeeze very lightly," he whispered to himself. Bang…boom, bottles four and five disappeared. Only one left, then it was gone. "Not bad, six out of nine hits for an old coasty," he joked.

His confidence came soaring back the more rounds he fired. Facing back towards the barn he spun around on his good leg and fired. "Almost. Okay spin, raise, acquire, squeeze," he whispered. On the third spin, he hit green. Then it dawned on him he was killing little green men again, but this time they weren't firing back. Hey maybe this could be a good dream therapy, he thought.

Getting bored, he got creative and fired from various angles lengthening the distance, improving his marksmanship.

"That was a hell of a shot," someone yelled.

Startled Lucky spun around towards the voice ready to fire. Quickly he lowered his gun when he saw the green state police uniform.

"Thanks, what the hell brings you way out here sir?"

"Trying to find you…you're a hard man to find."

"You could have called."

"I did…obviously you never answer your messages, so I forced your salesman Ryan to draw me a map," he paused glancing around the quiet farm. "Actually your owner leaned on him a little."

Lt. Brooks grinned while he watched Lucky go back into a zone. Expertly he spun around at ninety feet and splattered the last bottle all over the dock.

"You got me, I couldn't make that shot."

"Yup, not bad for one good eye and one good hand," he kidded.

"Where'd you learn to shoot like that?"

"Key West. Courtesy of Uncle Sam," he grinned knowing Lt. Brooks probably already read his military jacket.

Then he cleared the chamber making sure the gun and clip were empty, before he tucked it into his waistband. Slowly he plucked the empty brass casings off the ground and tossed them into the trash bag. Before he left, he kicked the remaining green glass off the dock into the water.

"So what brings you out here?" Lucky asked eyeing the gold bars on Lt. Brooks' immaculate dark green state trooper's uniform. "Obviously you're on duty."

"I needed to update you. Hector's been very busy, we tapped his phone and bugged his apartment. You do know there's a contract on you? Ten grand plus a 'Vette," he said concerned watching closely for a reaction.

"I heard something like that…but I'm still here!"

"Well I wanted you to know. It looks like you can protect yourself, but I'd be real careful. His gang of thugs is real busy looking for you. We overheard them talking about a missing shipment of cocaine," his eyes narrowed on Lucky's face. Still no reaction.

Be cool. "Really?" *Sure I stole their shit, so what?* "Hey how 'bout some good coffee Lt?"

"Sure if it's as good as your shooting I'm game," he responded walking beside Lucky at a very slow pace towards his apartment.

He filled Mr. Coffee with Starbuck's finest gourmet vanilla bean. "Hope you like Starbucks. It's the best I can do way out here in the boonies," he joked.

"It'll do just fine," he said checking out the apartment. "At least your face looks a little better and you're off your crutches, but you still look like shit, obviously you're still using."

Lucky ignored the barb and put out the half and half, Sweet-n-Low and sugar cubes. They sat at the table sipping the delicious smelling coffee. "Oh Lt. Brooks, by the way, I found out this morning that a load of 'Vettes will be in from Florida late Saturday night. I was gonna call you later today and tell you." *Sure I was.*

"Wow, that's great news…we sure didn't know that. How the hell did you find that out?"

"I'm a salesman remember? I had a cash buyer call City Corvette and ask," he lied smiling. "They were more than glad to share the information once they heard the magic word cash."

"Why didn't we think of that?"

Lucky shrugged, "Because you're cops."

Lt. Brooks laughed sipping his coffee. "You'd make a good detective," he joked dryly. "You're gonna spoil me with this wicked good java. It beats the hell out of our lunch room brew."

Lucky still on guard waited him out.

"So Lucky things are really heating up. I hope you're going to be smart and not become a liability. Because if I was smart, I'd lock you up till all this shit blows over," he bristled studying Lucky's reaction intensely. "This is how we're gonna play it. I want you out of sight, the last thing I need is you getting hurt worse or dead."

"Why, do you think they can find me way out here?"

"I don't know. Who else did you say knows you're out here?"

"Two, no three people actually including Ryan. But the other two are very close friends and would never tell."

"Then you should be alright. But stay alert and don't hesitate to call me," he told him. "You want some protection at night at least through Sunday?"

"No…hell no. I don't need a cop sitting outside, advertising where I'm at. Besides I don't think my landlord would be too pleased." *Since he's got a crop of pot growing in the back pasture.*

He stood up to leave setting his empty mug in the sink. "Be careful Lucky, don't go shooting someone by mistake or on purpose. You might get yourself in more trouble."

"No problem sir. If I have to shoot anyone, it will be because they left me no choice."

"Okay then, I'll let you know as soon as we take them down, so keep your cell phone close by. And hey, thanks for the Florida tip." *You're welcome, now get lost.*

Lucky watched out the window while Lt. Brooks walked to his cruiser with his smokey hat smartly on his head. He climbed into his green and silver striped cruiser with supervisor printed boldly on the side with white letters.

Great now he knows where I live.
Shit he knows about the tute.
I wonder how much they've overheard?
What has Hector figured out?

SIXTY THREE

LUCKY CALLED ROMEO to find out what was going on. "Man oh man there be a lot of shit goin' down. Them Kings are wicked pissed off," he snickered. "I got the whole hood cornered with all this premo shit you sold me," he bragged.

"Shit I even wacked the hundred ozees with ten ounces of cut and it's still the best shit these junkies ever seen. Can you believe I'm getting low already? The whole city is wired."

"Holy shit."

"Ya but the heat is on. We're gonna have a get down turf war soon. They can't take it much longer, but hey the strong survive and the weak go someplace else," Romeo said alarmingly.

"So Romeo you have my pizza money yet?"

"Yup Gringo, fifty large. You want it?"

"Sure it would be nice with all this shit goin' on," he scowled. "Fuckin' state police. Just left my crib...you won't believe it...they came to warn me about Hector's bounty...you believe that shit or what?"

"Oh man Gringo the heat...shit...you didn't say nothin'?" Romeo demanded.

"Fuck no. They want Hector's ass, not mine. I guess my old man's got 'em scared to mess with me." *Besides he'll be out of the way soon enough.*

"You better hope so Gringo, the word is the price went up. Twenty grand for your ass. They really must want you bad, cause they got every low life strung out on crack tryin' to find your hideaway and now you tell me the state Gestapo is on the scene," he whistled nervously.

"Hey at least I told you, right! And we know what they're up to."

"True that."

"Clean your face on the last pizzas and we'll do the same deal again."

"What? Shit Gringo, man you loco, you thinking big for a car mouthpiece," he kidded amazed by Lucky's brass balls.

"Hey the man said move this shit. I could make a call out of state and be done with it, but we're doing good business and you've been straight up plus you also stepped in when I needed a friend. That all weighs heavy with me so run them Kings out of town. Let's do this."

Romeo hesitated. "So I give you fifty I owe plus twenty-five down on the same count?"

"Yup and we can meet in the same place today when you're ready!"

Two hours later he pulled up to his back door with seventy-five grand in nice new Ben Franklins. Once he got back inside he was very excited eyeing all that cash. He just couldn't believe it was all his. Eagerly he grabbed his notebook and updated it adding deal.

WHO	SALE	PAID	OWE	TOTAL
Romeo	6K	5K	1K	5K
R	15K	16K	0	21K
Julio	1.4K	200	1.2K	21.2K
J	1.28	1.926	560	23,126K
J	0	560	0	23,686K
Sam	1.5	1.5	0	25,186K
J	500	500	0	25,686K
Sam	10	50K	0	75,686K
Sam	25K	25K	0	100,686K
R	21K	21K	0	121,686K
J	450	450	0	122,136K
R	75K	25K	50K	147,136K
R	75K	75K	50K	222,136K

Even though the math showed he had $222,136 dollars, his actual count was $68,000 under the living room rug and when he added the seventy-five grand to the seventy-five grand already hidden down in the barn, he'd have a $150,000 total downstairs and plus the $68,000 upstairs, for a grand total of $218,000. He only lost or spent forty six hundred that he could see.

He snuck back downstairs to the barn and dug up his stash like an old pro. He added the new money to the hole along with the last two kilos. After he tied the bags up tightly he reburied his treasure.

Satisfied, he sipped a frozen mudslide out of his favorite Boston Celtics mug his father bought him at the last game Larry Bird played in a green shamrock uniform. Being an ex-mixologist he took pride in creating a perfect cocktail. Baileys, Absoloute, Kaluha and lots of crushed ice blended perfectly in his Black and Decker Turbo blender. A scoop of cool whip on top made his mouth water. Carefully he stuck the glass blender into his freezer to preserve the rest.

On impulse, feeling a bit better, he called Laura who had just gotten home from work. "Would you please spend the night with me tomorrow night at Hampton Beach?"

"Where are you taking me, to your dungeon or is it a surprise?" she giggled obviously in a silly mood. "Never mind all that, I'll cancel my hot date, just pick me up at six and don't you dare stand me up Mister Lucky Sullivan."

"No way Angel, I'll be there."

"How are you feeling anyway?"

"Much better thank you…the teacher's back," he kidded sexily.

"Mmm sounds like school's back in session."

"Pack accordingly."

"Oh I will Professor, I will."

Ryan stopped by after work and apologized about telling Trooper Brooks where he lived.

"Don't sweat it, I know he didn't leave you much choice," he tensed. "But don't you dare tell anyone else, and I mean anyone, where the fuck I live!" he yelled angrily making Ryan take a step back.

"Okay okay, I tried to warn you off but your damn phone was off."

"Shit I got enough damn problems right now," he declared trying to calm down.

After they each had a frozen mudslide, they indulged in a few lines of powder before Ryan threw a hundred dollar bill on the table for a to go pizza. Of course Lucky gave him a great deal cutting off a three gram chunk off one of the ounce boulders for him and his wife.

After Ryan left, Lucky started stashing all his loose drugs and cash, and only brought the two gram vial with him when he packed his overnight bag for Hampton Beach.

Carefully he hid the five loose ounces of powder into his L.L. Bean winter down survival coat with a zillion pockets, another expensive gift from his parents over Christmas a few years back. Then he hid a few grand inside the coat's plentiful pockets. Walking over to his bureau, he spread out the rest of his crack inside a few pairs of athletic socks, careful not to make them too bulky. He shut the sock drawer mixing them in with the rest of his socks. He knew he needed to stay straight or lose Laura for good. After all, it was only one night.

The following afternoon, about two pm, Lucky pulled the big Lincoln into Johnson's Chevy. He parked beside his favorite ride on the lot, a 1972 Mercedes Roadster.

Before he could even get out of the car, Ryan was there beside him to transfer his backpack and overnight suitcase. "Don't forget my plate," Lucky said with a smile pleased by Ryan's attitude and enthusiasm.

"Got it boss," Ryan grinned eagerly.

Very, very slowly Lucky limped into the showroom to collect his paycheck and switch out car keys. He was surprised at how friendly and concerned everyone was including the owner.

"You're looking much better Lucky, glad to see it."

"Getting there sir, hope to be back on Monday."

"Only if you're up for it, just don't rush it, Lt. Brooks said you're lucky to be alive."

Great. "You can't get rid of me that easy. If I can limp, I can sell," he responded with a smirk, waving goodbye on his way outside to the Mercedes where Ryan helped him drop the top and said their goodbyes.

SIXTY FOUR

LUCKY PULLED OUT in the old Roadster feeling pretty chipper with a pocketful of money. He headed for the small local bank to cash his paycheck. Casually, a dark green van with magnetic signs that said Sweeny's Plumbing & Heating pulled out and followed him to the bank.

After he cashed his check, he realized he'd forgotten to slide a hundred dollar bill under the landlord's door and he had no idea if he'd be spending the whole weekend with Laura.

He glanced at his watch. "Fuck it I got plenty of time," he mumbled enjoying the sweet sunny September afternoon, while he cruised back out to his apartment.

The van kept a safe distance back. Lucky idly glanced back in the rearview and didn't give the trailing van a second thought. His mind wandered to Laura dressing up in a sexy school outfit and he couldn't wait, his shorts were getting uncomfortable already. He pulled in and checked his mailbox. Empty. Then he started climbing the steep stairs to grab a rent envelope when the green van passed by slowly.

Five miles out in the sticks there wasn't a heck of a lot of traffic passing by, so automatically Lucky eyed the familiar van suspiciously when it passed by. Still he didn't pay any mind.

After he sealed a crisp Ben Franklin in the yellow envelope provided by the old farmer, he wrote in the date and his first name then slid it under the landlord's door, satisfied he climbed back in the old car.

Now he was relieved. His father always told him to take care of your bills first, and he knew that would have bothered him all weekend knowing he was late, especially having access to all that cash.

Casually, he pulled back out on the lineless country road after lighting his favorite cigar, a Cherry Tijuana Small. He eased the seat back, glad to be rid of the crutches as he accelerated gently in the old roadster.

He glanced back nonchalantly into the rearview surprised to see a dark colored green van closing rapidly. Instinctively he floored the twenty-five year old Benz, feeling the adrenaline surge through his veins.

A heavy cloud of blue smoke burst from the dual exhausts of the high mileage tired V-8, as the old tires squealed loudly on the loose sand trying to gain traction.

Closer and closer the van came. Where have I seen that van before? he asked himself. Johnson's?, The bank?, A few minutes ago? He wondered eyeing the hostile plumbing van gaining quickly in his rear view.

Forty…fifty…sixty…now the van was only ten feet back. Seventy… eighty…five feet back and a long country five miles back to civilization.

The van closed up on his bumper. Awkwardly he yanked the Baretta out of his backpack trying to keep control of the old roadster. Man I wish I had the damn Mustang, I'd be gone already he thought just as the van tapped his rear bumper letting him know he'd never make it back to town. *Oh shit, not again.*

The old Michelin Radials squealed in protest when he skidded sideways around the first sharp curve almost losing control. Fucker's got a suped-up motor, he told himself clutching the oversized steering wheel.

Nervously he approached the sharpest corner on the whole road glancing down at the speedometer. Ninety. "Shit I'll never make it, not in this car," he muttered. At least take him out with me he decided.

Spontaneously he swerved into the left lane to help cut the corner. The suped-up van accelerated in the right lane trying to make the pass. His cigar still clutched firmly between his teeth burned bright red from all the wind fanning it.

"Oh shit," he mumbled seeing the plumbing and heating van pull up aggressively beside him in the right lane keeping him pinned out in the oncoming traffic lane. He hit a patch of loose sand and skidded wildly praying for tar. Halfway through the dangerous corner the Michelins caught howling loudly. Directly in front of him in the right lane was an oversized load of hay being slowly towed by an old farm tractor who had just started turning into his field.

They were going way too fast, there was no time to react. Suddenly they were directly beside one another when the crazy driver of the van screamed wildly at Lucky waving a gun.

Swiftly, Lucky raised his Baretta in defense but he never needed it. The van crashed recklessly into the big hay trailer at better than eighty miles an hour.

"Holy Shit," Lucky screamed losing his cigar. He was blinded by flying bales. Immediately he slowed down and pulled back in the right lane shaking, as he watched with horror in his rearview mirror. The road was covered, hay was everywhere, and the old wooden trailer was scattered in a million pieces. Looking around he spotted the van upside down in a ditch tangled in the farmer's barb wired fence, with the Sweeney's Plumbing and Heating magnetic sign hanging off the side.

The shock wore off when he spotted the angry farmer still sitting on his tractor shaking his big fist wildly. Lucky roared with laughter, "Wow, what the hell was that?" *This is getting serious.*

A mile closer to town, he spotted the blue lights closing rapidly. TheHillbro cruiser zoomed by Lucky in a rush towards the farmer's house. He quickly grabbed his Nextel phone and dialed. "Hey Lt., Lucky here, just wanted to let you know they found me."

"How?"

"Don't really know. I think they followed me from the dealership. A van full of Northern Kings, or wannabes trying to collect that big bounty, tried to run me off the road but they crashed. Hillbro;s finest should be on the scene now," he paused. "They might need some backup; they're armed and pissed off. Just thought you'd like to know."

"Yes, I'm glad you called me. Watch yourself."

"I am."

"You better! The price on your head went up to twenty grand."

"So I heard." *Don't forget the 'Vette.*

"Where are you headed?"

"Out of town."

"Good…stay in touch."

"I will, adios sir."

SIXTY FIVE

H E MET UP with Romeo on the way to Laura's and picked up fifty large in brand new bills. Relieved, he stopped at an old watering hole, because it was only four thirty and he was only five minutes from Laura's. This was one date he would definitely be on time for.

Cautiously he locked the cash in the trunk, parking directly out front, so he could eye the Roadster from inside. He wasn't going in empty handed. His Baretta was tucked in his waistband in the small of his back, covered by his Red Sox jersey. And even though it was a locals' hangout, Lucky felt very comfortable there because of the country atmosphere. Besides the bartender, a hot looking bimbo that served the coldest and cheapest draft beer around, always let you get a good eyeful of her well developed chest, that were scantily covered to increase her tips.

He shot pool with a few locals beating them on their own table. Feeling generous, he splurged and ran a tab for an hour on pitchers of Bud for all fifteen hardcore happy hour drinkers. He figured it was cheap insurance in case someone unwanted showed up unexpectedly. After all, he was only a half mile out of Manchester.

At five-fifty pm, Lucky paid his fifty dollar tab and handed the smiling bimbo twenty bucks for the free show. He left to a lot of friendly pats on the back from all his new friends. Another sucker with a Mercedes they most likely thought watching him leave amongst all the four by four pickup trucks.

Smiling, he pulled up right on time, six pm sharp. Laura was eagerly standing beside her Lincoln looking extremely hot in black leather pants, matching pumps, and a sexy white blouse. Her long black hair looked radiant.

Strutting she stuck her thumb and butt out provocatively. "Hey stranger in the cute car, going my way?" she asked licking her red lips beautifully.

"Yes. Yes I am," he said smiling back; excited he reached over to unlock the passenger door for her. "Here, let me put that in the trunk for you."

"Relax, I got it. I'm not helpless you know."

She climbed in, giving him a light kiss.

"You look a lot better," she purred squeezing his hand. "So where am I getting kidnapped to?" she asked not expecting an answer.

"To the beach, my angel," he chuckled realizing how happy he was to have her back beside him. She was the perfect woman and he knew he didn't deserve her.

Serenity entered his mind. Peaceful, content, everything felt so wonderful. The company, the weather, the gorgeous sun setting behind them. He realized what it was he'd been missing the most. Her smile. They held hands while Tracy Chapman's big hit 'Just Call Me' boomed out over the stereo cassette deck as they cruised towards Mother Nature's playground; the Atlantic Ocean.

Boy I'm so damn happy.
I've got a natural high.
God how I love her.
Then why do I keep taking the devil's highway?

"You okay?" she asked out of the blue, like she knew exactly what he was thinking.

He smiled and nodded giving her hand a light squeeze. *Got me again, didn't you?* It took over an hour to reach New Hampshire's biggest salt water playground, Hampton Beach. Their excitement grew the closer they got to the boulevard. The summer season had passed with Labor Day come and gone, but you wouldn't know it by the volume of cars heading for the strip for Friday night fun and frolicking. They cruised the strip both enjoying the sights of fancy waxed cars, beach waves crashing on one side of the street, and vendors taking advantage of the nice September weather to, peddle their food and wares for another day, before the cold fall weather set in for good.

He pulled the old Roadster into the oldest hotel on the beach, Wentworth by the Sea, a beautiful historical first class resort. Lucky, living large, rented the presidential suite and even managed to get it at the off season rate.

They were escorted to the ocean view room by a professionally dressed porter. The large suite was magnificent, they sipped a glass of complementary champagne out on the balcony overlooking the beach.

"You know, all the big shots over the years have stayed here. The Kennedys, Fords, Bushes, who knows how many others, probably right here in this room since it is the presidential suite," he laughed thinking of President Kennedy sneaking off for a secret rendezvous with Marilyn Monroe.

Like kids, they ordered everything. Shrimp cocktail, oysters on the half shell, oysters Rockefeller, Cape Cod Bay scallops wrapped in bacon and brown sugar. Then turning the page on the enormous menu, he added two cups of their famous New England clam chowder, two pound boiled Maine lobsters, and sauted jumbo garlic prawns. Laughing he eyed the extensive champagne list, going right to the most expensive he added two bottles of Don Perignon. "My God Lucky, that's awfully expensive. What's the occasion?"

"You are," he beamed. "I had a record week and I'm celebrating that I'm still alive." *Just barely.*

Enthusiastically, he raised his champagne flute in a toast. She saw the old Lucky and she loved it. After their toast she dimmed the lights and disappeared into the palace-like bathroom. When she came back out she looked like a model straight out of Frederick's of Hollywood. The expensive silk lingerie clung to her classy body like they were made especially for her.

Tastefully, she covered herself with a silk robe which only teased his desire more. She lit candles and paraded around in six inch fuck me heels, not realizing how gorgeous she looked. The sweet innocent

Greek goddess. My student, my lover, my wife. Don't I wish, he told himself in a daze of lust.

The porters showed up with a world-class food cart fit for six dignitaries. It looked magnificent all in sterling silver with matching hot plates and warming ovens built right in.

"Wow," Laura smiled having the servers set up a table for two on the large balcony where they set up using fine linen, sterling silver, and expensive china.

This was strictly a cash affair, so while Laura was busy with the porters, Lucky discreetly grabbed the enormous room service bill out of the fancy black leather book and went over to his backpack.

"Holy shit," he muttered noticing the third bottle of Moet they had already finished off was conveniently added on. The three bottles of champagne totaled four hundred and fifty dollars.

"No wonder I don't drink this shit very often," he mumbled. The total bill was just six hundred and fifty dollars. Lucky stuck eight one hundred dollar bills in the leather book and glanced out towards the balcony, while the fancy dressed studs were drooling over Laura's luscious body. He grinned watching her innocently blush.

He handed one of the two servers the booklet and stuck an additional two twentys inside the book. "Thank you sir, if there's anything else, please call on me personally, my name is Kevin."

"No this is great, thank you."

They feasted under candlelight with the sound of breaking waves crashing off in the distance. Like lustful kids they fed one another bites of all the delectable dishes. The food was five star, just as advertised, and the electricity in the room was highly explosive. Once they finished eating they pushed the fancy cart out into the hallway making sure they stuck out the fancy do not disturb sign on the gold door handle.

Giddy and full from all the expensive bubbly and world class food, they slow danced, careful not to bump his healing injuries in the candle lit room with the sweet ocean breeze blowing briskly in the open balcony doors.

It had been too long for both of them. They couldn't wait to make love on the satin sheets in the stylish king size bed.

W.C. SCOTT

"You know I love you, when you're like this. My little boy, my stud," she whispered rubbing her long nails through his curly hair.

On the bed, he started very slowly, teasing her unrobed body with cold drops of champagne and his hot tongue. He teased and teased her entire body till she shook with frustration as a long version of "Stairway to Heaven" filled the room adding to the special moment they were sharing.

He entered her extremely slow, teasing her womanhood. Within minutes their lustful lovemaking became a frenzied sound of moans and groans, especially when both felt it building and building. With perfect timing they climaxed together. He collapsed into her waiting arms smelling the fresh salty air blowing inside the room.

Minutes later, after they both recovered, the gas fireplace flickered romantically, while they soaked themselves naked in the powerful Jacuzzi located in the center of the big room, relaxing in each other's arms, enjoying their last glass of Don Perignon.

His defensive mechanisms were too relaxed to prevent the feelings flooding him all at once. He couldn't help himself. The tears started slowly, then they poured down like a summer thunderstorm opening up.

He tried to catch his breath.

"Talk to me baby – talk to me."

"I…I…miss my daughter…I…I…hate my life. I've been so stupid… so damn miserable," he rambled on. "I just keep fucking up…It's like I'm on the devil's highway and I can't get off."

She rubbed his back. "Aren't they still down in Palm Beach?" she asked sweetly knowing just what to say and when to say it.

He nodded. "Yup as far as I know, my parents are handling all that," he sniffled wiping his eyes. "Thank God she's got such a great mom. At least I did one thing right when I picked her, but man I put her through hell and she gave me anything I ever asked for," he cried. *What a jerk I am.*

"Hey it's okay honey. Go ahead, let it all out." *It's about time.*

"Oh I just don't know anymore, everything is happening so fast. People are after me, shooting at me, trying to run me off the road. It's like I'm in a fuckin' nightmare or something."

"Something else has happened hasn't it?"

He nodded not ready to tell her. "Shit,even Lt. Brooks told me there's a twenty grand price tag on my head, along with a used 'Vette, unbelievable, can you believe that shit? I'm just so messed up, and my body's wrecked," he exhaled slurring his words exhausted. *What am I gonna do?*

"I guess I just needed to talk about it, it's been building and building," he said clinging to Laura's arms as he rested his head on her breasts while she kissed away his tears.

"I'm here for you Lucky, you know that. And you can tell me anything because I love you, we're soul mates." *More than you'll ever know.*

"Marry me then."

Surprised Laura looked into his eyes deep into his soul. "You're serious aren't you?"

"Of course I am. I love you, you know that you'd make a perfect wife." *But I don't deserve you.*

Stunned she responded carefully, "Lucky I'd love to marry you. But only if you can get your shit together and get off drugs," she paused trying not to hurt his feelings. "I mean it, get some help. I'll wait for you…but not forever…you have to do it for yourself baby." *And I don't know if you can.*

"Okay…okay," he whispered. "Let's go to bed and cuddle." *I'm totally exhausted.*

"Come on baby, come to mama," she said trying to cheer up his somber mood. They made love again and fell asleep with their legs intertwined cuddling romantically like cubs. He slept dream free and very soundly, for the first time in well over a month.

SIXTY SIX

AFTER, THEY ATE at Richard's Waffle House where they feasted trying to quell their expensive hangovers, before they headed back to Manchester to deal with reality.

He dropped her off at two pm. "Thanks Lucky," she smiled sincerely. "I had a wonderful, splendid, enchanting time, you can kidnap me anytime," she said giving him a sexy kiss goodbye. "Call me okay. I'm here for you and please be careful."

"Aren't I always?" he answered smartly when she closed the door. "Bye Angel." *Hope I see you again.*

"Bye Lucky," she smiled blowing him a kiss. Damn, what a woman, he sighed, watching her leather pants walk up the sidewalk.

*   *   *

He pulled up to his apartment a little after three pm eager to watch the Florida Gators play the Florida State Seminoles in the swamp. Once he undid the dead bolt he opened the door and froze, "Fuck."

The place was trashed. Quietly he pulled his Baretta out of his backpack and entered carefully. The sliding glass door was shattered and a cement block sat on his living room rug.

He shook his head angry. The sofa cushions were slashed open and pulled apart. Dinner plates were smashed. The refrigerator severely dented, was tipped over upside down and spoiled food was everywhere.

Startled he edged towards his bedroom, right away he noticed his expensive L.L. Bean cold weather down jacket was gone and so was the five ounces and five grand hidden inside it's pockets. He saw his

Timberland boots where he had also stashed five grand in each boot. Relieved he picked one up. "Fuck me," he muttered irate.

Eyeing the bed his mattress was cut open and thrown everywhere. Then he remembered his socks, surprised they were still full of crack. Quickly he stuffed the six pair of athletic socks and vials of powder into his backpack.

The old antique dresser was destroyed, broken into firewood. He peeked into the bathroom, not expecting to find anything. But immediately he saw the spider webbed mirror over the sink. In pigs blood it said "You're dead amigo and so is your girl," he followed the blood arrow down.

He screamed violently when he saw a picture of his precious daughter stuck to the mirror defiled in pig's blood.

I'll fuckin' kill him. He's dead.
No one messes with my Boo.
Motherfucker you're dead.
The hunted just became the hunter.

"Lt.," he barked urgently. "It's Lucky. Listen my place is trashed and there's a gang message on my bathroom mirror in pig's blood," he raged. *Hector you're dead.*

"Don't touch anything. I'll be there in an hour," he ordered concerned. "Get somewhere safe and I'll call you on your cell, go on move it. Get out of there, it could be a trap."

He started to leave fuming then he remembered the rug. Violently he pushed the smashed TV out of the way and tossed the cement block over to the side. Then he pushed the destroyed sofa off the rug. Carefully he pulled the rug back sending shattered glass everywhere.

"Yes," he cried out eyeing the sixty-eight grand flattened safely to the floor. "Unbelievable." As fast as possible he started stuffing wads of cash into a small suitcase. Fives, tens, twenties, and fifties went into the suitcase.

He heard a noise. "Oh my God," the farmer yelled clutching a shotgun, he stuck his large head through the smashed slider. "What the hell happened here?" he demanded, extremely angry.

Lucky glanced up grabbing the last few handfuls of cash off the floor. "Someone broke in here while I was gone. I called the state police, they'll be here in about thirty minutes," he said firmly picking up his Baretta off the floor while he pulled the rug back in place.

"Don't worry, Lt. Brooks has a good idea who did this."

"What the hell," he hollered upset. "What about my furniture, my stuff?" he demanded stunned walking around the room. "Jesus Lucky, who the hell's your enemy? What the hell's going on?"

Lucky ignored his questions and pulled out a wad of money. "Lucky I want you and your shit out of here and I mean it," he barked angrily shaking his head absolutely disgusted. "Jesus Christ Lucky, what the hell is this?"

"Don't touch anything, Lt. Brooks wants to see everything the way it is so they can take prints."

"Then what about the rug?" he said sarcastically.

"Hey I had to get my money and so did you," he barked right back at him. "Listen, I'll be back tomorrow morning to get my shit."

Lucky pulled the rug back and put the broken TV and cement block back in roughly the same spot. When the landlord came out of the bedroom shocked at all the pig's blood from his dead pig he had found out in the pasture. "Who the hell did this, you read that shit, you're dead? Jesus Lucky who's after you? What are all those squiggly lines and is that your daughter?"

Lucky was getting really irritated. "Those are gang warfare signs and the police know who the hell they are, and they'll take'm down." *Or I will.* "Listen I'm sorry about your place, but at least I paid for the damage," he shouted back pulling his daughter's picture off the mirror and tossing it angrily.

"What pisses me off,is they did this shit while I was home and I never heard them," he yelled smashing his oversized fist into his hand.

"It's probably a good thing you didn't catch 'em. They're crazy and very violent, believe me I know." *Just look at my body.*

"Shit, I'd put my old twelve gauge up their fuckin' ass with a load of buckshot," he said with an angry smirk. "No one gets away with this shit. Hey here…here let me help you."

Lucky started towards the door with two suitcases. Knowing he was still injured he carried one of the suitcases down to the Roadster.

"Shouldn't you wait for the police?"

"No...no, he told me to go, he's got my number," Lucky said hurrying behind the wheel. He couldn't leave quickly enough, thinking about the stuff hidden in the barn. At least that should be safe, he hoped. *Here I come motherfucker, payback time.*

SIXTY SEVEN

H IS FIRST STOP was Johnson's. It was deserted as usual on a Saturday afternoon. He needed new wheels. Something different, something fast.

He left five minutes later in a late model Ford lightning supercharged pickup with an enclosed locking bed. Lucky didn't know much about engines, but he did know this truck was the fastest production street truck made, according to his Motor Trend car magazine he faithfully read each month. And with an aftermarket Paxton supercharger added on just like the Mustang it had to be badass.

The custom headers and special modified cat back high flow exhausts gave it an awesome rumble. The aftermarket ground effects and sticky Yokohama racing tires only added to the wow effect.

After filling it up with Sunoco racing fuel, he took off for the highway like a bat out of hell. "Fuck it," he screamed tromping the accelerator to the floor board. "He wants me…Well here I come," he roared eyeing his Baretta. "Fuck, they stole my damn shotgun those bastards."

Aggressively, he raced the hot truck onto Interstate 89 South bound towards Bow Junction. The speedometer quickly reached one twenty. The further away he got from his apartment, the angrier he became, he was quickly losing control. Nothing else mattered, but Hector threatening his baby girl. Oblivious to everything, he yanked out a two gram vial and did a blast at one-twenty.

"Here I come motherfucker," he screamed, hitting the dashboard as he accelerated/ AC/DC "Hell's Bells" cranked full throttle out of the Pioneer supertuner which only fed his insanity. 125…130…135…140…145…150…he laughed crazily blowing by cars like they were standing still…155…158…160…162…164. "Fucker's got some balls," he declared excitedly taking his foot off the gas.

"Now I know what you got," he mumbled slowing to one hundred. Then his escort radar detector started chirping loudly. Quickly he took his foot off the gas peddle and slowed to eighty-five then seventy-five as the signal grew stronger.

"Shit…fuck," he screamed seeing the speed trap ahead. He hoped they hadn't clocked him at one-sixty. There were eight shiny State Tooper cruisers lined up on the side of the highway working the speed trap, with a small Cessna airplane circling above. *I'm screwed.*

The first trooper pointed sharply at the truck telling him to pull over. He hesitated. "Should I?" he mumbled. "Nope I better pull over and pray. He stopped about a quarter mile down with a blue flashing cruiser in hot pursuit.

The trooper jumped out aggressively with his hand resting boldly on his 357 service revolver, while he eyed the fancy truck and the New Hampshire dealer tag stuck to the back by a magnet which read "Live Free or Die" N.H. Dealer 21-14x."

"License and registration," he demanded angrily.

Lucky handed him his New Hampshire Driver's license and sales manager's card from Johnson's. "Sir there's no registration; it's one of my dealer's cars."

"Lucky Sullivan, where have I heard that name?" the trooper asked staring at his license suspiciously. "So what the hell's the rush, Mr. Manager? You know they clocked you at well over a hundred?"

That's better than felony one-sixty. "Yes sir, my place up in Hillbro just got ransacked by some Manchester street gang and Lt. Brooks, who I'm sure you know out of Troop D in Bow told me to get the hell out of town sir. So I was pushing it pretty hard," he said honestly hoping for a break.

"That's the biggest bullshit story I've ever heard Mr. Lucky Sullivan, who do you think you're dealing with huh?"

"Okay I don't blame you sir, listen, I'm calling him right now on my phone because he's on his way to my apartment and he should pass by here any time."

"Go ahead hot shot, call. But you're still getting a ticket. I should haul your ass in because before they could clock you, they said you were really moving like one-fifty. So go ahead and let me see you sell your way out of this expensive ticket." *Salesmen, I hate 'em.*

Lucky was already dialing. "Hey Lt. Lucky here, listen sir I got another problem, um I'm here with Trooper Bean, southbound on 89, they got a speed trap with a plane and of course I was trying to get out of town swiftly like you told me to, I was pushing it sir." *He's pissed.*

"Jesus Lucky you're a real pain in my ass. Slow the hell down. Stop making my job harder than it already is. You hear me?" he yelled loud enough for Trooper Bean to smirk. "Put Bean on."

"Yes sir Lt. Trooper Bean it's for you." *Asshole.*

Bean took the phone and stepped away from the truck and talked to Lt. Brooks, who told him to chew his ass and let him go, because Sullivan was involved in Operation Snowstorm.

"Is that an order Sir?"

"Bean, just do it."

"Yes sir, I'll do just that, but you owe me one sir."

"Bean you don't have to like it, but that's a direct order from a supervisor who's overseeing a large investigation. So write it up if you want to, but in the mean time you'll follow a direct order, is that clear enough?"

"Absolutely sir, loud and clear," he said handing the phone back to Lucky.

"God damn it Lucky. I can't keep saving your ass, and your place is a disaster, I'm in it now," he explained.

"We're gonna take prints and pictures so go find yourself a rock to hide under. I mean it. Stay the hell away, you got that? We're down to the wire now, so don't make me lock your ass up, cause I will," he threatened.

"Yes sir, I will sir, I appreciate it."

"You damn well better, now slow the fuck down, that's no damn race track you're on, you got that," he fumed hanging up.

Lucky glanced over at Trooper Bean, who was still pissed off and held his license and business card busily writing a ticket.

"Shit," Lucky sighed under his breath. *Oh well, I gave it my best shot, fuck it.*

"Here," Trooper Bean said handing him a ticket with his license.

Lucky eyed the ticket. "Warning speeds in excess of 100 mph. No ticket issued per order Lt. Frank Brooks."

"Now slow the hell down. Next time I'll nail your ass. Brooks or no Brooks, you got that?"

"Yes Trooper, loud and clear, thank you sir."

"Don't thank me hot shot," he snipped. "Brooks saved your ass again, by the sound of it. Now get the hell out of my sight," he stormed off.

Alright things are starting to go my way he thought pulling back onto the interstate knowing if he was running one-sixty he wouldn't have stopped, not with all the drugs and cash in the back. He did another blast of coke to celebrate his change in luck setting the cruise control at seventy-five.

Ten minutes later his phone rang. It was Laura and she was bawling. "Oh Lucky," she cried hysterically. "Someone killed my Taffy, oh my God Lucky, who would do such a terrible thing?"

He knew exactly who, Hector. "When?"

"Well I was in the laundry room down the hall, so I put Taffy out on the patio for about an hour and I just found him with a big knife sticking out of him with a bloody note attached," she whimpered crying.

"What did the note say?"

She sobbed trying to catch her breath. "It said you're dead amigo."

"Motherfucker's dead," he exploded flooring the truck.

"Who did this to my baby boy?" she cried.

"Hector and his gang who work for the old man. Call your father and don't touch Taffy okay. Listen, call Lt. Brooks, he's at my place now. You have his number, it's on the fridge."

"Why is he there?"

"They trashed my place and ripped me off."

"Oh my God, what are we gonna do Lucky?"

"Stay inside, I'm on my way."

"Fuck, fuck, fuck," he roared. "You're dead motherfucker, you're dead." He tromped the gas pedal, ignoring every internal warning sign. Speed was the only thing that mattered.

Fifteen minutes later he raced up to Laura's condo. He comforted her while she waited for her dad and Lt. Brooks to show up. He covered Taffy with an old blanket.

"Listen baby, you'll be safe inside. No one can get inside," he said confidently,knowing he had already reinforced all the doors and windows months ago.

"I gotta go baby," he said anxiously wanting to leave before Lt. Brooks showed up.

"Where are you going?"

"You know where I'm going. That motherfucker threatened my daughter and killed Taffster," he raged in a tantrum.

"Oh please don't get in trouble or get hurt, please."

He stared at her hard. "He's going down Angel," he told her dead serious. "And don't you dare tell Lt. Brooks what I said."

"No...I won't, just be careful please, and please call me okay. Don't make me worry," she pleaded.

"I will...promise...go to your dad's," he said hugging her goodbye, hoping it wasn't for the last time.

SIXTY EIGHT

H E PULLED INTO Riley's Gun Shop in Hooksett, just down the street from Laura's condo. Ten minutes later, he walked out with two boxes of Black Talon hollow point cop killers using his Coast Guard petty officer's I.D. to buy the restricted law enforcement ammo. The bag in his other hand had the latest second chance bullet proof vest and three new empty clips for his baretta.

On a mission, he raced straight to Romeo's and pulled up directly in front. Sliding on his new vest and grabbing his pack and new purchases, he went up the stairs flying, forgetting all about his knee.

There were six Columbians in the living room along with Romeo. "Hey what the hell you doin' Gringo, tryin' to get yourself killed comin' here?" Romeo blurted out.

"Fuckin' right I am. Where is he, where's that asshole live?" he challenged boldly.

"Easy bro…put that shit away before you shoot someone," Romeo ordered pointing at Lucky's gun. "Now what the hell happened?"

They all listened while Lucky told them all about his apartment being trashed, the missing money and drugs, his precious daughter defiled with pig's blood and threatened, then his girlfriend's dog killed with a butcher knife and the nasty note.

"Holy shit Gringo, no wonder you're so pissed," Romeo responded, eyeballing his gang waiting for a reaction. "Man Gringo, you can't take this dude on by yourself, he's got too many armed crazed goons addicted to the devil's pipe."

"I don't give a fuck Romeo, I'm an expert shot, I've been in combat," he boasted to the hoods. "Shit in the Coast Guard I wasted five dudes on a ship and I can pick off a seagull at fifty miles an hour bouncing around in a boat. I'm sure I can pick off his punks one by one."

"Shit Gringo, you've been holdin' out. You never told me you was a federal water cop."

"You never asked. Fuck yeah, Key West, Florida drug enforcement." *And tiny green men* he laughed as they were all shocked he used to bust drug runners.

"Can you really shoot Gringo?"

"No joke man, I can shoot lights out."

"Man you know you got twenty gees on you head bro?"

"True that, and don't forget the used 'Vette."

"Gringo every scumbag down here has seen a picture of you and won't hesitate to take you down, twenty large sure buys a lotta dope."

"Fuck it Romeo, he crossed the line when he threatened my baby girl. Just do me a favor and point me in the right direction, I'll take my chances."

Romeo shook his head offended. "Shit Gringo, you might be real good, but you can't take down fifteen, that's right fifteen wired dudes by yourself," he pointed out clearly turning towards his home boys.

"We be makin' a whole pile of coin off this Gringo's generosity. Boys are we in or what? This the same dude me and Baby Boy been shoutin' about. He's blood as far as I'm concerned. I'm in. You guys call your own shot. Hector's shown his hand, he's desperate, and he's goin down hard," he stated enthusiastically standing up.

"Make up your own mind, you backin' this action?" he demanded knowing they would.

Lucky watched surprised when all seven of them made gang signs and chanted a war cry swearing an oath till death.

"I gotta grand cash for each one of you as a bonus," Lucky told them hoping to inspire them further.

"Where you parked?"

"Right out front, mean ass Ford truck."

"Baby Boy hide his ride," he instructed tossing Lucky's keys to Baby Boy who quickly moved towards the door.

"Okay! Now let's make a plan. Bring the map," he ordered all business like. He eyed the detailed map spread out on the kitchen table talking to himself.

Lucky looked on amazed as every detail was carefully recorded. Gang zones, hot areas, pickups, neutral streets were all labeled. Color coded with highlighters and markers with tiny monopoly game houses and hotels.

"Listen Gringo, we be in, but you gotta do this our way," he stressed. "These be our streets and we know every ant and crackhead within a mile, you be out of your element."

Lucky agreed with a nod.

Romeo pointed all serious. "Here's Hector's crib over here and the cops most likely feds got their eyeballs all over it."

Lucky looked up surprised that they knew.

"Yup, we spotted them plain wraps over a week ago. They ain't foolin' nobody, but they ain't makin' no play, so they must be listening with ears through the phone and walls. So we hit 'em over here," Romeo pointed, circling a plastic red Monopoly hotel glued to the makeshift map. "At his clubhouse."

He explained, "This is how we take 'em. We go in late, strapped, and silent, taking out his looking posts first," he paused thinking. "Hey Gringo, how good a shot are you really?"

"Put it this way, I got twenty large and twenty pizzas, I can outshoot anyone in this room. I can drill anyone or anything I can see," he said confidently. *Especially Hector.*

"How 'bout say two hundred yards through a laser-guided night scope on a rifle equipped with a silencer?"

He hesitated while all seven Columbians silently waited on his reply. Somehow he knew this was some sort of test.

"Depends, if I got my choice of a military grade sniper rifle or your basic M-16 which I'd be a lot more comfortable with, then I'm your man."

"That's settled, me and Gringo will set up here on the hill behind the old stone wall, long and silent, while you six will split into three teams of two," he told everyone studying the layout.

"Beetle Juice will wire us all with headphones – but all voices will be code only, unless you have to break, which means trouble and operation clubhouse ceases to exist, while we just disappear."

He turned to Baby Boy, his Lt. "I want everyone in night darks, face paint, vests, the works," he demanded eyeing Lucky's new five hundred dollar second chance bullet-proof vest.

"Baby Boy, you and Fast Lane take care of all that shit. We should have enough shit in the armory."

Baby Boy nodded knowing what time it was.

"Then we burn Hector out of his castle," he roared with evil laughter. "Revenge amigos. The truce is over, there ain't no room in the hood for both of us."

Rapidly Romeo's switch blade snapped open. He cut his thumb drawing blood. All the Columbians did the same staring at the outsider as they raised their bloody thumbs together.

"Fuck this," Lucky responded grabbing Romeo's sticker he cut his thumb. They all roared crazily, a blood oath declaring war. Violently they pressed their eight bloody thumbs together and shouted in Spanish, while their combined blood dripped over Hector's clubhouse on the map.

"Midnight tonight," Romeo announced insanely, "and Paco make sure we got plenty of your special cocktails to bring him out of the devil's den."

Paco just grinned.

"Meet here at ten thirty sharp. Everyone keep it cool on the streets. Don't tip no one off. Just business as usual," he ordered as the gang immediately separated.

Lucky wasn't sure what the hell he'd just gotten himself into, but he really didn't care. Revenge was the only thing that mattered.

"Come on Gringo," Romeo motioned him into the back hallway where Baby Boy was already removing a secret panel off a wall.

"Holy fuckin' shit Romeo," Lucky responded surprised by the organized hidden room full of weapons.

Romeo proudly grinned. "What you think we do with all that green we be makin'," he laughed watching Lucky's eyes light up with surprise when he pulled back another panel.

"So Gringo, can you shoot lights out with this?" he asked Lucky seriously when he handed him a brand new military issue M-16 with a laser night scope and silencer attached. "It's single shot or full auto, not a three round burst like the new M-16 A but it's brand spankin' new."

Damn straight, he thought admiring the illegal machine gun. "Spent a lot of time on the range with this baby," he told them excited. *I'm coming Hector be ready.*

"Good that's your long, but this baby's mine," he grinned pulling a modified AK-47 scoped with a silencer out of the closet.

"Man oh man, you got some sweet weapons Romeo," he said noticing the various handguns with silencers, ammo boxes, vests, and different colored cammys.

"Okay Gringo, take off. See you back here at ten thirty. Keep it cool and we ride this train together. Here put this on," Romeo ordered handing him a black Tommy Hilfiger satin jacket and matching ball cap.

Romeo looked at Lucky while he tried to pose like a cool dude pretending to be a gang banger. Romeo and Baby Boy howled with laughter breaking the ice. "Now you don't stick out so much Gringo, yo be lookin' like you belong."

"Right on man," Lucky said as Baby Boy led him covertly back to his hidden truck. He decided he had some shopping to do before the big party.

SIXTY NINE

AT TEN THIRTY Lucky showed up dressed in dark night swat fatigues. He had his face expertly painted and had shocked Alexis when he came out of her bathroom dressed for war.

"Holy shit Lucky, oh my God...never mind...never mind...don't tell me...just go before my boyfriend gets here. Will you please hurry," Alexis pleaded.

He did a quick blast of coke before he got out of the truck to get his endorphins amped. When he finally was let inside the Columbians' fortress disguised as a rundown apartment building, everything had changed inside.

All Romeo's crew were decked out in black fatigues with new non-reflective black face paint nervously waiting for Operation Clubhouse to commence.

"Jesus Lucky, you look like the Soldier of Fortune magazine. No shit," Sasha teased turned on.

He grinned. "Here hold this for me," he told her seriously, handing her his backpack full of a hundred and ten thousand dollars,

He had bought the latest police utility belt at the Manchester army-navy store. Sixty foot MD-60 military grade pepper spray, handcuffs, an A.S.P. (expandable aluminum wand) and three full clips of 9mm Black Talon Hollow Points hung from his belt in the proper black pouch accompanying his familiar Baretta in it's new black nylon holster.

"You expecting trouble Gringo?" Romeo asked eyeing his serious get up.

"Never know bro...but I'll be ready."

Then he asked again, "you ever kill anybody Gringo?" The room went silent waiting for his answer to the question they've all been wondering, but afraid to ask. Will he freeze when it's time to get down?

Do tiny green men count? "Yes…yes I have, five to be exact," he said honestly. "But didn't I already tell you that earlier tonight?" Immediately he felt the room temperature warm up considerably.

"You sure did, good you gave us the same answer. Now listen up guys, this is gonna be a total silent takedown, till we draw heat from the Kings. Nobody's packin' noisemakers including you Gringo, so give me your gun and clips," Romeo demanded, showing he was still running the show.

"Why? This is my last line of defense, my right hand," he argued removing the deadly bullet from the chamber.

"Use this instead," he ordered handing him a 9mm Smith and Wesson with a silencer screwed on.

"Like I said everyone goes in silent, one bang and we'll have major heat from the cops and the Kings."

Romeo took charge and went over the plan once again. "Me and Gringo will take out the two outside lookouts from here at the stone wall. Team one and two will move in and take down the two outside corner eyes."

Team three had outside perimeter and on Romeo's code they would send in decoys to act like junkies, who needed to make a buy, distracting the corners till they could be taken down silently letting team one and two slip inside the perimeter undetected to the hiding doorman packing heat.

Once team one and two disposed of the four outside club security gang bangers, then Baby Boy would try and remove the heavily armed outside guard posted up at the top of the stairs where all transactions took place through a sliding panel in the door. Together team one and two would try to break down the heavy door and toss in Paco's flaming gas cocktails to bring Hector and company outside. If they couldn't take down the heavy door, Lucky and Romeo would shoot the second story windows out so team three could toss the deadly fire water into the devil's den.

Then everyone would scatter covering every exit and they'd wait till the rest of the scumbags came running out.

Eleven fifty pm it was time.

The latest word from the street was that Hector was spotted entering the clubhouse. Excited, they took two Cadillac's, parking one on each end of the dark street labeled hostile, out of bounds on the map so that would leave everyone two alternate escape routes.

Everyone knew exactly where they were suppose to be, so no conversation passed over the multi-channel Radio Shack walkie talkie head sets. Romeo and Lucky loaded down with their wicked hardware eased into position behind the old gray stone wall.

The headsets were the latest gadget put out by Radio Shack designed for competition commando paint ballers where you could turn off the mike and still listen.

"Hey Gringo, you think you can plug them from here?" he whispered handing Lucky a small vial he didn't recognize.

"Jump juice, try it," Romeo grinned wickedly. A cousin of mine in Maine got the biggest meth lab in all New England. State of the art, all underground, shit's potent."

Lucky hesitated already amped up on his own adrenaline and cocaine. "Fuck it, I might need the boost," he mumbled careful not to do too much. "Wow, burns like good crystal meth to me, whew."

Catching his breath, Lucky acquired a target with his new M-16 about a hundred and eighty yards. "Shit I can pop the dudes zit on his forehead," he bragged to Romeo, confidently eyeing the glowing green target illuminated brightly under a large elm tree.

"You ready Gringo?" Romeo asked knowing he was.

"Go ahead you got the honors Gringo, commence Operation Clubhouse, take him out. Stand by team one, two, three, it's party time," he said into his headset mouthpiece.

This is what I've been waiting for, revenge, and here's my chance, no more tiny green men, these are all grown up. Relax, breathe, concentrate, he told himself, going into a zone, exhale, squeeze gently, don't think… *revenge.*

Romeo watched eagerly through his night scope waiting for Lucky to pass his first test. Poof… "Target one down, team two stand by for second target."

"I got 'em," Lucky told him amped up, sighting the second target's chest posted up by the corner of the house.

"No he's mine, stand down Gringo," Romeo ordered as Lucky backed his index finger off the trigger and impatiently watched through his night scope. Then number two target's throat exploded with green blobs.

"Second target down, move in team two," he ordered while they both watched looking for more hidden targets. They watched team one drag target one into the bushes, while team two did the same to target two.

Lucky was back in a zone just like on the Panamanian freighter back in Key West, he sighted the second story windows where the main clubhouse was situated. *Where are you hiding Hector, come out…come out wherever you are.*

Team one and two moved into place by the back stairs knowing there was an armed Northern King sitting at the top of the stairs in the dark.

"Team one and two in place," Baby Boy whispered, clearly waiting for Romeo's command. He knew he had only one chance to surprise the shooter or he'd be hit.

"Take the garbage out. It's overflowing," Romeo told him.

Baby Boy tensed knowing everyone was relying on him to take out the main threat. *You can do it.* "Garbage going out," he whispered, pulling down his military night eyes, he spun into the dark stairway illuminating the gang banger smoking a cigarette, clutching a Tec-nine machine gun.

Poof…Baby Boy's Smith and Wesson barked softly. "Yes," he whispered excitedly. "Garbage is removed. Baby Boy boasted into the headset, as team two moved up the stairs quietly picking up the dead King.

"Check one, check two, move when ready," Romeo ordered.

Things happened fast. Baby Boy knew there was a coded knock to get the flap to open, which he didn't get out of the Tec-nine toting gang banger, so he was going to wing it.

Baby Boy rapped once, then twice on the thick door flap. Seconds later the panel on the door slid open. Baby Boy blasted the surprised dope server in the face sending him sprawling backwards into the den.

At the sound of the server's scream, the clubhouse came alive like a nest of angry red ants being attacked.

Baby Boy continued to fire suppressed rounds into the big room while King members returned fire with noise makers.

"I got one target upstairs," Lucky said concentrating on the King opening a bedroom window.

"Take him out," Romeo ordered.

Inhale, exhale slowly, lightly squeeze, focus, poof... "Direct hit bedroom window!" he announced excitedly.

"Nice shot," Romeo said listening to all the excitement through his head set. "Let's go guys, take down that door," he demanded.

"Almost," team leader two yelled, as they pried the sturdy wooden door with a huge pry bar while Baby Boy reached in with his non-shooting hand and slid the two by four brace holding the door securely from the inside.

"Two targets just dropped a rope ladder out the side window...now they're startin' down," Lucky declared rapidly.

"Can you hit both?"

"Probably but one might jump when I take out the other guy, so you take the high guy I got the lower one."

"Do it," Romeo agreed lining up his moving target.

"Ready?"

"Ready."

"Now."

Both targets fell hard to the ground below and didn't move. "That makes seven," Romeo said keeping track.

"Where in," Baby Boy screamed as all four Columbians unloaded their Smith and Wesson nine millimeter silent guns into the hostile room diving for cover.

Baby Boy saw movement behind the overturned couch. He fired three poofs into the couch till he heard a scream. "I'm hit, I'm hit."

The Columbians were under heavy fire from two different bedrooms and didn't notice the King hiding in the dark kitchen.

A shot rang out drilling Fast Lane in the calf. Baby Boy swung his big body wildly as a shot zoomed passed his head. He knew he was about to eat lead, so he fired off balance and shot the surprised King in the face.

Romeo glanced at his watch, "Times up teams one and two, threes on the way. Hold your positions till they toss our presents, then scatter."

Team three, Paco and company moved up the back stairs each clutching two gas cocktails with the rag fuses burning quickly up the side of the Budweiser quart beer bottles as team one and two backed out the door firing wildly at both bedrooms covering Fast Lane who was losing blood fast.

Paco flung the first glass present into the open bedroom door while Lucky shot out the windows pinning them down.

As soon as Paco heaved the last present, Baby Boy slammed the door shut and wedged the big crow bar between the door and wall so it couldn't be opened from the inside.

Then they heard the sirens off in the distance. The Kings' gunfire obviously forced nervous neighbors to call 911.

"Oh shit, we got company, all teams evacuate. Plan two now in effect," he ordered knowing his crazy amped up Columbians wanted to kill every last King who had invaded their peaceful territory a year earlier.

Romeo looked over at Lucky who was glued to the enflamed burning clubhouse waiting for Hector to come running out. "Come on…come on motherfucker, you gotta pay," he muttered searching hard. *Where the hell are you?*

"Okay Gringo, we'll wait a minute and see if he shows then we gotta haul ass, pigs are close."

"Holy shit, look at that burn, nobody can still be in there, no way," Lucky said shocked that the whole building was burning out of control.

"Yup, gas it's a wonderful thing. Come on let's go, we're outta here," Romeo ordered grabbing Lucky's arm aggressively breaking his trance as the sirens closed quickly.

They sprinted to the waiting caddy, Lucky's bad knee and all, he blew by Romeo like he was back running track at the University of New Hampshire, easily beating him to the unlocked car.

Four Manchester cruisers flashing blue lights came skidding to a halt blocking off the streets so the fire trucks following could get through.

"I hope the fucker burns crispy," Romeo mumbled deeply when they pulled away safely he tossed the vial of speed to Lucky.

SEVENTY

BACK AT ROMEO'S, the guys carried the shot up Fast Lane into the back room where Romeo sent one guy to get the unlicensed crackhead doctor who took up residence down the street when he lost his license to practice medicine for selling Oxycontin to anyone with money.

Romeo had used him before, he knew he wouldn't say anything and because of his reckless habit he could pay him in crack.

Ten minutes later, Lucky couldn't believe his eyes when an old haggard looking man with a straggly white beard and cracked granny glasses showed up lugging an old fashioned leather doctor's bag.

The Columbians had the place completely surrounded with security ready for any counter attack. There were two guys high up in the elm trees totally invisible and another hiding on the front landing behind a false one way mirror. They were all still wearing their head sets silently listening and waiting for trouble.

They knew it would come. The question was how soon.

Romeo eyed Lucky with admiration.

"What?"

"Man Gringo, you surprise the hell out of me, I thought you be a soft mouthpiece pushin' cars down people's throats," he snickered. "But man you're a hell of a shot and cool under fire, Amigo."

"Hey you fuck with my family," *you turn into tiny green men* "you... you...you...man I just hope we trapped him otherwise it's gonna get a lot worse for both of us."

Shit that coke shipment's coming in tonight
And Lt. Brooks will have it staked out.

If Hector ain't dead, maybe they'll nail him.
Yep he just might show up at City Corvette.
Wouldn't want to miss his precious cargo.

"Nice doctor," Lucky said changing the subject.

"Hey, he's a crackhead but he's damn good. Don't let his looks fool you, he was a Professor of Medicine at Dartmouth Hitchcock."

"No shit," *I guess the devil's drug doesn't discriminate does it?* "Look let me pay for the doctor, I got rocks."

"Okay but let him finish first before you give him any shit or he'll never finish."

"No problem."

"Get yourself cleaned up so you can get somewhere."

Lucky nodded, aggressively cleaning off his face paint in the bathroom mirror. Feeling drained now that his adrenaline rush had worn off. Man *what the hell am I doing?*

"Shit listen to this," Romeo yelled as he stuck his head set up to the small radio which amazingly had the Manchester police talking about the clubhouse over their radios.

He saw the expression on Lucky's face.

"Gave a crackhead ten rocks to steal the radio crystal out of a cruiser when they went in on a domestic disturbance that was all staged," he said still listening closely.

The neighborhood was being swarmed. They were searching for Hector and they had recovered twelve dead Kings around the clubhouse. The feds were now on the scene abandoning the stakeout on Hector's apartment.

"Shit he must have got away or he wasn't inside like we was told," Romeo said shaking his fist angrily. He alerted the security team posted outside and in the stairway, "He'll be coming, stay alert, and shoot him on sight."

He paced back and forth. "Lucky get your ass outta here," he commanded. "When the shit goes down you don''t need to be here bro." *You got that right.*

"Okay, okay," Lucky responded quickly grabbing his backpack from Sasha, he pulled out seven one grand bundles of cash and ten rocks for the Dartmouth doc.

"What the hell are you doin' Gringo?"

"Hey, I said a grand a piece and I keep my word. The cracks for the quack."

"Man you're fuckin' loco. Alright, I pay the guys later on. Here take your gun and Baby Boy will take you to your truck, now move," he said staring at Lucky strangely. "Adios Gringo, we'll finish this…good job Gringo." *Way to stand up white boy.*

"Thanks Romeo…I…uh," he stuttered lifting his backpack onto his shoulder seven grand lighter. "Thanks bro…you were right, I was out of my element."

"Get the hell gone, will ya!"

Baby Boy came running into the room wildly. "Man you hear that shit?" Baby Boy whined, "Damn stateies and feds are involved, shit Lucky, let's ride before they lock down the whole hood," he ordered, pulling Lucky back to the fire escape and down to his truck two blocks away.

Lucky was decked out in Romeo's Tommy Hilfiger clothes. He went outside under the watchful eyes of the elm tree Columbians.

Just as he climbed into the Ford Lightning truck, a Manchester police cruiser raced by with his lights and siren blaring. Time to get the fuck out of here, he thought. *Where are you Hector?*

First thing Lucky thought of as he nervously drove off in the loud truck is that Lt. Frank Brooks might have put out a Bolo (Be on the look out) out on the truck because he hadn't checked in since the speed trap many hours earlier and now there were twelve dead Kings.

He headed north on I-93 towards Bow Junction and set the cruise control to exactly seventy miles an hour, the posted speed limit. He glanced back skittishly into the rearview reaching for his Nextel phone. It was one forty am and he dialed his answering service and listened.

The fist message was from Lt. Brooks who had just left Laura's and was extremely upset that Lucky was in town. He told him that if he didn't hear from him by midnight he'd activate the warrant on him.

"Shit."

The second message was from a frantic Laura, warning him that the police had been by twice looking for him, and that she'd be at her father's for the next few days because Lt. Brooks thought it was a good idea. *Great.*

The third message was from Alexis. "I'm so fuckin' pissed Lucky. I caught my steroid stud fucking my roommate when I came back from my sister's early. Where the hell are you? I need you…"

"Man oh man, shit's heating up fast. Bastard's still alive. If they don't take him down tonight, I'm going to Palm Beach. He's gotta kill me before he messes with my Boo," he told himself driving towards theHooksett toll plaza.

Nervously he eyed the brightly lit toll plaza expecting the police to be close by; he paid the toll with tokens and pulled away just as his phone rang startling him.

It was one fifty am.

He hesitated, should *I? Maybe it's Alexis.* "Hello?"

"Damn you Lucky, you're in deep shit now," Lt. Brooks screamed.

"What do you mean?"

"What I mean is that I found cocaine on a dinner plate in your cupboard. It tested very pure, but even worse we found a Juan Valdez Columbian coffee wrapper in your trash can still caked with cocaine residue in the shape of a kilo," he spit out disgusted.

"Oh, oh," he whispered. *What am I gonna do now?*

Silence.

"Maybe the Kings planted the dope and the wrapper when they tore up my place," Lucky suggested hoping he'd buy it.

"Yeah sure, I almost believe that," he answered distracted. "I'm in the middle of your big tip, but I just hope for your sake you weren't anywhere near the Northern King's clubhouse tonight."

"Why what happened?" *Everything.*

"Twelve dead bodies. Six shot expertly from a long distance away by someone obviously very skilled with a rifle, then the place was torched with gas bombs. That's right, unbelievable Lucky, all on the same night the Florida 'Vettes are due in," he said accusingly. *But can you prove it?*

"Wow, holy shit sir ... is Hector still with us?"

"He's still alive, but missing. We figure he'll make an appearance over here tonight since some one ripped off his last shipment, Lucky," he implied sarcastically. He paused very upset. "So Lucky where the hell have you been hiding all evening? Hope you got a rock solid alibi 'cause I know you weren't anywhere near your worried girlfriend."

"It doesn't matter does it?" he snapped back irritably.

"Okay smart ass, play it your way. Just know that every damn cop's lookin' for you in that fancy Ford truck you're driving. That's right, a 1995 Blue Ford Lightning New Hampshire dealer plate number 21-14x. You're not as smart as you think!" he warned. "Stay the hell away. Let me know when they lock you up. I'll come see you when I find the time. I gotta run I think I see a car carrier coming down the street loaded with 'Vettes."

Click.

"And fuck you too," he yelled into the dead phone.

SEVENTY ONE

O H GOD, IT'S really happening now he told himself. His mind raced while he nervously snorted the evil cocaine steering with his good knee.

It was two-thirty am when he eased into Johnson's vacant parking lot. Immediately he went inside and grabbed the extra dealer plate he had stashed in his desk drawer off the old dealership wrecker sitting out back with two flat tires. Pulling open his middle drawer, he yanked out the spare set of keys to the supercharged Mustang. *Party time.*

He switched plates putting the wrecker plate on the 'stang and his dealership tag Lt. Brooks knew so conveniently well on the back of the wrecker. Once finished he pulled back out to the quiet deserted streets of Hillbro.

Next stop the barn.

On his way back out to his apartment, he spotted a similar year Mustang sitting in a driveway under a garage spotlight. Quickly, he shut off the loud Mustang and coasted to the side of the peaceful country road.

Armed with his Leatherman toolkit, he snuck across the grass and unscrewed the front plate figuring it would be days before they noticed their front plate missing.

Next stop the farm.

SEVENTY TWO

THEY HAD CITY Corvette completely surrounded. The Narcotics Joint Task Force made up of both Feds and New Hampshire's finest had been waiting impatiently for ten days now. And finally Lucky's tip had paid off.

The 'Vettes had arrived.

Because it was Lucky's tip, Lt. Brooks was allowed to observe the takedown courtesy of the D.A.'s office. He was not part of the takedown team. Over the next hour seven 'Vettes fresh from the Orlando, Florida auto auction, were unloaded and locked into the back lot just like last time. Except this time there was an armed guard sitting in a Dodge Dakota pickup truck watching the off-loading.

The lot boy drove up and dropped off King and Queen inside the fence then departed while the armed guard satisfied turned back to his Hustler magazine.

Immediately unmarked cruisers sped after the empty car hauler and lot boy pulling them both over once out of the area where they were held in case they needed to answer questions or to remove the dogs.

Everything was quiet until the team spotted a dirty dark colored sedan pull into the twenty-four hour self-service carwash.

"We got company at the carwash, two males," went out over the secured frequency. One guy, the passenger got out and started washing the dirty old Ford Ltd,while the driver carrying a black nylon bag walked off towards the backwoods.

"One suspect on the move, towards the woods," the team leader announced. "A-team has the carwash, B-team has first suspect on the move."

"A team copy's that, out."

"B team copy's that, out."

The suspect crept from car to car and snuck right passed the armed guard sitting in his truck busy with Miss September. Quietly he unlocked the back gate with a key provided from Hector and patted the familiar Dobermans giving them something from his bag.

Swiftly, he walked on straight to the third 'Vette in line and unlocked the car door with a second key. Thirty seconds later, he exited the 'Vette with a twenty-two pound bag.

"Stand by Team B, get ready to move," the team leader said watching the suspect through his binoculars across the street. "Wait till he gets back inside the bay, then both teams converge at once silently," he ordered, while Lt. Brooks stood by excited.

"Team A copy's that."

"Team B copy's that."

Two seconds after the suspect stepped into the self service wash bay with his package, both teams silently rushed the bay.

Ten fuckin' nights, Team A leader thought pissed off. Adrenaline, sweat, hatred, and excitement raced through him as he rapidly pulled the unmarked state cruiser in front of the bay blocking it off. *Gotcha.*

"Get down, get down, get down motherfucker," they screamed identifying themselves they threw both suspects violently to the wet cement pinning them down armed to the teeth.

The overall Team Leader, A fed, and Lt. Brooks pulled up quickly in another plain wrap cruiser, once the two were immobilized. The fed nodded at Brooks who picked up the contraband bag.

"Bingo," Lt. Brooks yelled frantically. *Finally, damn it.*

"Fuckin' pigs," the driver whined with a black swat boot firmly planted on his neck almost drowning in the soapy puddle.

"Shut him the fuck up," the fed ordered, as Lt. Brooks pulled Hector's latest mug shot from his pocket so he could see if he finally had his prize.

After a minute he shook his head disgusted. "Damn it, neither one is him." He was so sure Hector would come to collect his precious shipment after what happened to the last one.

"He's gotta be close by damn it," he said determined. Overtired, he crazily grabbed one of the punks by the chin, hurting him till he moaned, "Where the hell is he?"

"Who?"

"You know shit for brains…Hector…now where the hell are you supposed to deliver this shit to?" He loosened his grip a little. "You make the drop, you walk away, I got it in black and white," he said flashing the D.A.'s offer.

"No fuckin' way pig! I know nobody named Hecta," he grinned spitting on Lt. Brooks's polished boots.

Angrily, he slammed the gang banger in the gut. "Have it your way punk. Ten keys will get you twenty mandatory. Hope you like dick, shit for brains…last fuckin' chance."

"Fuck you honkey, I want my lawya."

Lt. Brooks nodded pissed off, and the big stocky team member elbowed the punk in the solar plexis, then tossed him handcuffed into the waiting cruiser, who pulled off immediately. After searching the old Ltd they found two illegal handguns with the serial numbers filed off, and a bag of weed, obviously stoners.

Thirty minutes later, Lt. Brooks had the driver in a small room off the Merrimack County Jail. The driver was already wanted on numerous charges, rape, armed burglary, and felony assault.

"No way man, I don't give up no Hector. I'd be a dead man inside or out," he answered scared. "I ain't sayin' shit, I was just washin' my ride, I don't know nothin'"

"We'll see about that lifer."

SEVENTY THREE

LUCKY BACKED THE low riding Mustang into the entrance of the back pasture and parked between the two stone walls barely off the street but not far enough to rip off the expensive spoilers and exhaust system.

First he snuck into his old apartment that had crime scene yellow tape across the back door entrance. He used his mini mag light clutching his Baretta because it was really creepy. Slowly he found his way back to his walk-in closet. He grabbed a manilla folder out of his London Fog rain jacket. Sssh what was that. A noise, there it was again. Quickly he shut off the light and froze with his back up against the closet wall and his Baretta held out in front of him waiting. Man not again, who the hell could it be this time of night…landlord…Kings? Who he thought just as Felix wrapped himself around his legs. "Jesus Felix you scared the shit out me," he whispered relieved giving him a quick rub. Rapidly he folded the envelope and stuffed it in his waist.

Down inside the old barn he found his hidden spot. With Felix looking on, he dug up his stash hidden in the dirt. The last two kilos of cocaine and seventy-five thousand in cash. Hurriedly he filled in the hole and dashed back to the Mustang.

With urgency he headed back down Interstate 89 towards Bow Junction. It was three am and he realized he had no idea where he was heading, but he knew if Lt. Brooks hadn't busted Hector yet, then he was driving down to Palm Beach in a hurry. Boo I'm coming. Don't worry baby girl, Daddy's coming, he told himself.

Motherfucker threatened my baby.
Hopefully Brooks nailed his ass tonight.

But what if he didn't…Jesus.
Plus I'm wanted…what should I do?

Lucky filled up the thirsty Mustang with Sunocco racing fuel outside Manchester and inside the twenty-four hour mini-mart he bought a box of plain white #10 envelopes and on a napkin he wrote.

Angel – I must leave. A lot has happened. You will find out soon. No matter what happens, I love you honey. He's after my baby, my Boo, you know what I must do. He's mine now, I will call you if I can from Florida. Envelope #1 for you + title to Camaro. Envelope #2 for Ryan. Call him, have him pick up all my stuff and bring it to you. Envelope #3 is bail money, use it if you need it. If I ever make it back, he won't. Always my Angel, Luv Lucky.

P.S. Loose lips sink ships – no Lt. Brooks.

P.S.S Flush this note. Revenge for Taffster, pray for me.

He put the right amount of cash in each envelope and pulled the Mustang out and headed for Laura's. He pulled right up front still packing his Baretta, he got out quickly walking up to her dark condo.

The Northern King spotted him right away. He'd been waiting for Lucky to come back since Lt. Brooks left hours earlier. Now was his chance. Lucky continued inside the building. He wanted to hug her and say goodbye but he knew she was probably at her Dad's and there was no time he thought, sliding the three envelopes under her door.

In the meantime the King jumped out of his old Lincoln and attached something underneath Lucky's car, just as Lucky came back outside he slide back behind the wheel of his car grinning as Lucky climbed back into the Mustang and pulled off.

The King glanced down at his GPS surveillance grid tracking system as it lit up. "Gotcha Lucky Sullivan." He waited about five minutes and pulled out following at a safe distance watching the screen. "Twenty grand and a 'Vette, all mine," he laughed hysterically. "Easy money."

SEVENTY FOUR

"ALEXIS IT'S ME."
"Where the hell have you been? I need you," she cried out, hurt and lonely.

A lot's happened since you saw me earlier tonight in my get-up. The gang that tried to run us off the road, well they trashed my new place and threatened my daughter in Florida," he told her in a zone.

"Oh now, what ya gonna do?"

"The head asshole responsible just escaped a police net," *and we burned down his clubhouse.* "Now he's on the loose and I gotta stop him or else."

"You're scaring me, or else what?"

"He gets to Florida before I do."

"Oh my God you poor thing, where are you?"

"On the Interstate just north of Manchester heading south towards Florida."

She hesitated realizing she had to get away from her boyfriend and slutty roommate. "Pick me up…I'm going."

"You sure? Could get dangerous."

"Damn right I'm sure. He fucks with your daughter I'll kill him myself."

"Ten minutes…be ready…we might be gone a while, a long while"

"I need a damn vacation, you can't talk me out of it, I'll be ready."

"See you soon, and thanks Alexis."

"Don't sweat it lover boy, together we'll nail his ass."

SEVENTY FIVE

L T. BROOKS WAS beside himself. It was already six am and he had no leads on Hector's whereabouts. Just when he was about to give up and catch a nap, he rubbed his tired eyes in frustration hoping someone on the street would jump at his cash no questions asked reward.

The call came.

One of their street snitches heard they were paying five grand cash for Hector's location, no questions asked.

Fifteen minutes later the snitch had five thousand in cash from an earlier drug bust and the tired team was back on the move to McGowan's Motel on the west side.

By six-forty five am they had the whole place surrounded. Everyone was focused on the end room where the scared manager said someone matching Hector's mug shot had rented the end room hours earlier with two good looking hookers in tow.

During the stake out Team C had raided Hector's apartment and found an ounce of crack and an illegal automatic machine gun.

It was enough for a sleepy judge to issue a warrant. They moved in expecting to face armed resistance even though he wasn't expecting any company and was busy entertaining two starlets.

They held the battering ram, while two team members waited outside the side window just waiting for the command from their leader. Lt. Brooks nodded at the fed letting him know the warrant was thumbs up. The leader gave his silent command. "Let's do it," he whispered through his headset. Simultaneously they knocked the cheap motel door off it's hinges and two SWAT members dove through the smashed window rolling to their feet.

Hector still wide awake, wired, and lying butt ass naked on the big bed with a nasty hooker on each side of him. He dropped the crack pipe and dove for his handgun sitting on the bedside table.

He never made it. They swarmed in like angry yellow jackets yelling get down, get down while a burly SWAT team member grabbed Hector hard by his long stringy hair and yanked him violently off the bed onto the old carpet.

After they cuffed him and the two ladies of the night, they slid his Sean Paul expensive sweat pants on him before putting him in the cruiser barefoot throwing his hundred-fifty dollar Air-Jordans into the trunk.

"Gotcha finally," Lt. Brooks mumbled exhausted but very relieved he knew he had Hector on multiple felony counts, maybe he could trade a few off and get him to give up the old man. Wishful thinking he thought on the ride to the Merrimack County Jail.

SEVENTY SIX

LUCKY AND ALEXIS continued south on I-93 towards Boston. By six am they crossed the border from Salem, New Hampshire into Massachusetts.

By seven am running on fumes, they pulled off the highway realizing he hadn't eaten since brunch the day before. After topping off with another tank of Sunocco racing fuel, he spotted his favorite breakfast sign. The bright yellow Waffle House sign. His stomach rumbled for covered, smothered, and smattered.

By eight am they were back in the Mustang both feeling much better after talking everything over, drinking three cups of strong coffee. Back on the Mass Pike he dialed Sam's private number in Westin.

"Hello," a groggy voice mumbled.

"Hey Sam, it's your new family."

"Jesus Lucky, what's up with you so damn early on a Sunday morning," he asked very irritated.

"Sorry I know it's early but I'm heading your way and I'm in trouble so I need a big favor."

Sam rolled out of bed after his wife gave him an evil look because she was trying to sleep. "Name it," he said, going inside the walk-in closet he shut the door. "If I can do it, I will."

"Can we meet at your shop?"

"Alright, how soon?"

"Thirty minutes."

"Shit – must be important okay."

Hector's Northern King second Lt. Mendoza also stopped at the Waffle House like Lucky and Alexis where he ate and then tried to check in with Hector, but no one knew were he was.

Lucky's Nextel phone rang startling him. He stared at it with fear wondering who the hell would be calling him this early on a Sunday morning. It couldn't be good news.

Maybe it's Laura.

No, it's probably Lt. Brooks.

Maybe it's Ryan.

Shit it's still early…I wonder.

He waited the required five minutes for the answering service to log the call in his Nextel mailbox. In the meantime, Lt. Brooks slammed down his phone angrily. "Damn him," he said wondering where the heck he was and what he had to trade for the cocaine he'd found at his apartment. "I knows he's holding back."

Lt. Brooks eyed all the paperwork on his desk sipping a big Dunkin' Donuts coffee trying to stay awake. "We'll pick his ass up soon enough, then we'll see what he's got to say."

Lucky checked his answering service. He was right, it was Lt. Brooks and he was really pissed off. The only thing Lucky heard out of the whole conversation that registered was "Oh by the way, I got him early this morning, Hector's locked up."

"Yes," he screamed excitedly, ignoring the rest of the message. "Call me if you know what's good for you. I want any info you got on the old man, till I get it you're a wanted man Sullivan. So don't play games, you can only hide-out so long. Call me," he ordered loudly.

'Sure pal, I'll get right on it," he replied sarcastically shutting off his flip phone. *Man oh man, no more Hector, unbelievable.*

SEVENTY SEVEN

AT SAM'S BODY Shop, they parked out back and went inside. "Hey family, what's up?"

"Shit you are. It's Sunday morning and you look like shit. You must've pulled an all-nighter. So who the hell's this beautiful babe?" he asked smiling, leering at Alexis's hot body.

"Alexis. Alexis Sam, Sam Alexis."

"Hi."

"Hi yourself."

"Listen Sam, I had a bad run in with these Northern Kings, they trashed my place, ripped me off, and threatened my daughter in Florida. I've been takin' matters into my own hands the past few hours and the good news is the cops just arrested the head scumbag, but now they're gunning for me hard, so we need a quick paint job and a place to chill out."

"Shit bro, you've been busy. Them some greasy dudes to be messin' with, they're wicked bad bro."

"Hey sometimes you can't pick your enemies."

"I hear you, so what do you want to do exactly?"

"A banana yellow colored Mustang, the same color as the one I stole a plate off last night."

"Shit, you are getting crazy aren't you?"

"Gettin' there brother, gettin' there," Lucky glanced at Sam's B-B-U t-shirt which stood for Boston Biker's Union which was a very well organized group of hardcore biker gangs that joined in a union with each other, each having their own specialty making them much more powerful and resourceful together than individually.

"Oh did I mention I got a twenty grand bounty on my head and guess what they're throwing in?"

"What?"

"A used 'Vette, you believe that shit?"

"What the hell you do, steal their dope?..." he asked kidding, then saw Lucky's expression. "Okay...okay nevermind."

Then he rambled on about the van trying to run him off the road and the five punks who beat him up. But what really caught Alexis and Sam's attention was him hooking up with the Columbians and torching the Kings' clubhouse.

"Shit Lucky, you're going off the deep end."

He nodded exhausted. *I'm in the deep end.*

"Jesus Lucky," Alexis spoke up for the first time breaking her silence.

"I know...I know, but the asshole made it personal."

"I can tell, it looks like you've been in the combat zone."

Beat, Lucky pulled out his tutor and hit it. Then he handed it to Alexis who casually did a bump before she passed it to Sam, who set his Dunkin' Donuts coffee down. Wake up call, he thought.

"Go ahead, take my car, there's a Holiday Inn a couple miles down. Register the room in Alexis's name and I'll make a few calls and get some boys in here to paint you a banana."

"How soon can you get it done?"

By tomorrow mornin' you'll be rollin' yellow."

"Good...good...Here this is for," Lucky told him tossing the silver lock box key. "That ought to cover the paint job. I'm sure you can put it to some good use in the future. Let's go Alexis, we're outta here."

"Hey you got any white left? Same deal as last time?"

He hesitated, "Yeah I can do that, but you got to lend me your digital scale, they stole mine. I'll have it ready for you when we pick up the Mustang tomorrow."

"Take it easy on her, she's got more power than you're used to," Sam said as they jumped in his bad ass Chevelle with their bags. "Hey make sure you call me with your room number so I can reach you."

"Will do," Lucky yelled mashing the gas, smoking the expensive tires on Sam's precious muscle car. He saw Sam's fist shake fiercely as he pulled out sideways down the road.

SEVENTY EIGHT

S ECOND LT. MENDOZA was confused when the signal stopped moving while he sat only a hundred yards down from the custom auto body shop with B.B.U printed proudly below the sign. Mendoza knew what it stood for so he stayed put. "Shit," he mumbled, turning the alarm back on so when the Mustang moved again he'd wake up. He'd also been up all night and never expected Lucky to take him out of state. But he needed a catnap and now was a perfect opportunity. This big reward was turning into a much longer deal than he first thought. "I still gotcha Lucky, I still gotcha."

He tried once again before nodding off and still couldn't get a hold of Hector. He figured he was still busy messing with the new dope shipment.

It was now six pm Sunday evening when Lucky awoke to a loud tractor trailer pulling his noisy rig into the Holiday Inn. Dazed and definitely confused, he rubbed his weary eyes and felt Alexis's warm naked body close by. "Holy shit," he muttered pressing the light on his Casio 'G' shock watch.

He woke her up with his tongue. She responded slowly with light moans edging him on till he climbed on top of her tanned sexy body and entered her wetness. Eagerly, she met his thrusts, thinking about her ex-boyfriend fucking her roommate. "Asshole," she mumbled. *At least he could've asked me.*

"What?"

"Oh nothing lover boy…harder baby harder…yes give it to me…oh yes I need it…so bad." *Make him pay.*

Her dirty talk drove him crazy and he increased his frantic pace seeking release. The look in her eyes did it. He exploded willingly inside her moaning loudly while she groaned back in her own pleasure. Spent, they held each other for a moment and after they cleansed themselves in a nice hot shower for two they called Sam.

"Hey sleepy head, wait to see your new ride," he laughed heavily.

"Can't wait, I hate yellow! Hey how about Alexis and I spring for some pizzas and beer for the guys?"

"Shit that sounds wicked good. They'll love that. I'll order the pies from here, we gotta local place that makes the best damn pizza in Boston and they deliver so…just pick up some beer and smokes."

"Okay, we'll see you soon."

While he got dressed he admired Alexis's adorable outfit, sure to be a hit at the body shop. Out of one of the socks he pulled a ten gram chunk of cocaine and threw the socks back into his backpack and he was sure to take it with them when they left. He wasn't leaving a hundred and seventy-eight thousand dollars in cash anywhere. Even though he knew Hector was in jail, he had no idea how many bounty Rambos were still after him.

*   *   *

Early that morning after Alexis and Lucky had split for the Holiday Inn he had called four of his biker buddies who were in on the 'Vette heist and offered them a grand a piece to knock out the Mustang on a Sunday.

Now he eyed their hard work and dialed McKenna's Pizza House making sure to order enough for everyone. He was sure the guys would be very hungry after they got a good look at the hot babe Lucky was with. "What was her name?" he wondered. "Oh yeah, Alexis man, she's hot, smokin'. How's he do it?"

*   *   *

Lucky really not thinking clearly, pulled up to a busy corner market in a very rough looking neighborhood. Cautiously he parked Sam's seventy-one Chevelle close to the door with Alexis locked inside holding his Baretta.

He knew the classic muscle car was being sized up the second he stepped out. After all a car was stolen every eight seconds in the great State of Massachusetts, giving them top billing in the whole U.S. of A. But Massachusetts also had the toughest gun laws in the country. A handgun possession, out of state permit or not, carried an automatic one year in prison.

Quickly he entered the store obviously owned by foreigners. "Jesus fuckin' sand niggers got a monopoly on beer and smokes," Lucky joked with himself, buying two cases of Bud, two huge bags of Lays potato chips, and a carton of Marlboros and Marlboro Lights.

Three minutes he was back outside with his arms full. A wild looking group of greedy admirers had boldly surrounded the Chevelle ogling Alexis and the car lustfully. They backed off when Alexis boldly raised the Baretta like Lucky taught her; Right up to a guy's face on the other side of the window.

"Fuckin' broad's packin' heat," the sleazeball yelled backing away allowing Lucky to pass by.

"Nice neighborhood, wonder if they have anything available for rent," he joked firing up the powerful Chevelle.

Alexis just grinned clutching his gun. "Thought I was gonna have to splatter one of those creeps. God they said some disgusting things."

"Forget about it, we be gone baby."

When they pulled up to Sam's shop, McKenna's Pizza truck pulled in beside them. A cute redhead smiled over at them clutching three big pizza boxes while Alexis and Lucky followed her inside.

"You all having a party?" the redhead pizza girl asked, smiling at Alexis.

"Yup, we sure are you wanna join us?' Lucky asked her wishing she would.

"Wish I could. I gotta work."

"How much for the pizza?"

"Forty-five."

"Jesus, must be good shit."

"It is, don't worry."

"Okay, I believe you," he said handing her three twentys. "Keep the change."

"Why thank you kind sir," she flirted recklessly eyeing Alexis's healthy body.

Alexis and Lucky watched the cute red head leave. "You're too much Lucky," she laughed.

"What?", he grinned, knowing she'd known him for ten years and had seen it all good and bad, while he watched the redhead's cute ass strut out the door.

Lucky set everything out on the big table as Sam stepped over smiling. "Let's eat," Sam yelled to his four guys who were busy on the Mustang.

Lucky lit up two fat joints and handed them to Alexis to pass around. He knew she loved the attention she was getting in her sexy tight Daisy Duke jean shorts and skimpy bathing suit top, making all the guys trip over one another with lust.

"Man bro this pizza's wicked," Lucky mumbled, hungrily taking another big bite.

"Double meat deluxe, the fuckin' best," Sam told him hitting the joint and passing it.

"Wow, holy shit, the car looks so different…it's so…yellow."

"Sure the hell is, but that was the idea right!"

"Yeah, sure was."

"It's called triple yellow Corvette Emron banana paint," he laughed sipping a Bud. "Just happened to have some left over from our last job with 'vettes…so you're getting the good shit."

"Great." *Wonder what the dealership will say? Fuck 'em.*

"Yup, you'll be ready to roll first thing in the morning. We just got to shoot on some clear coat later tonight and you'll be good to go."

"Okay."

"Just don't wash it for a few days, hey you need to check out the Sunday late edition of the Boston Globe Lucky," Sam said grinning when he handed him the paper opened to the article circled.

Lucky glanced at it which read:

Gang warfare in New Hampshire's Queen City. Twelve dead. Allegedly Northern King gang members were executed late last night in Manchester, N.H. as their clubhouse was burned to the ground. A state police spokesman said an ongoing investigation into a rival gang, over a turf war and stolen cocaine, is currently in the works and that more information would be released soon.

"Shit," Lucky said eyeing the article realizing he was in way over his head. "Here read this Alexis so you know what time it is."

Everyone was still munching on pizza and beer. Stuffed Lucky said, "Oh I did bring some dessert for you guys," he grinned heading to Sam's office while Alexis willingly entertained the boys.

He pulled a large St. Pauli Girl Beer mirror off the wall and started chopping up monster lines for everyone. "That ought to keep you guys awake for awhile," Lucky laughed, walking back out to the shop toting an old triple beam scale in a wooden case that looked like someone stole it from some high school science lab. "Nice scale, where's your digital at?"

Sam shrugged, "At the house, but that'll work."

Lucky nodded. "Hey we're out of here guys," he said motioning to Alexis. "Sam there's a chunk in your desk drawer for later, we'll see you in the morning…later bro."

"Bye Alexis, keep him out of trouble if you can," he teased her.

"Now that's a full time job, but I'll give it my best shot," she teased the guys swaying her hips sexily as they went out the backdoor. "Bye guys."

"Bye Alexis," they all said sadly.

Inside the Chevelle, he looked over at Alexis. "Whew that's enough to drive a girl insane," she joked excited, fanning her face.

Lucky grinned cranking up the car knowing how turned on she was. Good less work for me he thought eyeing her excitedly.

SEVENTY NINE

THEY STOPPED AT a corner liquor store and bought a half gallon of Absolute Vodka and a gallon of Tropicana Premium fresh squeezed O.J.

Impulsively he grabbed a twelve pack of Michelob Light, Alexis's favorite and a box of Tijuana small plastic tipped cherry cigars to go along with a box of Glad sandwich bags.

Back at the Holiday Inn, Lucky anxiously filled the ice bucket over and over filling one of the bathroom sinks to chill the vodka and o.j. while Alexis slid into something a little more comfortable.

"Shit," he yelled impulsively. "I'll be right back." Ten seconds later he was on his way to a strip mall he saw earlier. Keenly he hustled into the Stop-N-Shop grocery store and bought four key limes for their cocktails. "Have it your way at Vodka King," he hummed standing in the shortest check out line; he grabbed a pack of Rolaids.

When he returned, he eagerly cut up a lime with his Leatherman tool and put the rest in a sandwich baggy. "Time to party," he boasted. "Hector's in jail, let's celebrate baby, yes sir."

She came out of the bathroom all dolled up, he immediately handed her a potent screwdriver. "My, don't you look delicious."

"Why thank you kind sir. Feeling pretty good are we?"

"Yes ma'am, very good in fact."

They drank scewdrivers while Lucky broke out one of the last two keys. "Honey you mind giving me a hand, we gotta make up thirty-five ounces. Twenty five go to Sam tomorrow morning for twenty-five grand."

"Holy shit lucky, where the hell did you get all that?" she asked amazed at the huge amount of cocaine in front of her.

He shook his head, "What's this twenty questions?"

"Okay, okay never mind lover boy let's do it, so you can give me some much needed attention, I'm uh so hot tonight," she purred teasing his neck.

"Good. Listen I'll cut out chunks and put 'em in baggies. You weigh 'em. If their under thirty grams add a little, if it's over thirty grams take some out with this spoon here."

"Oh okay. Just like baking my cookies," she laughed.

"Yup exactly, but these are very expensive cookies."

They both drank and drank, did lines, and smoked pot. The more they partied, the hornier they got. He was so relieved at Hector's capture that he over did it and continued to party at a blistering pace. Alexis with her own agenda, matched him drink for drink, line for line drowning her own heartache and memories of her roommate riding her boyfriend on the couch when she came home early. Ugh.

By midnight, thirty-five ounces were lined up on the dresser. He counted out twenty-five ounces for Sam and put the other ten away.

Over the next hour they took turns licking cocaine off one another's body, watching the pay-per-view adult viewing channel. Again and again they brought one another ever so close to orgasm, but stopped in time letting it build up and up till they both polluted on vodka, very turned on with the help of the evil love powder, finally needed to stop the teasing. It was time for some serious sex. They both needed it, wanted it, craved it, had to have it now.

Release.

Again and again, they abused one another's drained bodies, until they both passed out from exhaustion and satisfaction some time around five am.

Four hours later, around nine am they both woke up to a loud phone ringing. He stirred with a vicious vodka hangover. "Oh Jesus my head's killing me," he mumbled reaching for the annoying phone.

"Yeah?" he sighed into the phone.

"Hey family, your bananas ripe and ready. We're all waitin' on those twenty-five white blankets. What gives?"

"Man what time is it?" he demanded irritably.

"Shit bro, it's nine am, Tuesday morning. Thought you were in a rush?"

"Okay, okay we're just wakin' up. We'll see you in a while," he told him, dropping the phone back in its cradle. "Shit baby, we gotta get up and get out of here."

"Oh Lucky, I don't feel so goood," she moaned trying to raise her aching head.

"Me neither, come on we'll go pick up my car and go rent a nice suite somewhere, besides you gotta call your work."

"Shit you're right, I almost forgot."

EIGHTY

MENDOZA HAD UNCOMFORTABLY napped in his big car, getting very aggravated that he couldn't reach Hector with the good news. Frustrated, he pulled out his wallet and dialed a number he had never used. *Only in case of emergency do you ever use this* Hector told him two months ago. "Well I think this should count as an emergency," he muttered dialing the number.

"Sir, this is Mendoza. I been tryin' to reach Hecta all night about your boy but he don't answer. I'm wonderin' if he be okay sir cause I'm tailin' your boy waitin' on instructions." *So I can collect your twenty gees.* "So after I follow him to Mass, I sit here all night. I finally decide to call you figurin' this counts as an emergency."

"That was very good figuring Mendoza. Our beloved Hector got caught in a motel late last night with his pants around his ankles and two hookers jerking him off," the old man said sarcastically. "He's sitting in jail, but it looks like he'll be making bail any minute now."

The old man looked at his Rolex nervously, "So where's our little friend hiding at now?"

"Well sir, I'm about thirty minutes south of Boston in a town called Hanova. I got me a GPS signal tracka stuck to the belly of his Mustang. The car's been inside a body shop since yesterday mornin', looks like a crew has been in there all night workin' on it. He and some hot lookin' blonde are holed up in a Holiday Inn down the street."

"Very good Mendoza, very good indeed. Listen, give me your phone number and I'll definitely get back to you shortly, once I decide how I want you to dispose of our problem. You do know what happened last night?"

"No sir, whas up?"

"Well, they busted two of our amigos in the carwash next door with ten kilos. They also impounded all seven of my new 'Vettes and late Saturday night someone torched your clubhouse and killed twelve of your brothers, he told him solemnly. "I can't prove it Mendoza, but if I were a betting man, our friend you're following had something to do with all of it, you understand me?"

"You bet I do sir. This asshole's history," he said pissed off.

"Thinking about breaking Lucky's neck," he told the old man. "Mendoza keep your cool, don't lose him no matter what. There's a five grand extra bonus on top of the other just for you, don't let me down."

"No sir, I got 'em. I'll follow him to hell and back till you tell me otherwise." *For twenty-five large and a 'vette, I'm on it.*

"Good, now wait for my call and as soon as Hector's out on bail, he'll send some reinforcements your way," he told him angrily thinking about how Lucky had cost him two shipments of product and a quarter million in impounded 'vettes that'll take months to get back through the courts. *You're dead Lucky, you just don't know it yet.*

EIGHTY ONE

L T. BROOKS COULDN'T get Hector to roll on the old man, but he at least had ten kilos of uncut cocaine and seven top of the line late model 'vettes sitting outside in his impound lot. He could feel things were starting to go his way; it was just a matter of time and a little more luck.

The F.D.L.E (Florida Department of Law Enforcement) was working with the informant on the Orlando end of Operation Snowstorm. They were discretely tracking who had access to the 'Vettes prior to loading, who actually loaded the 'Vettes and how the money changed hands. It was obviously a very tight knit group handling the cocaine on the Florida end, because very few loose ends if any could be traced.

Both the car carrier driver who made the delivery regularly up to City Corvette and the attack dog owner were sitting quietly in their own cells at county jail not saying a word to anybody, Lt. Brooks knew somehow someone had already gotten word to both of them to keep their mouth shut and talk only to the lawyers so conveniently provided and they would stay alive to be well compensated.

Lt. Brooks had it all working at the same time. Tired and exhausted, he knew no matter what the D.A. said Hector was going to probably make the million dollar cash bail the state attorney had formally requested, hoping it was high enough that Hector couldn't meet bail. Somehow he had his doubts and it was very frustrating after all he'd been through to catch this piece of slime, and now less than twenty-four hours later he'd be free again. Oh what a system he thought irritated.

His phone rang bringing him back to reality. "Lt., word down here at the court house is Santiago's expensive mouthpiece somehow already secured the money for bail just a few minutes ago and a bail bondsman's already standing by."

"Great," he said dejected knowing it had to be the old man.

"Just thought you'd want to know sir."

"Thanks, thanks a lot Sgt." *Jesus what else can go wrong?*

∗   ∗   ∗

Nine-thirty am Manchester Municipal Court House. Hector Santiago's high priced mouthpiece Jeffrey Simms in his two thousand dollar custom tailored suit stood arrogantly beside Hector in his bright orange jump suit with prisoner boldly stenciled across his back. His night in jail didn't do much for his haggard looks as the judge listened to the assistant state attorney argue why Hector was such a high flight risk and should be held with no bail.

The judge didn't buy it. Santiago wasn't being held for murder and although he was charged with some serious felony violations, the evidence wasn't overwhelming. But he also knew he was facing an election year in the conservative Republican Granite State and if he were to lower the bond amount he would be ripped apart in the Concord Monitor and Union Leader. "I need a bail figure from the state," he said full of authority.

"The state of New Hampshire requests a minimum of a one million dollar cash bond for his release limited to within the borders of the Granite State, your honor," the Assistant D.A. announced strongly.

A minute passed. "Bail set for Mr. Hector Santiago at one million American dollars in cash bond as recommended by the Assistant State Attorney. The bond will be forfeited in full if your client fails to show up for his scheduled court date counselor," court adjourned."

The bail bondsman called in earlier by the old man was already starting the necessary paperwork to sign for the million dollar note guaranteeing payment if Hector disappeared. His cut, a hundred thousand free and clear. He only took the risk because the old man had promised him Hector wouldn't skip. "He'll either be in court or he'll be dead, either way you won't have to pay off on the promissory note," the old man said.

By ten am, Hector Santiago was released with the condition he couldn't leave the state without permission.

Lt. Brooks pissed off at Lucky, knew he should at least warn him about Hector's release. His parents would crucify him if he didn't at least try. So he called his cell phone and left the bad news on his answering service telling him to stop hiding and talk to him. *There, covered my ass.*

Forty-five minutes later, Hector was picked up in a limo outside the jail, and led to a private room at the Manchester Country Club where a waiter politely took his drink order. Five minutes later the old man entered the private room dressed in his Arnie Palmer golf attire smiling.

"Well, well, well. Look what the cat dragged in – geez fuckin' too busy partying with hookers when you're supposed to be taking care of my business," he barked angrily. "You read the papers Hector, you and your boys are all over it. Twelve dead, burned drug house, man oh man, you really let me down this time. Costing me a lot of money to say the least."

Hector knew when he was like this, he was better off just keeping his mouth shut and let him get it off his chest, because he knew he wouldn't have put up the bail money if he didn't need him. Things were happening too fast.

"Shit, you know you've cost me six hundred grand in under a month," he yelled. "And don't forget seven 'Vettes I just lost." The old man knew things were getting desperate. He needed the other eighty kilos of cocaine off his toy, the Fast Lady that was moored at the Palm Beach Yacht Club in Florida. But things were so hot right now he wasn't sure what to do or when to do it, and the sharp businessman he was, he recognized an oncoming disaster from a mile away. It was time for damage control.

"Your boy Mendoza, he's got Lucky's tail down in Hanover, Massachusetts about thirty minutes south of Boston. I want you to send your best team down there and eliminate the problem permanently. No more fuckin' games with that asshole Hector. He's cost us a lot of money; I probably shouldn't have fired his ass in the first place. Believe me, without him around everything will be a lot easier. Besides from what I hear he helped the Columbians raid your clubhouse."

"What?"

"That's right, Lucky's an expert shot and according to my sources he killed at least four Kings all by himself."

"He's dead meat," Hector said fuming.

"So you know what to do now?"

"Yes sir, I'll take care of it right away."

"Damn right you will," the old man muttered leaving the room.

EIGHTY TWO

H E TROMPED THE gas popping the Hurst shifter on the big block Chevelle, leaving a cloud of blue smoke as he raced through the gears towards Sam's Body Shop.

She pointed at the golden arches and he saw it barely in time chirping the fat tires downshifting he swung the loud Chevelle into the drive thru lane where they loaded up on Egg McMuffins and hot coffees for the whole body shop.

They pulled in under the tired eyes of Mendoza who was outside his car pissing in an alley. "Shit showtime," he mumbled seeing the Chevelle. *About fuckin' time.*

"Hey open the damn door so I can pull inside and we can unload this race car," he yelled over the motor to Sam who nodded looking his baby over quickly before he went back inside.

His Nextel phone was off. But his message light flashed when he shut off the Chevelle. His headache was still kicking and he wondered who the hell it was this time. He sat there for a few minutes watching Alexis hand out Egg McMuffins and coffees to the crew. Boy she sure looked good in a pair of jeans he thought reaching for his phone and dialing his service.

"Lucky, I've got bad news, Hector just made bail. That's right he's back on the street. So watch your ass you better get smart and call me before I find you. You're already in way over your head. Your only chance is to help me nail the old man."

"Fuck, fuck, fuck," he yelled wildly spilling his hot McDonald's coffee all over his bare legs. He hopped out of the Chevelle and slammed the car door. Everyone turned and saw the look on Lucky's face.

"The fucker just got out on bail. I'm going to Palm Beach right now," he roared. "Come on let's do this Sam in your office."

They went into his office and three minutes later Lucky came out in a hurry clutching a bag with twenty-five grand in cash.

Alexis had all the guys help load their stuff into the bright yellow Mustang and she was ready when he came out sitting in the passenger's seat with her seat belt on. The look said I'm going with you, no matter what.

"Thanks family, thanks guys, we're outta here," he yelled thankfully jumping into the very yellow Mustang. Lucky roared out of the shop and headed for the highway, driving right past an alert Mendoza who did a double take at the new color and different license plate attached to the back. *Motherfucker thinks he slick.*

*   *   *

As soon as they started moving the GPS tracker started beeping. "Finally," Mendoza said watching them drive past. Impatiently he let them get a ways ahead before he pulled off in his big Lincoln and started to follow. Don't lose him he heard the old man tell him.

Within a half hour Hector finally called Mendoza and told him he had company on the way to take care of the problem. Once Mendoza told him Lucky was on the move on the Mass Pike heading south, Hector told him to stay with him no matter what. "I got it man he's only a half mile ahead, it's like followin' a deer leavin' tracks in the snow."

"Just don't fuck this up Mendoza, my ass is on the line on this, you got that! I wish I could strangle that shithead myself, but I gotta count on you to make it happen."

"Shit Hecta, I got this man, I ain't lettin' twenty-five gees slip through my hands and I always wanted a 'vette."

"Good! Just remember Mendoza, that asshole killed four of our guys at the clubhouse."

"What?"

"Fuckers good with a gun, don't try to be a hero, wait till help arrives, you hear me, you'll still get your dough."

"No problem Hecta, I'm just the tail. You know I'm good at this part."

"I know Mendoza I just need this asshole bad." *Real bad.*

"We get him." *Then I get the hot blonde.*

"Good. Later."

*   *   *

Lt. Brooks waited at Johnson's Chevy for Lucky to show up for work Monday morning. Within an hour after going through the vast inventory, the owners and Lt. Brooks figured out Lucky returned the Ford lighting truck and switched to the 1991 dark green supercharged Mustang Gt.

Fifteen minutes later, Lt. Brooks changed the statewide Bolo from the truck to the Mustang. He also listed Lucky as armed and dangerous, priority one suspect. Any contact with subject vehicle or subject, they were to immediately contact Lt. Brooks at the state police hotline or Troop D in Bow.

Before he got back on the highway, he swore frustrated, "Damn you Lucky, I need some information. Now I got to take you down before Hector kills you." *Where the hell are you?*

EIGHTY THREE

BEFORE THEY TURNED off onto Interstate 95 South towards Washington D.C., they pulled into a big truck stop to top off with premium gas, check the oil, tires, and use the bathrooms.

He bought twenty bucks worth of various types of beef jerky. It was a tradition with his second wife to load up on beef jerky for a road trip. He also bought an Igloo cooler loaded with classic Cokes and ice. They were both functioning on four hours sleep and Lucky had none the night before, making their severe headaches that much worse. They both had downed a handful of Advil and washed it down with a Coke.

Mendoza filled the thirsty Lincoln up directly across from the truck stop, where he grabbed a ten piece of pre-cooked chicken and two quarts of Colt 45 to wash it down.

Eagerly Lucky and Alexis buckled in and hit the road for the long direct journey straight down I-95 to Palm Beach. The only problem with the Mustang besides the GPS magnetic tracker stuck to its belly, was that it had a small gas tank and it only got about ten miles per gallon, because of the power boosting supercharger and performance parts.

Once on 95 Southbound, Lucky set his cruise control at eighty, then he started in on a piece of peppered beef jerky while they shared a cold coke.

Man this is crazy.
Hot chick, lots of money.
Lots of coke, altered car.
No Registration, stolen tags.
What a nightmare.

Hector you leave me no choice, you're dead.

Two hours later, they entered the notorious New Jersey Turnpike where he immediately sat up and slowed down to the posted speed limit, sixty-five. Tired and hung over with sore nostrils, he knew this was the toughest part of the trip. Jersey State Troopers had a ruthless reputation and were thick as mosquitoes in a New Hampshire swamp, on the Devil's Highway. Every ounce of his concentration was focused on driving carefully because they were watching.

"Pass me the tutor babe, I need a bump," he asked Alexis keeping his eyes glued to the road. She filled the silver spoon with the strong powder and eased it up to his right nostril while he swiftly sniffed it clean, stinging his sore abused nasal passage. "See I told you we should have gone to bed last night," she joked trying to break through the barrier he had erected, when he heard Hector was free he had changed dramatically.

*   *   *

Hector called Mendoza for an update letting him know that help was only a few hours behind and it was just a matter of time till this problem was permanently eliminated.

"After you take care of my problem, then do what the fuck you want with his bitch. But afterwards you got that?"

"Yeah, I got it, I just thought I'd make him watch us all take turns Amigo, before I do him."

"Mendoza, I'm counting on you. Everything is riding on this, so stay tight."

"I hear you bro later." *That bitch is all mine.*

EIGHTY FOUR

FIVE HOURS LATER, while Alexis and Lucky squirmed in the extra firm Recaro Racing bucket seats heading south towards the City of Brotherly Love, Philly, Lt. Brooks finally held another clue in his big hand.

After spending the past five hours going to Laura's, Lucky's parents, and back to Johnson's once again he ended up at Lucky's now vacant apartment.

First thing he noticed was all of Lucky's clothes were gone. He searched diligently, not sure why he was even there, maybe a hunch he thought running out of places to look, he peeked under the twin bed with his mag light and noticed something.

Carefully, he picked it up and went into the bathroom eyeing the spidered mirror. The picture in his hand fit perfectly in the missing spot, even the pig blood lined up running right through Lucky's daughter's cute face.

Curious, he flipped the picture over and read "Boo, 4 years, 1996, Palm Beach." "Holy shit," he said reading the message on the mirror again. Now it makes sense he thought racing back outside to his cruiser. He drove like a man possessed back to Bow from Hillbro breaking every law imaginable. He shut down his blue lights hidden in his grill once he turned into Hilltop Estates and turned onto Oakley Drive, Lucky's parents' road.

The Sullivans were horrified after seeing the defiled picture of their precious granddaughter. They had no idea how Lucky got involved with these gangs, but they assumed it was drug related. Yes they knew he had a cocaine habit, but they were praying he'd outgrow it before it did too much damage.

"Is your granddaughter still in Palm Beach?" Lt. Brooks asked, very concerned.

"No…no they just sold their townhouse and moved to California. They got sick of waiting for Daddy to come back home," Mr. Sullivan stated obviously upset.

"Does Lucky know?"

"No, his soon to be ex-wife, a doctor, didn't want him to know for a while," he responded sullenly.

"Would he go to Palm Beach if he thought his daughter was in any danger?"

"Absolutely nothing could stop him." *Including me.*

"That's what I was afraid of!"

"What the hell's going on Lt.?"

*   *   *

"Where you at now?" Hector demanded.

"Towards Philly. We just got off the Jersey Turnpike."

"Where the hell's he goin'?"

"Don't know but he's steady movin'. Get this, his dark green Mustang is now bright yellow! Can you believe that shit? He had it painted in Hanova at that Biker Body Shop."

"Shit I got a car comin' hard behind you. Probably three hours behind you. But if he's pushin' it, they'll never catch up," he yelled frustrated.

"Well the good news is, we never went over sixty-five the whole time on the turn pike. I think them Jersey pigs gottem scared, so they should catch up."

"Okay I'll tell 'em. Keep your phone charged and don't you dare lose sight of him…I'll think uh somethin'…he's gotta stop sometime especially with that hot babe along…" *I know I would.*

"No problem, my tracker's workin' like a charm," he laughed. "Him n' that hot piece of ass ain't goin' nowhere. He's drivin' like he's got a load of dope in the back." *Our dope.*

"You better hope so Mendoza. This time we take care of business. That punk's dead meat."

"Damn right he is. But when we catch him, she's my prize. I call first dibs on that hot piece of ass…boy am I gonna teach her to love Spanish meat. Yeah we're gonna have some real fun before –"

"Shut the fuck up Mendoza. You think I'm playin' huh! The boss is ready to rip my head off and shit in my neck. I don't give a shit about no high class broad, you hear me?" he raged. "Listen, afterwards once he's history, do what the fuck you want with the bitch. You earned it, but after…you feel me?"

"Loud and fuckin' clear Amigo." That sweet ass is mine."

EIGHTY FIVE

T WO HOURS FURTHER along they were in a road dazed state. Exhausted from the night before, but strung out on all the tiny bumps from the silver spoon and caffeine from the numerous Classic Cokes he was in a zone eyeing the gas gauge swearing to himself that he could actually watch the gauge go down and down. "Man, would you look at that. Fuckin' engines thirsty, it's almost empty again!"

"Good I got to pee," she giggled.
"Okay, we'll stop soon or we'll be walkin'."

The next exit he pulled off into another service plaza and let Alexis off by the front door leading to the shops and restaurants while he pulled over to the full service pumps. "Fill it up hightest and check the oil," he told the pimple faced kid as he got out and locked the doors. Stretching, he eyed a spot to pee. On the way back to the car he grabbed a gallon jug of blue windshield washer cleaner and a can of fix-a-flat. After he paid, he drove back over to the restaurants and waited for a ten year old black Lincoln with New Hampshire plates to back out so he could pull in and park right out front.

Mendoza glanced back surprised. "Shit," he muttered not believing his weary eyes. There was Lucky ten feet behind him inches from his bumper. I could get out right here and blow him away and take his bitch and go collect my money he thought greedily backing out letting the bright yellow Mustang pull in. *But I better wait.*

Only for a quick second did Lucky hesitate when he eyed the familiar green and white Live Free or Die New Hampshire plate motto. Another Granite Stater on the move he thought putting it out of his mind.

He got out to stretch, but didn't dare leave the hot looking Mustang with all that money and cash in it. He'd heard nightmares about a lot of cars getting ripped off at these types of rest areas. After all he was just outside New York in South Jersey somewhere with out of state plates and a new banana paint job. A carjacker's dream. Not today motherfuckers, not today. At least not me, he thought tiredly.

Alexis strutted out the door with her arms full of food, while four teenagers gawked at her holding the door, they followed her outside with their eyes all over her backside.

He smiled realizing she didn't even know she was being stalked, and he knew he wasn't very hungry after all the cocaine he had ingested, at least not for food, but Alexis was looking awfully tasty. But he'd try to eat, even if he had to force himself to keep his strength up. Besides he loved McD's Quarter-Pounders with cheese and extra onion and pickles which Alexis had so thoughtfully bought with fries and chocolate shakes.

*   *   *

"So what the hell's going on? You come here demanding answers, but not sharing many facts. Are you suggesting that our granddaughter, our pride and joy is in some type of danger?" Mr. Sullivan demanded.

"No...sir I don't believe so, especially since you told me they moved?"

"Okay Lt. what the hell has Lucky gotten himself involved in this time?" he asked visibly upset.

"Sir, I'm not sure I can really answer that honestly. All I can really say is it has to do with City Corvette and at least one New England based gang called the Northern Kings."

"Are you telling me he's part of all this nonsense in the paper, part of this...this gang of hoodlums in Manchester?"

"No sir, it's more like they're after him for various reasons based on revenge of course, most likely related to drugs which probably all started at City Corvette."

"Tell me Lt., where is my son right now?"

"I have no idea sir. But if I was a betting man, I'd say he's on his way to Palm Beach to protect his daughter," he responded truthfully. "I should have locked him up for his own protection while I had the chance."

"If something happens to him Lt. Brooks you'll wish you did."

Lt. Brooks let the threat go by ready to leave. He said, "Thanks Mr. and Mrs. Sullivan for your time," handing Mr. Sullivan his police card. "Sir I will call you and keep you updated as soon as I hear anything."

"You damn well better. This whole thing has gotten way out of control Lt. Your control. I don't need to remind you who I work for. You've kept us in the dark way too long as it is…good day Lt. I'll be waiting for your call." *And you better call.*

Lt. Brooks wished he'd never decided to stop by the Sullivan's. Even though he got information he needed. *Shit now I've got to straighten out this mess…where the hell are you Lucky,* he thought.

"Jesus Christ Lucky what the hell is going on son," his father yelled, loosening his expensive silk tie aggravated, concerned, and embarrassed. *I hope you're okay.*

EIGHTY SIX

ROAD VISION. THEY'D been driving and driving since ten am. It was now ten pm. "Over half way there," he mumbled looking at Alexis's curled up cute body sleeping uncomfortably in the racing bucket seat.

Steering with his good knee he did another blast, spilling some onto his lap while he kept his eyes glued to the tractor trailer he'd been following.

He was in a zone.

Hyper focused Lucky clutched the Classic Coke bottle between his legs. Telling himself he could make it. Only ten or eleven more hours. If only I could go faster, he thought already running eighty-five behind a line of big rigs.

My baby Boo.
I'm coming Boo.
Daddy's coming.
Hide Boo, Hide
Daddy's coming

By midnight he was wiped out on cocaine as they raced into South Carolina pulling off into another truck stop for gas.

A mile back, Mendoza noticed the red dot slowing down so he drove past the exit and took the next one filling up the big Lincoln while he called the trailing car full of five Kings racing to catch up.

They were only an hour back now, because Lucky was still being cautious with a car full of cocaine, cash, and illegal plates. He'd been following the loaded down tractor trailers heading south.

He tiredly used the men's room, buying a large coffee with milk and sweet-n-low. He paid the attendant silently watching the other attendant clean the windshield over and over hungrily eyeing Alexis's exposed sleeping body through the windshield.

God she gets all the attention where ever we go he told himself. Back on I-95 Southbound he sipped the old coffee, chain smoked Marlboro Lights and abused more cocaine. He started in on himself.

I should've slept instead of partying all night.
Can I make it…I gotta make it.
I won't sleep till I see my baby girl safe.
No way Hector's ahead of me…no way.

He punched the Mustang up to speed and passed by a black Lincoln and fell in behind another group of truckers making time, the later it got the more the big rigs owned the open road.

Lucky drove on without his cruise control on so he would pay more attention to his driving. He followed a Wonder Bread truck keeping his eye on the cute young girl on the bread wrapper as they started to pass another Wonder Bread truck.

Two more big rigs closed up rapidly behind Lucky, one in the left lane and one on his right. Annoyed, Lucky flicked the knob on the rearview mirror blocking the trucks bright lights that were blinding him.

Then it happened fast.

He never saw it till it was too late. Anxiously, he felt boxed in looking to his left, then right. The only thing he saw was the Wonder Bread girl's face and white sheet metal everywhere.

An uneasy feeling crept over his worn out body, when the two big rigs following moved in tighter creating a box, while at the same time the truck in front slowed suddenly causing him to take his foot off the gas pedal. "Shit," he sighed starting to panic. Seconds later, the big rig right on his bumper hit the Mustang in the tail pushing it easily into the trailer in front, smashing one of the Mustang's headlights.

"Fuck," he screamed trying to control the car as he bounced off the trailer's steel bumper.

Alexis screamed, smacking her head against the passenger window. "What the hell is going on?" she yelled groggily looking around. "Oh my God Lucky!"

"Put your belt on now," he shouted, while the trucks started moving again. This time, the two rigs on his sides squeezed in closer and closer leaving him no room at all.

"What the hell are they doing?" Lucky cried out, when the truck on Alexis's side, collided with the passenger's side, slamming it into the big rig on the driver's side.

"Do something please," she pleaded pinning her strong shapely legs up against the dashboard. They bounced from one trailer to the other while the two trucks in the front and back sealed off any escape.

Immediately his mind raced back, way back, remembering something about the old man owning some type of trucking company. "Fuckin' Wonder Bread, shit I've seen it on his wall," Lucky tried to explain frantically as the two side trucks suddenly widened and the rear truck accelerated ramming them hard into the steel tailgate bumper of the front truck.

He fought the wheel wildly, trying to steady the battered Mustang. Things were desperate. He needed time to think. He had no time to plan, they were trapped.

We're trapped.
In the devil's den.
Gotta be the old man.
But how did he know...
Damn him...Holy shit...we're...

Swiftly, the truck on the right pulled up evenly with the Wonder Bread truck directly in front of Lucky leaving the right lane open. He glanced to the right seeing the opening, but then he spotted the reinforced guard rails. He turned left wide eyed as he felt the big rig literally push him into the right lane.

The trailing truck in the center lane followed the Mustang into the right lane boxing him in again. Then it dawned on him there was no breakdown lane. We're trapped.

They were on a long bridge.

Too late, nowhere to go, the truck on the driver's side turned aggressively into him, slapping the Mustang violently off the bridge rail. The truck behind him smashed his rear end shaking the pancaked Mustang fiercely.

Before he could recover, the Wonder Bread truck beside him swerved harder into Lucky's space bouncing them viciously off the cement guard rails crushing the passenger's side in worse. "Aaahhh," Alexis screamed crying while the car started coming apart.

"Get in the back, now!" he ordered her. "And get down low."

She dove into the back seat frantically pinning herself between the two front bucket seats. Then it happened, just like in the movies. The bridge was coming to an end and the trucks moved in hungrily for the final kill.

He braced for it, but he was powerless, clenching his shoulders and grinding his teeth. There was nothing he could do, as the heavy Wonder Bread rig slammed him from the side once again, pinning him against the guard rail sending metal and sparks flying.

Just as quick, the strong bridge rail was gone, and the truck behind him under a full head of steam smashed into the ass end sending the Mustang flying down the steep banking towards the dark river far below.

EIGHTY SEVEN

HE SPUN THE wheel and pumped the brakes rapidly, trying to slow the car down as the water raced toward them quickly, mowing down hundreds of shrubs and bushes. The battered Mustang with only one headlight bounced and skittered down the long steep banking.

Alexis never stopped screaming. Lucky thoughtlessly running out of options, slammed the Mustang into reverse and revved the motor just as they went airborne. The tachometer raced into the red threatening to blow the supercharged motor.

Lucky screamed into the darkness waiting for the river water to come flooding in. Instead they were slammed into a huge cement drainage culvert that drained into the wide river below.

The rear Goodyears squealed loudly pouring out clouds of smoke as the tires tried to stop the forward momentum when the car continued to crash into both sides of the rocky culvert. It didn't matter, they were going too fast. The Mustang plowed into the retaining fence, setting off the driver's airbag, slamming Lucky in the face blinding him.

He fought with the bag, feeling the car teetering on the fence, he reached for his Leatherman tool on his belt and popped the airbag. He couldn't see anything, but he could sense danger knowing they were rocking on top of the last barrier to the dark river down below.

"We gotta get out of here now," he screamed loudly into the dark silent car that was starting to slide forward inch by inch.

"Don't move," he ordered, tossing his backpack blindly out his shattered window, then he pulled the rear hatch lever and climbed out the windowless driver's door making the car react by the shift in weight leaning backward then forward it skidded a few more inches.

"Shit," he yelled, grabbing the heavy louvered rear hatch and yanking it open, he latched onto Alexis's outstretched arms and yanked her hard over the back seat into the hatch and out the back.

She fell hard on top of Lucky onto the slimy culvert just as the car rocked back and forward, then it was gone.

Stunned they waited clutching each other. The next thing they heard was a loud grinding splash, followed by silence.

"I can't believe this is happening," he mumbled holding Alexis's whimpering body closely. He glanced up towards the Devil's Highway two hundred feet above the deep culvert.

No big rigs loomed.

Only a large dark colored car sat pulled over on the shoulder, just past the bridge. It looked like a big Lincoln, but he couldn't be sure.

Why would he be pulled over there unless, then an alarm went off somewhere in his memory bank. "Come on we gotta get out of here now," he said pulling her to her feet. He reached out blindly trying to locate his backpack which was stuck in the banking.

Crazily, he searched for it finally finding it, he yanked it open, feeling for his Baretta.

Move now…they're coming.
How did he know where we were…
Doesn't matter now, someone's up there.
And they want me dead.
Boo I'm coming, Daddy's coming.

Cautiously they moved up the steep slippery culvert. He kept glancing up towards the highway expecting trouble. A second car pulled up behind the Lincoln and stopped. Five hard looking guys hopped out swiftly and started down the steep banking armed with flashlights and guns, they followed the tire tracks down and down.

Lucky spotted them, his mind raced thinking if we can only get above where the Mustang entered the culvert, maybe we'll be alright.

With a burst of adrenaline, he pulled Alexis up higher and higher with the valuable pack on his shoulder.

The mosquitoes swarmed them and they kept tripping over all the loose boulders scattered inside the drainage ditch from the Mustang bouncing off the rocky sides.

Finally, they were up to where the Mustang entered. They were coming closer and closer he could hear their voices. *Move now.*

Madly, they used the loose rocks to climb up the eight foot opposite side. He stood behind her and pushed her higher and higher as the flashlight beams closed in. She reached the top. He still had at least three feet to go but the sides were slick with green moss covered rocks. Panicking he couldn't get a hold. Come on come on, he told himself knowing he had only seconds.

"No," he sighed, "don't quit." He ripped off his pack and flung it up past Alexis into the dark, lightening his load by thirty pounds.

With a last try, he dug his nails through the wet moss feeling for roots, he pulled himself recklessly up towards the top, just as the flashlights hit the culvert.

Shit I'm dead meat he thought clinging to the side when Alexis cleverly bent a flexible young pine tree over the edge smacking him in the head. Violently he snatched it and pulled himself up. The tree held. Madly he climbed to the top just as the flashlights moved toward the sound and shined their lights into the empty culvert stumped.

Alexis was crying still in shock. "Ssshh," he whispered covering her mouth as he eyed the roaming lights and loud voices.

He watched as one light followed the tire tracks down the steep culvert to the crumpled retaining fence. Someone else said something in Spanish and another flashlight lit up the talker's face.

"Oh my God," Lucky whispered into Alexis's ear amazed he was looking at the driver of the van that tried to run him off the road back in Hillbro. "I've seen that guy before."

"See the two sets of footprints," an accented male voice cried out shining more light into the culvert while they followed them up the culvert with their lights over the loose boulders towards the opposite wall.

"Where's the pack?" he demanded quietly.

"Over there," she pointed.

"Come on," he murmured.

"Hey, over there! There they are," someone screamed. "Shoot 'em."

EIGHTY EIGHT

BULLETS SAILED OVER their heads, they ran and ran through thick marshy woods into a mass of hungry mosquitoes, trying to eat them alive. They continued to bump into obstacles, trees, rocks, and branches, slapped their exposed arms and legs. It didn't matter, they were running for their lives, prickers, mud, water, nothing could stop them.

Finally, after an hour running and hustling parallel to the highway, Lucky spotted the next exit lit up by a passing trucker's headlights through the trees.

Exhausted, he jammed his Baretta into his shorts and covered it with his wet, sweaty, dirty shirt. Carefully, they continued working their way up the long off ramp to the all night truck stop.

Hidden behind an old Texaco sign, he looked everywhere for the dark Lincoln and Wonder Bread tractor trailers. "Okay, okay let's go," he said pulling her along. "Hey you okay?" he asked her seeing her bloody face under the light.

"Oh, I'm just great," she weeped sarcastically.

Bringing her back to reality, he grabbed both her shoulders firmly. "We gotta get out of here, it's not safe. Come on I need you, so pull yourself together." *Easy for you to say.*

They walked up the grass to the truck stop and entered it, carefully looking around. He pointed at the ladies room. "Go ahead, I'll meet you right there," he said pointing at the abandoned 24 hour restaurant.

She nodded silently and limped into the ladies room a mess. He watched her go before he entered the empty mens room clutching his waistband. He cleaned up quickly washing off dirt and dried blood the best he could. Pulling the woods out of his curly hair, he exhaled heavily looking at himself in the mirror.

Hang on Boo.
I'm coming…I promise.
Shit that was close.
Too fuckin' close.
We need a car…fast.

They took a booth near the back of the restaurant so Lucky could watch the door. There was only one waitress and one cook on duty. It was one-forty-five am. He glanced out the big glass windows overlooking the gas pumps and parking lot. Only one lonely car parked over on the side in an employees spot, a twenty-five year old Karmann Ghia convertible.

He ordered them both steak and eggs with O.J. and coffee. Alexis was quiet. Too quiet. "Nice old car, is it yours?" he asked the overweight middle aged waitress named Shirley. Her red dyed hair with black roots, and gnawing on a wad of Bublicious, she smiled realizing he asked her a question.

"The car, yup sure is," she grinned looking out the window at the rusty faded Volkswagon with a big rip in the worn out convertible top.

"Want to sell it?"

She turned back laughing. "Now why would I do a foolish thing like that sugar? Hey it ain't much honey pie, but it's all I got," she stated walking off shaking her head.

"What are we gonna do now?" Alexis whined wishing she'd stayed at home.

Determined he grabbed her hand looking right into her scared eyes. "Well we're gonna eat, then we're gonna ride out of here in that," he pointed at the old Volkswagen smiling.

"But…but she said-"

"No, she said she's not interested right, well I'll make her very interested, trust me on this." *Bitch is sellin' she doesn't know it.*

"Okay lover boy, show me."

She brought the hot coffee and O.J.

"How's it run?"

"What? Oh…my car…it runs pretty good I guess…why?"

"Well if you won't sell it, how bout you rent it for a few days?" he asked slapping three grand on the table.

"Shit y'all crazy or somethin' mister?" she asked ogling all the cash.

We're dead serious, Shirley. Our car is gone…and we need wheels like now. See how serious we are, here's two more grand that makes five grand, easily ten times what your car's worth. It's all yours, all you have to do is bring us the keys with our breakfast and in a few days I'll call you from Florida and tell you where your car is."

Her eyes wide open in disbelief, she stared at the cash, eagerly. "Mister for that much cash you'all can keep that fuckin' car."

While they tried to eat, they watched Shirley waddle out to her car and clean out her stuff. "Here," she smiled dropping the keys and signed title on the table. "Just send me back my plate when you get to where you're going."

"Absolutely, nice doing business with you Shirley," he said sliding the five bundles across the table where she quickly grabbed up the money and stuffed them sneakily into her apron pocket like she was stealing. "Mister…you're crazy…y'all have a safe trip," she grinned dropping the check on the table.

EIGHTY NINE

I T WAS TWO-FIFTEEN am and they were back on I-95 Southbound into Georgia. Alexis hadn't said one word since the truck stop. "You okay baby?" he asked concerned.

She nodded, now tearless obviously feeling better. "Did that just really happen?" she asked confused.

"I know…I know…unbelievable."

She nodded dazed, "you aren't gonna stop till you get him, are you?"

"Nope."

"Good."

"Hey get the tutor."

"Yeah…let's do it."

The old Karmann Ghia with a hundred and fifty thousand miles on it ran like a champ. They raced through Georgia being blown all over the road by the big-rigs. They continued southbound both chain smoking Marlboro Lights and hitting the silver spoon full of magic powder. The new bond, the new commitment to see it through, grew between them, hour after hour as they continued southbound towards Palm Beach.

She burst out laughing, "What about all my clothes?"

"What clothes," he grinned laughing at his own filthy ripped shorts and tee shirt.

"The ones you're gonna buy me silly," she joked.

"Oh…those clothes." *Go ahead get all you want, you deserve it.*

By six am, Lucky was really dragging. He pulled into another service center to check the red oil light that had just come on breaking him out of his road trance. The attendant checked the oil and told him he was down three quarts. *Shit that's all we need.*

Lucky snatched the attendant's rag out of his hand and latched onto the oil filter which was so loose it almost fell off in his hands. "Shit fucker's loose as hell," he swore tightening it with his two hands. "Hey get me an oil filter wrench will ya?"

"I guess," he mumbled eyeing Lucky's clothes and beat up face, hesitating, thinking this guy's broke. Just look at the shit box he's driving.

Three quarts of Valvoline and a couple of turns on the wrench and the oil mystery was solved. Alexis came out carrying two large coffees and a box of Krispy Kreme honey dip donuts only a day old. "Are we ever going to stop and rest, you know, hotel, shower, sex, and sleep," she demanded knowing the answer.

His hands still covered in oil he responded wearily, "Honey as soon as we make sure my Boo is safe, we can go anywhere, do anything you want, promise."

"Good cause this wicked sucks."

"You can say that again…"

How the hell did they follow us?
They knew exactly where we were…
But how…are they watching right now?

The Karmian Ghia ran much better with oil and a tank of high test while they both enjoyed the wind blowing in their faces with the top down. It was ten am and they were a little more than an hour north of Palm Beach. Alexis handed Lucky a pair of cheap dark boy sunglasses that she bought at their last stop.

"Thank you," he said smiling.

They were very buzzed on cocaine and the cold Classic Cokes she had in the cheap Styrofoam cooler Shirley so generously left behind chilled their dry throats. The Florida sun even at ten am was beaming down on them while they cruised in the convertible wearing dark boys trying to prepare for what might happen in less than an hour.

The dark Lincoln and old Cadillac both with New Hampshire tags were no longer following Lucky. They were thirty minutes ahead of

Alexis and Lucky and knew exactly where they were heading courtesy of the old man who found out through tax records that Lucky's wife and daughter lived in Palm Beach out in the Polo grounds of Wellington.

The sun beat down hotter and hotter the higher it shined on the devil's highway. Finally Lucky started catching his third wind, he sped up pushing the old convertible faster and faster...70...75...80...85...

I'm coming Boo, Daddy's coming.
Come on hide Boo, hide.
Only forty minutes more Boo.
Then we can go feed the fishes like we used to.
Yeah that's what we'll do, feed the fishes.

NINETY

T HE OLD MAN paced back and forth impatiently on his two million dollar, sixty-five foot Hatteras yacht waiting for the phone to ring.

The highly exclusive Palm Beach Yacht Club was where his expensive toy "The Fast Lady" was moored. With everything that was happening back in New Hampshire, he was very disturbed knowing there was still eighty more kilos hidden inside his port fuel tank.

Ever since the police had raided City Corvette, all cocaine shipments had stopped completely. As a rule, always within twenty-four hours of Fast Lady's return to port after meeting the drop plane seventy miles off the coast of Florida all drugs were removed discretely to a Wonder Bread warehouse in Orlando. He continued to pace clutching his Dewars Scotch sipping nervously when the shipboard phone rang breaking his frustrated thoughts.

"Sir I just landed at Palm Beach International, your driver Ricky just picked me up. Nice wheels sir," he said glancing around the expensive Cadillac limo.

"Fuck the car Hector, just get your sorry ass over here now," he demanded.

Thirty minutes later, the limo pulled into the exclusive Marina and Ricky the driver escorted the overdressed hood, past all the expensive yachts to the Fast Lady's slip.

"Nice fuckin' toy boss," Hector said ogling the first class layout. *Cheap bastard.*

The old man just leered at him. He was more uptight than he could ever remember; his whole empire that took him years to build was falling apart in front of his own eyes. "Fix yourself a drink, then tell me what the hell's going on for Christ's sake. I still have eighty packages on board and you got six of your best men still chasing this asshole all over Florida. When's this nightmare going to end Hector, tell me?" he yelled, guzzling his scotch.

Smoothly Hector dropped a handful of cubes barehanded into the expensive glassware skipping the ice tongs. Greedily he eyed the top shelf liquor selection and grabbed the only bottle he recognized, Jack Daniels Black Label, filling the rocks glass to the top. Hector stalled on purpose, just to irritate the old man and let him know who was really running things.

"Relax boss, they're about thirty minutes ahead of our friends, who are now driving a real piece of shit, an old Volkswagen," he boasted laughing.

"Where the hell did he get that?"

Mendoza says he bought it off an old fat broad who works as a waitress at some truck stop, get this, for five grand cash. Yup, she told my boy after a little friendly bribe that home boy's backpack was slap full of green money...our green money."

"Shit, what about the stuff?...He couldn't have sold ten keys that quick for Christ's sake, he's a damn car salesman, not a drug dealer," he shouted angrily at the thought of Lucky with all his cash and cocaine.

"You're right. Hopefully it didn't end up in the river with the car," he barked back letting him know what he thought of the Wonder Bread stunt the old man had ordered without telling him.

"Fuck you, if he was dead we wouldn't be going through all this shit now would we?" he said gulping his double olive Martini that he switched to after the scotch.

"Listen Hector, this kid has caused us so many problems," he went on taking a deep breath, running his big hand through his thick white hair. "But," he smirked, "you lured him down here for a reason...you used the one card he couldn't or wouldn't resist...his kid! Now don't fuck it up, kill him and bring me the body," he demanded pointing towards the ocean. "And we'll make sure no one can find the asshole." *Ever again.*

NINETY ONE

L T. BROOKS AND F.D.L.E. took up residence in a vacant town house for sale directly across the street from Lucky's ex-wife's former residence.

The tactical unit had already setup two wireless remote mini cameras. One in the front and one in the back and every twenty seconds the laptop screen changed from one camera to the next, or it could be set on split screen.

Thirty minutes later the Lincoln and Cadillac pulled into the nice polo ground development. "It's number 311," Mendoza mumbled into his cell phone as they slowly cruised the quiet middle class neighborhood.

"Got it three-one-one. It's the place with the Re-Max sold sign on my right," the caddy driver responded.

"Yup I see it. Pull in, keys under the front mat, there ain't no one in the crib, so pull your ride into the garage and shut the door, then do what you been told," Mendoza ordered.

"Ten four boss man."

"Hey knock off the bullshit. This here little fucker is slippery as hell, or have you already forgot he killed four of our brothers. Now remember if he can see you he can hit you, man's deadly with a Baretta, so watch your ass, let's do this right," Mendoza yelled.

"Fucker's one dead hombre," was the somber reply in the caddy.

"Get inside, out of sight, he'll be here any time…and we wanna surprise him don't we?" *I want my money and his high class broad.*

"Fucker's mine."

"Good I'll be close by, I think he might know my car, so I'll hide it up front somewhere and give you a heads up when I spot him…out."

NINETY TWO

"COMPANY," LT. BROOKS said alertly watching a thug grab a key under the doormat and open the front door. Thirty seconds later the garage door started to open letting the caddy pull inside. Quickly the door started back down.

"Bingo, the Northern Kings have arrived," he said enthusiastically to the F.D.L.E team. "I counted five total across the street…but I bet there's more."

"And I bet they're also armed and dangerous right Lt.?" the team leader added seriously.

"Definitely and if we play it right Sgt., we can take down all the Kings and our prize guest all at the same time without firing a shot," he gleamed hopefully.

Mendoza pulled the big Lincoln in beside the plush tennis courts and watched two bimbos try to play tennis in their tiny Anna Kournikova tennis outfits. He kept one eye on the bimbos and one eye on the entrance to the polo run.

His phone rang. "You in place yet?" Hector demanded watching the old man squirm.

"Yup, just waiting for some company."

"Good it's about time we took care of this problem."

"Yeah it is." Cause I want my reward. *His blonde bitch.*

"No cops?"

"Nope place is wicked quiet, deserted just like he said," Hector told him. "We'll be waitin. ."

*   *   *

Lucky pulled off I-95 at the Palm Beach Airport exit and continued following it to the airport.

Alexis looked over eyeing the airport signs. "Where are we going?"

"The airport," he smiled trying to stay in control.

"Why?"

"Two reasons…first to see if you've had enough and want to fly home first class of course, and second to rent a storage locker, I'm not taking all this to a possible shoot out. Not me," he paused looking her in the eyes. "So what's it gonna be pretty lady? I'll give you plenty of money if you decide to go home."

She didn't even hesitate. "You done?" she asked irritated.

He nodded.

"Good, I'm staying. This asshole tried to kill me too you know… let's get 'em."

"Okay partna, I'll be back shortly. Ten minutes later he was back carrying a shopping bag, he climbed back into the convertible Ghia. "Here take this…it's for you…you know in case anything happens… you know…so you can get home okay."

"Don't say that, didn't you tell me you were badass with that thing?" she demanded pointing at his gun.

"Yeah but I'm pretty beat."

Don't give me that lover boy, if they're there you will go in and kick ass, understood?"

He nodded.

She smiled. "Good let's get this over with, so we can go to bed. Holy shit Lucky, this is a lot of money."

"Twenty-five grand Sam gave us," he said pulling back out of the airport while she stuffed the twenty-five bundles of cash into her cheap Florida beach bag she bought at one of their many fuel stops, after losing her pocketbook in the sunken Mustang.

W.C. SCOTT

"Thanks I think."

"So Alexis's decided to ride it out."

"Wouldn't miss it for the world," she said sarcastically.

"Well you're a good sport and a hell of a partner."

"Thanks I think," she laughed.

They left the airport with the top back up even though the old Volkswagen didn't have any A/C, and they were getting very close to the polo grounds which acted like a magnet; the further west they went the faster he drove.

She's okay...you're just paranoid.

How would they know where she lives?

Then why are you here?

If anything happens to Boo...I'll

"Hey you okay?"

"Huh...yeah...yeah...just thinking."

"You really think they're down here waiting...don't you?"

"I hope the hell not," he exhaled heavily at the red-light grabbing his vial of courage, doing a couple of bumps, then glanced at his Casio 'G' Shock. It was high noon when he turned into the familiar polo run development. His heart raced in unknown anticipation. Please be okay Boo, please he begged nervously talking to himself clutching the slippery oversized steering wheel with sweaty palms.

Slowly, cautiously he pulled down memory lane and the old memories came racing back. He couldn't help but smile to himself thinking about Boo learning to swim at the pool and the many times she took him over to the small stream to feed the fishes with bread. His heart ached heavily. I'm an idiot he thought. Beautiful daughter, smart wife and I'm using drugs. What's wrong with me? Then he saw a Barbie jeep sitting outside someone's house. The wonderful feeling came rushing back when he thought about Boo's big smile the Christmas he bought her the 12 volt jeep. They put it together, together. She handed him every bolt and nut. *Here Daddy* he could hear her sweet voice. It was killing him. *Why oh why.* Just watching her race around in her jeep made him so happy. *What have I done...*

Reality came screaming back and his heart sank when he spotted the Re-Max sign in the yard. "Oh my God…it's…it's sold," he declared not believing his eyes glaring at the townhouse looking for any sign of life.

They drove by very slowly; every window in the house was covered with heavy blinds his wife had put up. He felt it deep inside, "Something isn't right."

"What do you mean?" *Looks okay to me.*

"Look around, there isn't one person outside, no kids, nobody on the street, it's just too quiet…kind of creepy."

"Maybe everyone's at a parade or sale or something."

"Heads up, our package has arrived, be still he's checkin' the place out right now," Mendoza barked over his cell phone.

"Gottcha Amigo, we're still," was the reply.

At the end of the cul-de-sac, Lucky pulled over and climbed out of the Karmian Ghia. Stuffing his Baretta into his shorts sticking an extra clip into his pocket.

"Our prize just drove past gentlemen, pass the word he's driving a beat up Karmain Ghia," Lt. Brooks said determined. *Gotcha now Lucky.*

"What are you going to do?" Alexis asked concerned.

"I've got to check it out with my own eyes," he decided looking back down the deserted street.

"Can you drive a stick?"

"Not well."

"Do the best you can…go to the pool house and wait fifteen minutes," he told her gravely. "Now if I don't show up…then…go to the Ritz-Carlton Hotel in Manalapan and get a room."

"Where the hell is that?"

"Just head east till you hit the ocean, then just ask someone. It's a huge five-star resort," he told her trying to encourage her. "My friend Marty runs the concierge desk. Find him and mention my name and he will look after you, okay?"

"If you say so, I'd rather see you in fifteen minutes." Lover boy.

"Here."

"And what am I gonna do with this?"

"Hold onto it…and you know if I don't come back…well it's in locker 311, just like Boo's house number," he joked nervously stalling. "And make sure she gets her share okay?"

"God you're unbelievable. Of course she will, but you'll be the one giving it to her, not me, so go on, get going if you don't come back I'll kill you myself."

"Okay take off, remember fifteen minutes, then go."

She nodded starting the car, nervously she pulled off burning the clutch. *Go get 'em lover boy.*

NINETY THREE

LUCKY FINALLY ARRIVED. Now I can save my ass Lt Brooks thought rubbing his tense hands together.

The cops were watching Lucky through the high powered binoculars waiting for Lucky to show up on the laptop screen. "Team two, second party is on scene. I repeat, second party is on scene wearing black torn shorts and a dirty white ripped polo shirt," the F.D.L.E. Swat team leader crackled eagerly into his walkie-talkie.

"I say again, second party is on the move in your direction, looks like he's come to crash the house party. Subject Lucky Sullivan, white male, age twenty-five black shorts, off white dirty polo shirt is armed and should be considered very dangerous. He is an expert marksman, prior military, very familiar with Swat tactics. Use all precautions and any level of force necessary...but he is considered a key state witness and was cooperating with Lt. Brooks, that's all stay alert, team leader out."

"Team two copies out."

Lucky walked back down the quiet street observing with every hair on his neck standing up. Everything felt wrong. Not one car had come down the street, nor one person had come outside.

Boo are you hiding too?
Daddy's here, you'll be safe.
Hide baby, just like Daddy taught you.
That's my girl, peek-a-boo.
I see you.

He cut across the tall grass which was usually very well maintained, but hadn't been cut. His heart sank when he eyed the sold sign boldly displayed. Cautiously, he observed the silent house moving into the tree garden for cover. I hope she's not inside, he told himself not wanting her to see him spying with a gun. That's the last thing he needed. But he had to see for himself. Slowly, slowly he tried to peek into a window and see his precious Boo watching one of her Barney videos. Then he'd leave quietly.

Twelve minutes he sighed looking at his watch. Carefully he followed the privacy fence around the back to the enclosed backyard each townhouse was afforded. Silently, he lifted the latch and pushed the squeaky gate open quickly sliding inside in a crouch. "Shit," he mumbled at the noisy gate.

Both teams of cops watched eagerly. Team one inside the house with Lt. Brooks watched on the second camera, while team two behind Lucky, were close enough to see without glasses.

"We got company, our hens out back sneaking around," a gang member upstairs peeking out a bedroom window muttered into his cell phone.

"Wait till he gets inside," Mendoza ordered. "No shots unless you have to, trap him inside. Remember, keep him alive we all get a bonus."

"True that."

The curtains in the back were all closed tightly. He stuck his ear up to the slider trying to listen for any noise, TV, radio, but nothing.

Something's wrong. Everything feels so wrong.

"Shit," he mumbled. It was creepy quiet. No birds, nothing. Too damn quiet he thought. Sweat ran down his back. Instinctively he yanked out his Baretta and tried the backslider. Locked…slowly he edged over to the kitchen window and spied the engaged lock.

"Unlock the front," the thug whispered to his amigo nodding at the front door. Soundlessly, the King unlocked the deadbolt and disappeared. Above the doorway on the second floor, a two hundred and twenty pound gorilla whose cousin died in the clubhouse fire, waited patiently to pounce on his prey from the railing above crushing the hen.

With his Baretta tight to his side he eased around the windowless garage and tiptoed towards the front door. He glanced at the time on his stopwatch, seven minutes to meet Alexis. *Come on Boo, where are you?"*

"Team one second subject Sullivan is out of sight, should now be on your side, team two standing by," team leader two said into his headset.

"Team one copies, he's moving towards the front door with his gun held in a two handed combat grip. Close in slowly two, should have fireworks shortly."

"Copy two, moving in."

Lucky peeked through the thick glass squares on either side of the front door without success. It was too dark inside. He kicked the doormat over and looked for the hideaway key he had so cleverly embedded in the thick grass mat.

It was gone.

Not good he thought. Slowly he edged over to the door and put his ear up to the wooden door.

Nothing.

"Fuck it, here I come Boo," he whispered raising his trusty steel friend as he twisted the chrome door handle. It turned easily in his sweaty hand which he wiped on his shorts. Hesitating, he took a deep breath and exhaled then pushed the door open stepping back he raised his Baretta.

Nothing but darkness.

His heart was beating very fast, the living room was empty. "They're gone," he sighed realizing the place was empty. His heart sank heavily and he dropped his guard exhausted. *My God they moved but why?*

"He's going in everyone stand by," team leader yelled.

"Copy that."

Shocked, he stepped into the foyer and immediately he sensed company in the house, movement on his right, it's so dark he thought trying to see. Man it's a trap, he told himself hearing a sound on his left he swung his gun to his left ready to fire. Automatically, holding his Baretta in a two-hand combat grip. Something moved fast and he fired a shot into the master bedroom missing just as the gorilla above launched himself off the railing above crushing the hen to the floor violently.

The front door slammed shut and that sound was the last thing Lucky heard when a King whacked him in the head with a pistol, his world turned black.

"We got'em," the excited King yelled into his phone pushing Lucky's lifeless body onto his back.

"Is he alive?"

"Yeah, I think so."

"Good Amigo, now tie him up and put him inside the sail bag in your trunk. We got an expensive package to deliver. Yes, then we'll party," Mendoza said grinning for the first time in days. He finally knew the old man would kick in an extra bonus. *Now where's his blond bitch?*

NINETY FOUR

THE F.D.L.E. SWAT Team eagerly moved to the garage ready to explode onto the unsuspecting townhouse. The Swat Team leader inventoried his gear. A Colt 45 semi-automatic pistol in a fast release thigh holster with a backup Colt inside the pocket of his tactical bullet-proof vest. Clipped to his utility belt were flash bangs, smoke grenades, and other diversionary devices. He wore a ballistic assault helmet and a Motorola two way secure radio headset with a cheek microphone on a breakaway strap. The whole team both inside the garage and outside the target zone were in full B.D.U – Battle Dress Uniform.

Two members packed Heckler & Koch MP-5 9mm submachine guns capable of firing up to eight hundred rounds per minute on full automatic. While two others were packing the deadliest assault rifle on earth, the Spencer Super 90 M3 Twelve gauge pump shotgun – they were ready to kick some ass.

"Wait," Lt. Brooks pleaded just as they were ready to open the garage door. "Let's follow them, they already got Sullivan and there's only one person who really wants him…the old man, the person behind everything."

The F.D.L.E. Sgt. didn't like it. "Lt. this is my operation, I make all the decisions, you are to observe sir."

"I know but –"

Frustrated the Sgt. cut him off. Team leader two move in on the house and we'll follow the Cadillac."

"Two copies."

"You better be right Brooks," he barked angrily. "Team one load up both trucks move now." They piled into the two unmarked four door limo tinted Chevy Trailblazers that barely fit in the two car garage and started after the fleeing Cadillac.

Alexis glanced at her Mickey Mouse watch nervously. Twelve minutes, I'm not leaving she thought. "Come on Lucky please," she sighed.

The Lincoln pulled out of the tennis courts catching Alexis's eye. She leered at the familiar plate and remembered Lucky saying Lincoln. "Oh shit, they're here," she cried out not knowing what to do.

She watched as a Cadillac also with New Hampshire plates fell in behind the Lincoln. Suspiciously they sped over the speed bumps not slowing down. "Oh my God...Lucky what's happening?" she said glancing at Mickey Mouse. Fourteen minutes. Undecided, confused she pulled out towards the townhouse as two dark tinted trailblazers raced past.

Her intuition told her something was definitely wrong. Slowly, she drove past number 311 and spotted the open garage door. "Oh shit, they were waiting for him," she said as a cold chill ran down her spine. *Oh lover boy where are you?*

On her next pass by she spotted the Swat Team swarming the house. "Oh my God," she whined wide-eyed. Not knowing what to do, she accelerated shaking and crying.

"Oh Lucky what am I gonna do, where are you?" Go to the Ritz Carlton, ask for Marty, just find the ocean she heard him say calming her a little. *Okay lover boy.*

Bound and unconscious Lucky rode inside the sail bag in the dark hot trunk. Thirty minutes later the car caravan of hoods pulled into Julie-Anne's restaurant directly across from the ritzy Palm Beach Yacht Club.

"We got em...and he's breathing," Mendoza told Hector who pumped his fist wildly.

"Where you be at Amigo?" Hector asked with a shit eating grin.

Mendoza snickered, "Across the street." Get *my reward ready.*

The swat team raced down A-1A right past Julie-Anne's.

"Damn it, we lost 'em," team one leader screamed frustrated.

"They've got to be somewhere, any other bright ideas Lt.?"

Two hours later, Lucky laid face down on deck of the Fast Lady not moving at all. "Put em below," the old man ordered feeling Lucky's pulse. He was so pleased he was still alive. "We get underway after dark, so get inside all of you and keep out of sight." *Finally he's mine.*

Frustrated and very upset they split up and started searching the A1-A area looking for two cars when Lt. Brooks's cell phone rang.

"Hey Lt. any luck down there?" the D.A. asked two-thousand miles away back in Concord, New Hampshire.

"You don't want a know. The King's have Sullivan and we followed them to the ocean, then somehow they vanished," he breathed heavily into his phone. I'm screwed.

"Well I don't know if it means anything, but I just intercepted a telegram addressed to you from Palm Beach International Airport," he told Brooks eyeing the Western Union priority sealed envelope. "You want me to open it?"

Damn you Lucky. "Yes open it."

The D.A. unsealed the envelope and read it. "Okay here goes:

Lt. I've got to do what a good father would do. Maybe you'll understand why someday. The last tip I know is check out his boat...the Fast Lady...it's moored in Palm Beach somewhere, he probably brings his dope in on his boat. So now we're even. Nail his ass...Lucky out.

"Holy shit," Lt. Brooks responded thinking. "Thanks Herb now we know why we're on the water, gotta go, I'll be in touch thanks." Oh Lucky I hope I find you in time.

"Good luck."

An hour later the Coast Guard, Florida Marine Patrol, Customs, and Palm Beach Sheriff's office knew exactly where the Fast Lady was moored.

"Let's move, it's at the Palm Beach Yacht Club," team leader one piped excitedly. "Get the Coast Guard on the horn; see how they wanna work it."

NINETY FIVE

MARTY CHECKED THE lovely distraught Alexis into an ocean front suite at the world famous Ritz Carlton using his employee discount card thankful that the snowbird season was still a few weeks away.

"Oh Marty, I'm so worried about Lucky," she cried out upset toting her cheap beach bag loaded with cash and nothing else.

"Well Alexis, I've known Lucky quite a while and if anyone can come out of this smelling like fresh baked chocolate chip cookies, it'll be him."

"I sure hope so…he…he told me to come here and wait…but I'm so confused…I need to buy some clothes," she stated exhausted collapsing on the big bed.

"What size are you?" *Where does he find all these hot babes?*

"Size five why?"

"I'll get you a few things and later if you want I'll take you to some killer shops on Worth Ave."

"Okay, we'll see…I'll just rest for now and take a hot shower and maybe he'll show."

"Call me if you need anything, don't hesitate. Just dial the concierge desk," he told her nicely, shutting the door and putting out the do-not-disturb sign.

"Jesus Christ Lucky, another bimbo and you're in trouble. Man oh man, I can't help you brother unless you tell me where you at," Marty the former army ranger mumbled getting back in the plush elevator.

She took a long hot bath in the oversized tub. Trying to relax she added complimentary bath oil to the water. Wrapped in a Ritz Carlton robe she finally fell into a deep restless sleep.

Darkness crept closer with the gorgeous bright red Florida sun setting in the west. A plan was struck by the team in cooperation with Customs,Coast Guard, and D.E.A. All agencies wanted in on this takedown.

Casually an unmarked forty-two foot black Scarab and a thirty-eight foot Mako sport fisher both confiscated in prior drug raids entered the restricted harbor at no wake speed. Docking was already pre-arranged with the Harbor Master who picked out two slips on opposite sides of the Fast Lady but in easy viewing. After both boats tied off, the sport fisher started cleaning their catch while the Scarab setup a grill on the deck.

Agents were now dressed in fishing gear and vacation attire drinking non-alcoholic umbrella drinks while the two medium endurance Cutters 270 feet long both out of Portsmouth, Virginia were in the area for scheduled helo operation training. Both Cutters, twenty-five miles off the coast of Palm Beach, were smartly equipped with Sikorsky search and rescue helicopters.

It was a quick sunset and it was going to be a dark night. The quarter moon was shaded by large rain clouds pushing in from offshore. At nine pm, the old man intoxicated, stumbled up to the bridge. He had been drinking all day, first in frustration, later in celebration. "Get under way Howie, time to offload the garbage," he slurred yelling at the boat's captain.

The awesome four engines cranked over alerting everyone standing by. "The Fast Lady is getting underway," the D.E.A. agent whispered into his mike while he fished off the end of the dock.

Within seconds, everyone moved into plan A. The Fast Lady with its running lights properly displayed pulled out slowly. Observing the no wake zone, it motored out of the private marina. Because of the heavy overcast cloudy visibility Captain Howie cautiously maneuvered the large sixty-five foot first class yacht around the free floating moored sailboats and aimed expertly between the two flashing channel markers barely visible in the thick wet air.

W.C. SCOTT

"It's working, we got 'em," the customs agent aboard the Scarab told Lt. Brooks who had hitched a ride. Lt. Brooks sat in one of the bolster chairs up on deck while he watched the agent in the long narrow stateroom below monitor the GPS tracking device that a Navy Seal had attached to the back of the Fast Lady's hull hours before.

"That was good thinking," he said pointing at the screen. "Especially in this weather." Finally glad to be moving, *I sure hope Lucky is with us for my sake he prayed.*

"Well it's not the fist time Lt."

"How long do we wait?"

This only has a range of two nautical miles so we can't wait long. The Fast Lady has a top speed of about forty knots so we have to stay close, but this black Scarab with those five 200 horsepower XP Evinrudes are pushing eleven hundred horsepower and runs oh ninety plus miles an hour.

"Holy shit!"

"Exactly."

Ten minutes to the second the black Scarab fired up, its powerful outboards followed the sport fisher sporting twin V-8 300 horsepower Evinrudes. The chase was on.

Little did they know the Fast Lady had four highly modified big block 'Vette racing engines pushing well over two thousand horsepower. Once it cleared the last no wake buoy it's engines roared to life sounding like four big block 'Vettes with straight pipes accelerating as the captain pushed the four throttles forward simultaneously.

NINETY SIX

T HE SEAS STARTED to get choppy as the offshore rainstorm blew inland coming down in buckets, while the Fast Lady cruised at 45 knots straight out to sea.

Once free of the harbor channel the Customs Scarab jumped out of the water when the driver pushed the four throttles to half throttle as the two mile GPS signal started to fade off the screen. "Fucker's faster than we thought," the officer yelled at the Lt. They were running at sixty knots when the driver was signaled to pick up the pace. Blinded by the heavy rain, he bumped the throttles to seventy-five percent pushing the go fast up to eighty knots.

The two Cutters five miles apart still closing went to General Quarters and launched both of their helicopters from the flight decks while both ships also launched their heavy duty Avon rigid inflatable small boats. Equipped with twin seventy-five horsepower offshore Evinrudes the light boats were fast and practically unsinkable. Both small boats were armed with an experienced boarding team and rescue swimmer slash medic.

The Coast Guard Choppers were equipped with the latest high tech tracking gadget available. The petty officer working the video display screen that showed their present location tracked via GPS and Loran coordinates superimposed over a moving live oceanographic chart. Heading, speeds, and distances to each target were clearly displayed on the screen in two letter digital readouts. On top of that the nose was equipped with infrared heat seeking signatures of humans or boat engines displayed in 3-D on the video screen.

Even with the hard falling rain once the first pilot tapped into the cutter's powerful radar memory seconds passed then the Fast Lady was illuminated on the green screen as hostile.

"Got her, Commander, she's running hard at fifty knots," the first class E.T. (Electronics Technician) called out to the two pilots who verified it with the Cutter Northland who was now designated as the command vessel.

Drunk and excited, the thugs completely soaked dragged Lucky's lifeless body aft, to the fantail and secured two ten pound York dumbbells to Lucky's body with half-inch nylon line.

From his perch, the old man watched eagerly wishing Lucky was awake so he could have the last laugh. "Fuck it, wake his ass up. I want him to see my face one more time before he drowns," the old man demanded loudly over the noisy engines clutching the bar rail in the solon with one hand and another martini in the other.

"Sixty knots. Unbelievable sir, they're doing sixty knots," the E.T. told the pilots who hovered high above.

"Pass it to the Go Fast and the Cutter techie."

"Roger that sir."

Ice cold water from an empty beer cooler drenched Lucky's face shocking his unconscious brain. Slowly his mind came back out of the darkness onto a vibrating deck. A piercing bright light hurt his eyes. Automatically he tried to move his hand to block it, but he couldn't, then he sensed rain and ocean air.

Oh shit! Fear came racing back. His senses were dulled but he knew he was in danger. Salt water he thought back. I'm still in the Coast Guard, Hurricane Andrew, what was that? Someone was bitch slapping him...yup that was a real hard one his mind registered.

"Wake the fuck up asshole," Hector screamed, kicking Lucky solidly in the stomach with his Timberland steel toed shit kickers.

Someone held his face hard. Hot burning tequila seared his nose and throat as they forced it down his throat choking him violently while he tried to breath.

"He's awake now," Hector laughed waving the old man over who was two sheets in the wind. "Slow the fuck down Howie, there ain't no one out here in all this shit," he yelled at Howie who was up on the flying bridge but could hear him clearly through the intercom, and had been pushing the big yacht for all she was worth wishing he was far away from what they were about to do, but hey a grand a week to be on call in a free beach front condo put in his name. He'd just have to look the other way once in a while he thought.

The big Hatteras slowed to thirty knots then twenty knots.

Slowly, Lucky tried to open his swollen dilated eyes, but the light was still so bright and now he knew he wasn't still in the Coast Guard. He heard it.

The voice.

Laughing madly, hysterically like a madman right in his face. Almost puking he could smell the heavy stale booze breath and even though he couldn't see his face in all the rain and bright light he knew exactly who it was.

The old man…no
And Hector too
Oh shit my head's killing me
I must be on the Fast Lady
Run Boo run, hide Boo hide.
Shit, where are you Lt. I told you…

NINETY SEVEN

T HE FAST LADY continued on unaware of the load of Coastys dead ahead. Both helicopters were high above the Fast Lady and were watching the action on the open deck far below on the screen. "Sir I think we found our first guest, looks like he's going for a swim sir."

"Get the rescue swimmer ready, stand by to move in."

Eagerly both 270 foot Cutters steamed ahead at a full 24 knots closing in on the Fast Lady, cutting off any escape. Both Coast Guard small boats cruised a hundred yards in front of their respective ships just waiting for the command, for a hostile boarding takedown, a Coasty's dream.

The open fisherman trailing the big Scarab still was pushing seventy knots, but with a top speed somewhere around a hundred knots, the bad ass 42 foot Scarab increased its speed now flying blindly in the pouring rain once they heard Lucky was alive and ready to be shark bait. *No hold on Lucky, we're coming.*

"So Lucky, no one fires you huh?" he bellowed sarcastically totally enjoying himself as the big Hatteras slowed down to two knots. "You stupid piece of shit, who the hell are you punk," he slurred angrily jabbing his fat finger into Lucky's bruised face while two Kings tried to keep the old man from falling on the rocking, slippery deck. "To fuck with me…" he laughed crazily getting soaked. "Hit the lights."

"This is Coast Guard cutter Northland, authorization has been granted for immediate hostile takedown. All parties involved move in at your fastest possible speed. Subjects are armed and dangerous and preparing to toss a former Coasty off the fantail with weights attached. Use all necessary force. Let's take them down now," the four striper ordered over the bridge radio aboard the quiet Northland. They were taking this personally once Lt. Brooks told them what time it was.

Both choppers running in blackout conditions swarmed down aggressively as each rescue swimmer in the back of the chopper checked his gear one last time.

The Fast Lady's exterior powerful spotlights shined brightly into the heavy rain. "Cut em then toss his ass, the sharks are hungry," he roared out of control. "Do it now. Hey have a nice swim Lucky."

Clumsily the four Kings who didn't have their sea legs and weren't use to the rocking boat, dragged Lucky roughly to the fantail while another King carried the two ten pound dumbbells attached to twenty feet of rope and Lucky's two wrists. Awkwardly they shuffled toward the aft gate steadying themselves in the eight foot rollers.

They pulled him through the back gate onto the big fiberglass diving platform then dropped him. Hector grinning took out his switch blade and cut Lucky's forearms from the wrist to the elbow. Blood gushed out dripping on deck as salt water washed it away. "You hear that?" Hector yelled over the four noisy 'Vette engines idling loudly out of the four back exhausts.

"Huh, hear what?" Mendoza yelled back. "Come on, let's do this –"

The sky lit up with two huge powerful beams of light. Over a loud speaker the pilot hovering dangerously close said, "This is the United States Coast Guard, you are completely surrounded. Shut down your engines and stop what you're doing or you will be fired on. You have five seconds to comply. Two boarding parties are standing by to come aboard, do you copy Fast Lady?"

"Waving his arms frantically the old man screamed at Howie to hit it. He hesitated for a second till he saw the look on the old man's face of total fear.

Howie floored all four six hundred horsepower 'Vette engines sending Lucky into the water along with three helpless Kings, two who couldn't swim. Everyone hesitated, chase the fleeing Fast Lady or save the drowning swimmer. One chopper stayed lighting up the water where three Kings were floundering. Lt. Brooks out of his element made the Customs *Go Fast* stop knowing Lucky was in the water. *Where is he?*

Everything happened fast. Rescue swimmer jumped into the water from the chopper above eyeing the last spot he just saw Lucky sink. Tangled in the two twenty foot lines the three drowning punks couldn't fight free especially with the two ten pound dumbbells pulling them down. Lucky a former rescue swimmer himself, managed a deep breath just before going under. He fought with all his strength to loosen his binds but to no avail, he was drowning.

Two separate rescue swimmers, one from the Coast Guard small boat and the other from above, raced in their fins and mask towards the big splash. Both were going for the former Coasty leaving the thugs who were drowning one another panicking. The rope wrapped tighter around their legs as they clawed and punched one another trying to push off their drowning amigo locked in a death grip of fear.

He continued to hold his breath, just like in the big pool at Coast Guard Boot Camp in Cape May, New Jersey. Four minutes and forty-eight seconds was the record he set.

Air was running out quickly.

Oh man Daddy tried Boo, I tried he pleaded ready to give up when a pair of hands grabbed him. Shocked he fought back till he saw the familiar orange rescue suit. A sharp blade sliced through the braided line freeing his hands.

New hope surged through him, but he needed air right now and he was still fifteen feet down. A hand found Lucky's mouth inserting a small mouthpiece, seconds later the mini bottle of oxygen never tasted so good.

The rescue swimmer freed Lucky's legs pointing up towards the bright light of the helicopter, out of the darkness. But the two Kings down below the surface worked themselves loose from the line attached and one dumbell smashed into the rescue swimmer's head instantly knocking him still. *Oh shit.*

Two more bodies struggling were pulled by Lucky bumping him as the other dumbbell dropped out of sight dragging them deeper. Then a hand shot out and grabbed his throat desperately. Lucky holding the rescue swimmer's body around the neck from behind in a rescue swimmer's towing technique turned the rescue swimmer's light attached to his mask toward the clutching hand that was pulling them deeper. Hector's face wide eyed was screaming "Fuck you Lucky."

Lucky full of fresh oxygen and adrenaline still clutching the Coasty jabbed out with all his might just like they taught him in Karate class fifteen years earlier on dummies. He jabbed both fingers viciously poking him in the eyes blinding him. Fuck you too Hector, I win," he mumbled pulling the rescue swimmer to the surface.

Shocked into action the huge eight foot swells disoriented him. He eyed the black Scarab twenty feet away dropping his mini air tank he yelled loudly until an orange floating ring was tossed towards them attached to a lifeline.

Once on board, delirious Lucky immediately started CPR on his fellow Coasty. Nothing else mattered. His years of lifeguard and Coast Guard training took over. Blood from both his arms flowed freely. ABC's he told himself. *Airway, check for breathing, circulation, come on don't die on me Coasty. You saved me, now I'm gonna save you.* Time was crucial, every second mattered. Chin head lift, head back, sweep mouth for obstacles, two quick breaths, watch chest for rise. Still has a pulse, no compressions. Breathe again. Violently the swimmer spit up sea water. Quickly Lucky turned him on his side while he coughed and sputtered but it was a wonderful sound and that was the last sound he remembered before he collapsed.

NINETY EIGHT

ONCE LUCKY WAS loaded into the stokes litter from the overhead Coast Guard helicopter and the injured but breathing rescue swimmer was loaded back onto his small boat, the Customs Scarab took off at full throttle after the fleeing Fast Lady. Lt. Brooks was so relieved Lucky was alive and Hector had drowned that he wanted the old man alive in the worst way.

The Fast Lady was running all out at sixty-two knots in eight foot rollers without running lights heading directly at the Coast Guard Command Cutter Northland who was at General Quarters with skilled gunner's mates standing by the 50 caliber machine guns. The Fast Lady was easy to spot with the overhead chopper lighting it up brightly as it tried to get away.

The Scarab closed quickly flying through the swells violently at ninety knots and the other Avon Coast Guard small boat that gave chase right away tried desperately to keep following right in the Fast Lady's smooth wake which broke the waves they were only fifty yards back.

This was it, hardball.

Howie knew he was screwed. Helicopter directly above, two huge white cutters dead ahead probably armed to the teeth and a pesky orange small boat on his ass. *So much for this fuckin job I'm in deep shit now.*

Then he saw it. A streak of black pulled up aggressively beside the Fast Lady rocking badly. It fired warning shots across the flying bridge then pulled away, seconds later the U.S.C.G.

Northlands gunner's mates let loose with a stream of 50 caliber tracer rounds as the captain gave the Fast Lady its final warning over channel 16 on the marine radio.

Howie heard it and knew what time it was.

On his way to the hospital via helicopter Lucky in and out of consciousness told the Coasty medic, "The boat's got drugs on it. I heard them talking, I think they said the port fuel tank's got eighty keys," Lucky whispered exhausted.

The Fast Lady was going so fast in such rough conditions the odds were not favorable for a clear shot with the 50 caliber machine guns, so the Northland captain ordered the sharp shooter slash medic in the helicopter to unload a clip from his M-16 A into the aft deck which housed the four big engines.

"Roger that sir."

Strapped in a harness the Coasty was pumped, he just got authorization to unload a whole clip into a two million dollar yacht. Who woulda thought I'd see the day, he told himself.

"Here we go gunner," the pilot yelled back swooping in lower. Hovering just above the deck the Coasty leaned out and took aim. On full automatic it took only seconds to quiet all four 'Vette engines. *Gotcha.*

The Coast Guard Avon swiftly pulled up along side with six angry Coasty's armed to the teeth. The four remaining Kings seasick didn't resist at all, and neither did Howie nor the old man. Once they put orange life jackets on each one of them they cuffed them, in front and transferred them to the Command Cutter where F.D.L.E, Customs, and D.E.A. members were eagerly awaiting their arrival. Then a team of mechanics from the other Cutter boarded the dead in the water Fast Lady and started repairing the quiet motors.

When at all possible all Coast Guard captains would much rather have a crew of his guys operate the seized vessel back to port instead of towing the vessel unless it's only a short distance. Besides being extremely slow long tows were a much higher risk that something could go wrong.

Four hours later at three am, the Fast Lady was tied up at Coast Guard Station Palm Beach alongside a 41 footer and the 270 foot U.S.C.G. Northland with the old man watching while the Coast Guard who had full jurisdiction of anything on the water tore his two million dollar yacht apart hoping they wouldn't find it and he could sue their ass.

Lucky and the rescue swimmer were transported to Palm Beach Hospital where both were admitted for observation. The next day, Lucky woke up blurry-eyed with a wicked headache handcuffed to the bed rail.

"Hey lover boy, welcome back."

Dry mouthed, aching all over he turned his heavy head towards the familiar sweet voice. "Hey M&M," he whispered trying to focus his eyes on Alexis's concerned face.

Then Lt. Brooks walked out of his bathroom ruining his vision. "Boy oh boy look who's back from the dead, just in time Lucky. You're in a world of shit," he scowled scornfully.

"You got him right?"

A nod.

"Was he dirty?" Lucky mumbled still burping up sea water.

"Damn right! He was very dirty," he paused feeling very pleased. "Just like you said, eighty kilos in the port tank. Your fellow Coasty's think you're a hero. They've invited you on board your old ship to eat with the captain. Imagine that."

"No shit."

"Exactly. I told him I'd let you know, but you'd be tied up with bracelets for awhile," he chuckled remembering the look on the old man's face when they held up his precious white powder so many people had given up life's dreams to chase.

"Oh and the eighty keys we confiscated matched the same ones we got at his dealership…so he's going down big time," he exhaled standing up to go, he turned back. "But it also matched the wrapper I found in your waste basket back at your apartment, yup. So you're dirty too!"

Lucky wanted to argue, but he knew it was useless. Alexis locked eyes with him pleadingly, then opened her small hand showing him the airport locker key. "We made a trade Lucky," she shrugged handing Lt. Brooks the key, who took it in his hand smiling.

"What the hell-?" Lucky said angrily. *I can't believe she just did that.*

"And a deal's a deal," he told Alexis, handing her back a different key. "Oh Lucky, by the way, thanks for the telegram, it saved your life." *And my ass.*

Speechless, thinking it had to be another bad dream Lucky watched the door slam, while Alexis nervously waited, then grinned, fumbling with the handcuffs. "I…uh…I…uh….had to Lucky. You're …you're freedom was worth the trade." *Lover boy.*

"I…I can't believe we went through all that shit…and now we're broke," he cried out unbelievably shaking his head disgusted, ready to cry.

"I'm so sorry Honey, but I tried to do the right thing." *You'll see.*

NINETY NINE

THE FOLLOWING AFTERNOON a hospital orderly wheeled Lucky outside all bandaged up to the old Karmain Ghia, while Alexis decked out in a classy hot outfit held the door open for him, "Your chariot awaits lover boy," she purred smiling.

God how can I stay mad at that, at least one part of me isn't injured he thought, wearing the cheap dark boys she handed him.

Minutes passed. "Where are we going?" he asked not really caring.

"It's a surprise, you'll see," she said all chipper.

Ten minutes later they were waved through the guard gate at small boat station Palm Beach. She turned the corner and there she was in all her white glory. His old boat. All hundred and ten crewmen and officers were on the Helo deck in dress uniform. "What the hell?" he muttered "is going on?"

Alexis stopped the old convertible right in front of the gang plank. Next thing he knew his door was being opened by Alexis and they're at the gang plank. "What are we doing here?"

"It's part of the deal with Lt. Brooks. Go on say it, they're all waiting," she whispered.

Say what oh yeah. "Captain sir request permission to board the Coast Guard Cutter Northland sir."

The next few minutes were a dream. A good dream. In front of the entire ship, the captain awarded Lucky the highest honor a rescue swimmer could ever wish for. The swimmers cross hung proudly around his neck, which was put there by petty officer Andy Wilson the rescue swimmer who saved his life, and he in turn had done the same.

The great lunch they shared with the crew on the helo deck was better than any cookout he could remember. When they finally waved goodbye tears ran down his face as they silently drove back to the Ritz Carlton where he was wiped out from all the excitement. She helped him to her ocean side suite.

"Guess we'll be moving out of here real soon, it's too damn expensive," he muttered while she unlocked the door; he clutched the swimmers cross.

"Surprise," Marty yelled jumping out of the hot tub scaring Lucky half to death. Shocked, then angry, Lucky stood in the hallway leering at Marty, his old best friend in the heart shaped Jacuzzi with a cute looking oriental chick naked. Oh what the hell, this could be fun, he thought.

Alexis grabbed his bruised hand and smiled pulling him reluctantly into the room. When he opened his hand there was a tiny key in his palm.

"What the-" *hell is going on here?*

"Hey James Bond is that how you treat all your old friends. I'd hate to see how you treat your enemies," Marty teased grinning.

"Hey Marty, who's your cute friend?" *With the killer body.*

"Sherri.Lucky, Lucky Sherri."

Lucky waved nicely, then continued to walk around the large suite slowly opening every closet till he found it.

The room safe.

Nervously he eyed Alexis then Marty. More friggin' games, he thought. But the key fit. Magically it opened and he stood speechless looking at his black backpack. "What!... How?...No way...you couldn't... you didn't...oh but you did!"

ONE HUNDRED

H E PULLED OPEN his backpack and did a rough count. Fifty bundles and eight ounces. "Wait a minute, what happened to the rest?"

"We had to give Lt. Brooks something good, so we gave him your last kilo and a hundred and thirty grand in counterfeit money you had."

"What do you mean counterfeit, what the hell are you talking about?" he demanded. *More damn games.*

"That most of that money you had was funny money. Oh it was really good stuff," she said. "Marty and I had to run every bill through the bill x-ray machine he borrowed from the front desk."

"No way."

"Yup, someone's been giving you a lot of funny money, so we bundled it back up, bought another black backpack, and gave it generously to Lt. Brooks," she giggled proudly. *For your freedom.*

"No shit, Romeo and his boys fucked me." *No wonder they were so damn nice.* He paused pissed. "Hey and what happens when Lt. Brooks finds out, what then smarty pants?"

"Easy one. He probably won't because the money and coke will be locked up in the property room, but even if he does we play dumb. Not real, what ya mean?" she laughed.

"Okay I get it. He's too busy with his big bust, right?"

"Exactly. Hey Hector's dead, the old man's going to prison, and your daughter is safe. Could be a lot worse," she teased taking off her clothes.

"How?"

"Two weeks vacation with me and seventy-grand!"

Coming soon...

THE DEVILS WEB
By W.C SCOTT
Another A Lucky Sullivan Novel
Spring 2000

"MAN, I GOTTA get out of here," Lucky mumbled out loud knowing they were looking for him. Stolen credit cards, bogus checks, fake prescriptions had finally started to pile up.

The paper trail led straight back to him, and the pressure of answering for his sins was too much.

He had boxed himself in with no place to hide burning the only two lifelines he had left, Lt. Frank Brooks and the beautiful Greek goddess Laura.

Lucky felt like a wild cat cornered in a barn with no way out. The safety barriers he had so deviously put in place months ago were now crumbling down leaving him exposed. There was no way he was ready to face the wrath of an angry Lt. Brooks. Shaking that scary thought out of his head, he reached over and cranked up the volume on the old Alpine stereo. "Bye-Bye Miss American Pie, drove my Chevy to the levy but the levy was dry and good ole boys were drinkin' whiskey and rye sing'n this will be the day that I die," Lucky sang along out loud to the old classic tune while he hurriedly packed his gear in the old Mazda.

Two hours earlier he had bought the old car off some guy's front lawn for five hundred bucks, slapped a dealer tag on the back and away he went.

He knew he still had two checks left to cash and his unsuspecting neighbor wouldn't have any idea he had cleaned out his checking and savings account until he was long gone.

The monthly statements from the bank had mysteriously disappeared buying him additional time to get out of town. Eventually his landlord would call the bank asking why he hadn't received his monthly banking statements.

The bank of course would apologize and immediately send out another statement which would show he was broke. And all the checks he'd written over the past few weeks were now bouncing all over the Granite State.

On Lucky's way out of town he would swing through two different bank drive thru's, leaving only a couple of pennies just enough for the checks to clear.

He pulled off satisfied he'd squeezed every dime he could steal and hopped on Interstate 93 south bound. The first green road sign he saw read Boston 110 miles.

The only place he felt safe was a long way away. Eighteen hundred miles south, the sunshine state was calling. He just hoped the old car with close to two hundred thousand miles on the odometer was up for one last trip.

Lucky knew once Lt. Brooks figured out he'd skipped town they would put a trace on his Nextel phone. *Might as well use it while I can!* Alexis popped into his mind. Damn he was going to miss her needy hard body. Impulsively he hit speed dial and waited. Her voice mail picked up so he left a message.

"Lexy you're the only one who knows I'm on my way to the sunshine state.....my only regret is you're not riding shotgun with me like last time", he paused thinking of how far and fast he'd fallen. "I'll miss you for sure-who knows maybe I'll be able to f ly you down for some fun in the sun. Adios Alexis... gotta go..."

South of Boston he switched to Interstate 95, The Devils Highway. Down the east coast all the way to south Miami. It was a long dangerous trip down the evil north-south corridor.

He ditched the phone, pulling the SIM card and battery. The further south he went, the better he felt. Twenty-nine hours later he crossed the border into Florida.

A f lat tire, leaky radiator hose and the on again off again red light oil sensor seemed a long time ago. The bright sunshine helped him forget about Lt. Brooks and his stack of felony warrants sitting on his desk eighteen hundred miles north.

After three long weeks in sunny south Florida, Lucky was exhausted. The late nights drinking and drugging till dawn had taken it's toll. Somehow he was almost broke. Over five grand had slipped through his greasy fingers and he had nothing to show for it except a wicked throbbing headache.

The cheap efficiency was trashed. Disgusted he stumbled into the shabby roach infested bathroom. The weekly rent was over due and the grumpy old alcoholic motel manager was hot on his trail.

Glancing in the cracked mirror, reality stared back at him. The old vanity mirror cracked down the middle left his head split open making him cringe. "What the hell am I gonna do now"? He asked himself rubbing his hand over his five-day stubble.

First shame then fear raced through him. He glanced away back into the one room efficiency realizing the party was over. "I need to get the fuck out of this dump," he mumbled shuffling back into the room.

Slowly he took it all in, disgusted he started rummaging through a pile of dirty laundry and old newspapers.

Eventually he found a week old Palm Beach Post Sunday classifieds, and sat down on the ripped divan smoothing out the crinkled pages until he found the help wanted section.

Deep down he felt it, desperation setting in. Reality reached up and slapped him in the face; he knew what time it was. Either work or starve.

One ad caught his attention. Something he could do so he could eat tonight.

HELP WANTED
Day Laborers Needed
CASH PAID DAILY!

On Lucky's second day at the temp agency, they sent him to work at a driving school out at Thunderfoot's mile. They were starting another four day class racing stock cars and corvettes.

His job consisted of setting up a hundred orange cones on their designated spots around the various race courses set up for the students.

Every time a student knocked a cone over or out of it's yellow f luorescent square he'd put it back in place. He also washed the cars before they were put up for the night.

The four days at the track flew by for Lucky. Finally Friday came, the last day. The twelve students had completed all their classroom video and simulator instruction each morning.

After a four star lunch catered by the Ritz-Carlton Resort where the class was staying, they would head outside to the track to put in seat time in both Monte Carlo stock cars and race ready C-5 Corvettes.

The wealthy students were dressed to the nines in brand new authentic white GMAC fire protective racing suits. The overalls were covered in racing sponsors patches just like the cup drivers.

Across the waist belt their names were written in cursive. In their hands, they carried white full faced Bell helmets with tinted visors. On their feet they all wore white Nike racing shoes and matching Nike racing gloves in their hands.

Out in the pit area Lucky could sense the extra excitement in the air. Today was the day they would race each other against the clock for the final bragging rights.

Their first race of the day would be to run five fast laps around the one mile banked oval in the Chevy Monte Carlo stock cars. No more babysitting. Today they would start out in the drivers seat instead of the passengers seat. The ace instructors were there to offer advice and support, but were not part of the equation.

The owner full of enthusiasm strolled outside to a shout of cheers and greeted his students. After all they were paying the big bucks to learn from the best and most expensive. Either way, they had been spoiled all week.

Now Thunderfoot, the owner would demonstrate how an old pro could still turn a few fast laps in a four hundred horsepower V-8 Monte Carlo stock car.

The NASCAR legend glanced around smiling. "Get Lucky a helmet.... he'll be my passenger," he shouted watching a big smile come over Lucky's surprised face.

Once Thuderfoot and Lucky completed two warm up laps the experienced pro accelerated hard underneath the big digital Coca-Cola starting clock. They flew into turn one, picking up more speed. Lucky instinctively grabbed onto the steel handle welded onto the roll cage over the passenger door.

Pumped up Lucky eyed the outside retaining wall only inches away. Five quick laps later they screamed across the finish line in a hundred and fifty seconds flat.

"Wow that was wicked cool," Lucky yelled out, while they coasted into the pits.

The owner caught up in Lucky's excitement grabbed him by the shoulder outside the car and smiled sincerely. "So you think you can handle the stock car safely without putting it into the wall"?

What did he just say? Stunned Lucky hesitated until he realized the old man was dead serious. "Yes sir Mr. Thunderfoot, absolutely sir," he yelled out smiling.

"Well you better son," he laughed joyfully eyeing the students reaction knowing they'd all taken a liking to the friendly New Englander. Before turning back to Lucky he bellowed, "because what I'm gonna do by popular demand is let you set an example for the class ... so don't let us down".

Lucky grinned still stunned. Quickly he walked to the next stock car in line putting his helmet back on before the owner could change his mind.

He turned and made eye contact with the owner across the roof. "No sir, I'll try my damndest not to let anyone down", he gushed pulling his chinstrap tight before he climbed over the fixed door. An instructor reached into the window to help him with the four point racing harness.

All the students were clapping and cheering Lucky on "Now don't forget class he's never driven these race cars before, so let's see if we can learn from all his mistakes", the owner guffawed smiling.

Lucky was glad he had his helmet on because he turned beet red hearing the old man make fun of him. Antsy he waited while another ace instructor climbed into the passenger's window with ease. Just like

NASCAR cup cars they were set up with full heavy duty roll cages, plexi-glass windows and side window netting.

The two main differences were the horsepower and the added passengers seat. Top speed was still a respectable one hundred and sixty-five miles an hour on the one-mile ovals straight aways.

Which of course would be considered a Sunday drive in an eight hundred and fifty horsepower number three Dale Earnhardt cup car with a top speed of well over two hundred miles an hour.

Near the end of the second warm up lap the ace instructor riding shotgun waved his left arm signaling Lucky that the finish line clock would start automatically on this lap.

Adrenaline rushed through Lucky's veins. The need for speed, the thrill of taking it to the very limit made his confidence soar. He raced into the sixteen degree banking in turn one still in third gear, holding the stock car steady as he watched the tach soar into the red. Quickly he speed shifted into fourth gear sling-shooting out of turn two picking up more speed down the back stretch. Glancing at the speedo he saw it hit one sixty-five and grinned. Turn three was coming up fast, out of the corner of his eye he saw the instructor latch onto the handle welded on the roll cage. Just like the owner did a few minutes earlier, Lucky wisely slid down low in the center riding the yellow line between turns three and four.

Keeping his speed, the car shot back outside in turn four inches off the outside retaining wall. Recklessly he gave a rebel yell feeling the stock car pick up more speed down the front stretch.

With his foot mashed to the floor he felt the thrill of pushing the race car to it's limit. Four hair brained laps later he screamed across the finish line freezing the big clock.

The digital clock read one hundred and fifty-five seconds. Giddy, Lucky slowed down and guided the stock car back into the pit area carefully. He watched as the first student accelerated off pit row onto the one mile oval.

"Holy cow," Thunderfoot yelled suspiciously. "Hey wait a damn minute, that's only five seconds off my time ... that's ... that's impossible"! "His hand automatically went to his goa-tee then he spun back around towards Lucky. "Hey, where the hell have you been racin' stock cars son"? Lucky locked on the first student still racing around the one mile oval just smiled sheepishly, "First time for me sir, and it was wicked cool".

The owner talking quietly to one of his instructors just shrugged his shoulders in disbelief. They watched the twelfth student cross the finish line in a hundred and eighty-two seconds, good for tenth place.

Everyone looked up at the digital scoreboard waiting for the final results to be posted according to everyone's time from fastest to slowest.

The students stunned realized Lucky ran the fastest time other than the owners by five seconds.

It didn't make sense. The kids first time..... They didn't believe it for a second. Next up was the difficult figure eight course. The students would be driving the race ready C-5 corvettes. Everyone eagerly watched one of the ace instructors flawless run through the tricky circular eight course without touching a single orange cone.

The small clock was frozen on eighty-eight seconds. Lucky paced back and forth in the center of the course making sure the orange cones stayed in place after each students run through the course. He had hoped the owner would offer him a chance to drive the tricky figure eight but he didn't.

So he shrugged it off grateful for the opportunity he'd been given. The fourth student, a rough looking dude covered in prison tattoos sported a ponytail and bulging muscles, ran a respectable ninety-two seconds. None of the other eleven students could best his time.

They all eyed the results overhead. The tattoo muscle head student turned and hollered over to the owner so everyone could hear. "Hey Thunderfoot let our helper give it a shot.... Five hundred bucks says he beats my time".

The owner stunned stopped and looked around realizing how quiet it was all of a sudden. Everyone was staring at him, daring him to say no.

Slowly he broke eye contact and glanced at his Rolex. He couldn't help notice the excitement coming from his young guns eagerly waiting for him to respond to the absurd challenge so they could make a quick buck!

The tattoo student's cockiness soared with the silence, quickly stepping into the roll of the class spokesman, he yelled "In fact a grand says he breaks ninety seconds and another grand says he beats your eighty-eight seconds".

The owner just smiled and shook his head-Christ there's always one asshole in every bunch. He glanced over at his instructors seeing the pleading in their eyes.

Max slung his ponytail over his shoulder grinning. "Come on guys don't tell us all you hot shots are scared of a lot boy?... shit what kinda Mickey Mouse school you runnin here ... huh"?

The four instructors got serious in a hurry glaring at Max. "Let's do it fat mouth, we call that bet", the ace jockey who ran the fast eighty-eight second time hollered out angrily before the owner could diffuse the situation.

Oh shit-why me? Lucky thought listening to them argue then he laughed, *Now I get to try it for real!* Little did anyone know that Lucky had been top salesman at City Corvette back in Manchester, New Hampshire where they always kept over a hundred used Vette's in stock for daring test drives.

And Lucky took full advantage of that opportunity taking plenty of long test drives pushing all those pretty Vette's to their limit through the winding on ramps and mountain passes of the Granite State.

He snapped out of his stupor surprised by the animosity between the two groups who had been getting along so well only a short while ago. The bet was on, and all eyes were locked on Lucky. "Shit I'm fucked if I do and I'm fucked if I don't", he mumbled walking towards the two groups.

The owner waved him over obviously very frustrated. "Put your damn helmet on Lucky ... your being put on the spot son," he whispered moving in closer.

"I suggest you remember who the hell you work for....shit never mind-it won't matter anyway," he laughed arrogantly. "Give it all you got you'll never break ninety seconds".

"That's what you think asshole," lucky muttered softly walking off quickly.

Thunderfoot spun back around shocked. "What, what did you ..... just say"? He demanded. "Huh?...oh nothin' sir, um I'll give it my best shot," Lucky blurted out quickly glancing over at his new very rich friends. That's when he and Max locked eyes for a few long seconds before Lucky smiled and gave him a thumbs up.

Tightening his chin strap he climbed into the Vette while an instructor helped him secure the racing harness and attach the steering wheel. Another instructor climbed into the passenger's seat not saying a word, he grinned smartly. Knowing he and his crew were about to get paid.

Lucky hit the toggle switch and the five hundred horsepower V-8 engine roared to life. Nervously he gripped the steering wheel slowly rolling the loud Vette up to the fat white painted starting line.

He held the heavy-duty clutch in half way and kept his right hand on the four speed Hurst shifter locked in first gear. Exhaling slowly he tried to control his breathing pushing everything else out of his mind he focused on the row of red flashing lights.

Anxiously he waited on the lights to flash yellow then green. *Come on I need a fast start,* he kept telling himself going over the difficult figure eight course in his mind.

Yellow lights, Flashing ...Green lights, Go.....go ...... Instinctively he dropped the clutch and stomped on the gas smoking the massive Good Year racing Eagles. He flew past the first row of orange cones at close to seventy miles an hour.

In second gear he braced himself for the long sharp left handed figure eight turn dead ahead. The owners arrogant laugh still rang in his ears making him push the light Vette harder and harder.

The Vette tried to break free. The rear end started to slide, feathering the gas just enough he kept it in contact with the hot pavement.

Wildly he skidded around the last turn flying onto the short sprint back to the finish line. The instructor reached over and hit the kill switch the second Lucky pulled back into the pits. Immediately he saw the class of students going crazy jumping up and down pointing at the clock and laughing at the stunned group of car jockeys.

His time, eighty seven point nine seconds. He realized he'd beat the instructor by a tenth of a second. Seconds later the students pulled Lucky out of the Vette like it was on fire, smothering him. Pissed off one of the instructors handed Max twenty five hundred in fifty dollar bills.

Max snatched the cash pumping his fist in the air smirking. "That was awesome," a student yelled slapping Lucky hard on the shoulder while Max stuffed fifteen fifties into Lucky's overalls.

"Great driving Mario," Max said laughing. "Thanks I think," Lucky answered back eyeing the instructors wearily.

Overwhelmed with all the attention he tried to go back over to the pit area quietly. He was still stunned thinking about the fifteen fifties Max had stuffed into his pocket when someone yelled out his name.

"Hey Lucky," causing him to stop and slowly turn around towards the voice. He eyed the group of hostile car jockeys obviously pissed off.

Everyone went quiet. *Shit here goes nothin'.* "Damn it man that was a hell of a run," the jockey acknowledged throwing up a quick salute before he spun around and walked off shaking his head still not believing he'd just been beat by a rookie!

It was time, the final test. The tricky obstacle course. Now it was no secret that so far no student had ever collected the twenty-five grand by beating the time set by one of the ace instructors on the final challenge.

But it was always there, part of the marketing strategy.

Thunderfoot'sMile shareholders advertised it everywhere!

BEAT OUR TIME!
WIN $25 GRAND
PLUS
2 VIP TX TO THE
DAYTONA 500

The final challenge was a combination of hard maneuvers so difficult that it took many practice runs to post a decent time.

The course made up of four very different skill sets. First a sprint from zero to one hundred mph, then onto the eighteen cone slalom course, followed by a run on the figure eight course, and finally onto the one mile oval for three fast laps.

A decent time by a student was around two hundred and fifteen seconds. Instructors ran a few seconds under two hundred.

The record, part of the hype at Thunderfoot's one mile oval, was that the NSCAR legend himself Thunderfoot Carlson held the track record of one hundred and ninety-two seconds.

Once the instructors were done explaining the course layout by having everyone watch a VHS video of Thunderfoot's track record setting run two years earlier, Max immediately jumped in to challenge the cocky drivers to another bet.

"Hey-I want Lucky to take my place," Max yelled pointing up at the big sign with twenty-five grand and two VIP tickets to the Daytona 500 boldly displayed.

No one responded Complete silence...... Everyone waited Max broke the silence again laughing. "What you hot shots don't want to win your money back"? Thunderfoot fed up with Max's bullshit responded immediately. "Well Mr. Max that's not gonna happen-he's not a student, you have to be enrolled to q u a l i f y... . . s o o b v i o u s l y w e c o u l d n ' t h o n o r o u r g u a r a n t e e d challenge.....But even if I did allow him, believe me when I tell you guys-Lucky is way out of his element on the one".

Thunderfoot ready to get on with the final stage before pictures and graduation, turned and walked over to the pit staging area. Max was having no part of it. He boldly stepped forward. "Oh come on-don't tell us the late great Jimmy Thunderfoot Carlson is backing down from a potential challenge on his own damn track"!

He continued on louder, "Shit just wait till the newspapers get ahold of the story-you'll be laughed out of business," Max sniped. "Yup I can see the sports headlines now.... NASCAR legend Thunderfoot Carlson backs down from challenge with lot boy on the difficult obstacle course at his own damn track...baff les rich paying students demanding their money back".

Everyone in the class got on board laughing nervously high fiving one another. All wondering who Max really was and how he was affiliated with the newspaper business. *Oh Shit* the owner realized catching his breath thinking, rubbing his goa-tee slowly he walked around his famous number nine Monte Carlo. *Who is this asshole anyway?* It didn't take him long to realize if this dickhead was serious and had media access, this little misunderstanding could turn into a nightmare.

He really had no choice. "Okay damn it, he's in, your out....but today boys and girls I've decided I'll be setting the time to beat", he stammered seeing the news surprise both the instructors and students equally.

"That's it"! He beats the time I set today he'll win the grand prize. If this makes it more fun for all of you, I'm sure you'll be telling all your friends about this crazy challenge. Everyone happy now"? He didn't expect a response. "Now please Max no more bullshit. I'll go first and set todays time and Lucky will go last in Max's spot".

Dazed Lucky backed up a little, very confused how all of a sudden he'd become the center of everyone's get back. *What the hell is gonna happen now?* He asked himself. "Maybe I can win some more money," he joked felling his pocket stuffed with fifteen fifties.

That's when everyone grabbed him and pulled him into their plush pit box. The rich students had his back. The sides were drawn.

Chaos, excitement. Building up.....

Everyone was on board. The sound of the throaty V-8 starting up made them all turn and watch. The old pro with his dander up was sitting in his shiny number nine Monte Carlo stock car with his name, track and driving school plastered all over it just like the cup car sponsors.

Seconds later Thunderfoot roared off pit road to warm up the tires. Even the instructors could feel the added tension in the air.

Boldly displayed overhead was the obstacle course record set by Thrunderfoot, and broken by Thunderfoot. One hundred and ninety-two seconds.

Curious even the ace jockeys wondered if the old man still had it in him. It had been two long years since he'd set that course record. Being pissed off could sometimes work against you inside a race car.

Thunderfoot roared back into the pits, ready. He rolled his number nine Monte Carlo up to the starting line.

Red light....blinking. Yellow light....blinking. Green light.....gone!

In a cloud of blue smoke Thunderfoot roared off. He flew through the first leg of the course zero to one hundred in a very fast time of eight point five seconds.

Not wasting a single second he powered his way onto the slalom course, flying around the cones. Quickly he turned a hard right fishtailing his way onto the tricky figure eight course.

Picking up speed he muscled the stock car onto the one mile oval quickly accelerating he power shifted through the four speed gear box pushing old number nine to its limit.

Three lickity split laps later he skillfully zoomed across the finish line freezing the big digital Coca-Cola clock on one hundred and ninety-five seconds.

Only three seconds off his own track record. It was the fastest time anyone had run in almost a year. "Holy shit Lucky you sure got your hands full...damn it man that was vintage Thunderfoot for sure," Max sighted heavily seeing all the cocky jockeys high fiving one another.

"Look at those fuckin' assholes will ya. So damn full of themselves," Max blundered getting more pissed off as they laughed and gloated pointing at him. Wrong move. The same cocky driver who handed over the twenty five hundred earlier.

They all kidded with themselves not really expecting a reply. Max sighed eyeing Lucky earnestly seeing he had his head down disappointed. "Damn right speed racer, in fact we got five grand says he breaks two hundred seconds".

Shocked he went for the bait so easily.

CPSIA information can be obtained
at www.ICGtesting.com
Printed in the USA
LVOW11*1707160418

573652LV00005B/75/P